I0072168

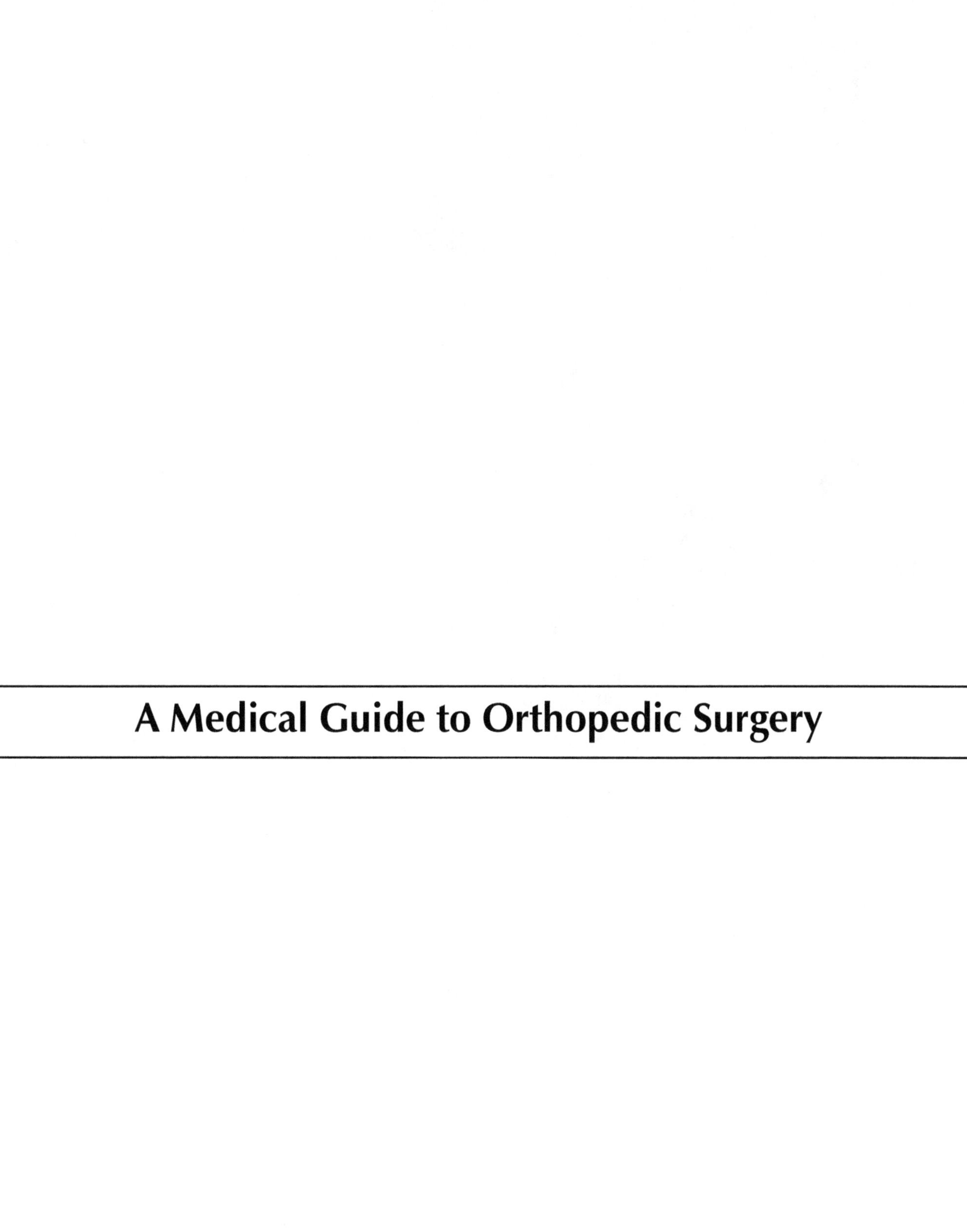

A Medical Guide to Orthopedic Surgery

A Medical Guide to Orthopedic Surgery

Editor: Solomon Willis

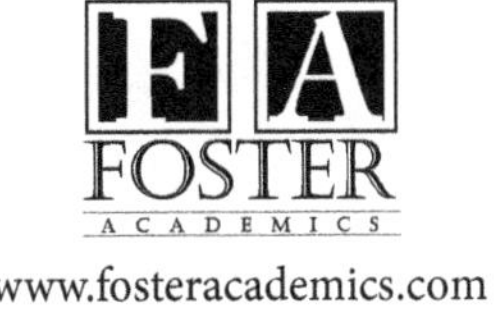

www.fosteracademics.com

www.fosteracademics.com

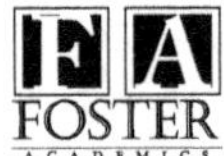

Cataloging-in-Publication Data

A medical guide to orthopedic surgery / edited by Solomon Willis.
p. cm.
Includes bibliographical references and index.
ISBN 978-1-63242-522-5
1. Orthopedic surgery. 2. Orthopedics. I. Willis, Solomon.
RD731 .M43 2018
61747--dc23

Foster Academics,
118-35 Queens Blvd., Suite 400,
Forest Hills, NY 11375, USA

ISBN 978-1-63242-522-5 (Hardback)

Contents

Preface

Orthopedic surgery refers to the practice of treating problems like spine diseases, degenerative diseases, congenital disorders, musculoskeletal trauma, sports injuries, etc. Some of the common orthopedic surgeries include knee arthroscopy, carpal tunnel release, hip replacement, lumbar spinal fusion, shoulder arthroscopy, low back intervertebral disc surgery, etc. This text is a compilation of chapters that discuss the most vital concepts and emerging trends in the field of orthopedics. It will serve as a valuable source of reference for graduate and post-graduate students. Through this text readers would gain knowledge that would broaden their perspective about orthopedics.

The researches compiled throughout the book are authentic and of high quality, combining several disciplines and from very diverse regions from around the world. Drawing on the contributions of many researchers from diverse countries, the book's objective is to provide the readers with the latest achievements in the area of research. This book will surely be a source of knowledge to all interested and researching the field.

In the end, I would like to express my deep sense of gratitude to all the authors for meeting the set deadlines in completing and submitting their research chapters. I would also like to thank the publisher for the support offered to us throughout the course of the book. Finally, I extend my sincere thanks to my family for being a constant source of inspiration and encouragement.

Editor

1

Variation in Planned Resection of CAM FAI Based on Surgeon Experience

Derek Ochiai,[1] Skye Donovan,[1,2] Farshad Adib,[3] and Eric Guidi[2]

[1] *Nirschl Orthopedic Center, Arlington, VA 22205, USA*
[2] *Marymount University, Arlington, VA 22207, USA*
[3] *University of Maryland, Baltimore, MD 21201, USA*

Correspondence should be addressed to Skye Donovan; jdonovan@marymount.edu

Academic Editor: Padhraig O'Loughlin

Introduction. Currently, there are no definitive guidelines for the resection of a cam lesion. The purpose of this study was to investigate factors indicating the potential differences in low and high volume hip arthroscopists in marking the area of resection in cam lesions using X-rays for preoperative planning. *Methods.* Thirty-nine surgeons with varying levels of hip arthroscopy experience participated in the study. Surgeons filled out a survey and traced the area of optimal resection on radiographs with varying amounts of cam FAI. Participants were grouped by number of hip arthroscopies performed, years of surgical experience, and number of surgeries performed. *Results.* Surgeons who perform osteoplasty as a high percentage of their total hip surgeries per year correlate to the total number of hip arthroscopies performed per year ($r = 0.412$, $p < 0.05$) and number of years of experience ($r = 0.72$, $p < 0.01$). Surgeons performing greater than 50 cases per year traced a larger resection area for 3 different patients' radiographs as compared to those performing less than 50 cases per year (117%, 143%, and 173%, $p < 0.05$). *Conclusions.* This study demonstrates that surgeons with less experience (decreased number of years operating and total number of surgeries) plan for resecting less cam than do experienced surgeons.

1. Introduction

The understanding of femoroacetabular impingement (FAI) continues to evolve. Preoperative X-ray and three-dimensional computed tomography scans are helpful to evaluate the extent of cam lesions [1]. Cam FAI is a structural, mechanical problem, necessitating symptomatic patients to have surgery. Surgery can be performed arthroscopically or by an open technique. Arthroscopic surgery has the advantages of most minimally invasive surgeries previously described in the literature. The advantages of open treatment include easy access to all hip structures and facilitation of intraoperative ranging of the hip at extremes of motions. In open surgery, the recovery time is longer secondary to the highly invasive nature of the operation and increased potential risk for avascular necrosis [2].

The use of hip arthroscopy for definitive treatment of FAI is increasing [3]. Arthroscopic management of FAI is improving, with excellent outcomes reported in the literature at early-term follow-up [4–7]. Despite the increase in FAI arthroscopy, the learning curve in planned resection of cam FAI has not been determined based on consistency and appropriate resection.

Despite availability of the advanced imaging techniques, the X-ray is still the cornerstone of preoperative planning for FAI surgery. Incompletely treated FAI is the number one cause of revision hip arthroscopy [8]. Appropriate cam resection is imperative to the success of the surgery. Martin et al. reported underresections of cam FAI, due to the learning curve for hip arthroscopies [9]. Learning curves for surgeons have been assessed in order to determine skill level and to improve existing education techniques. Shoulder and knee arthroscopy studies demonstrate that the number of surgeries and years of experience correlate with better surgical outcomes and decrease in operative time [10–16].

Currently, there is no description of the learning curve for preoperative planning for FAI osteoplasty using X-ray. By surveying surgeons with differing levels of hip arthroscopy experience and measuring preferred cam resection area on digital images, this study investigates factors that are associated with differences amongst surgeons in marked area of resection. Specifically the research question of interest is, do surgeons with more experience resect more in preoperative planning for FAI than those who are novice? Our goal is to identify survey characteristics that would eliminate variability in amount of resection preoperatively for cam FAI osteoplasty. This study intends to demonstrate a learning curve for surgeons (timeframe/performance standards) and to assess whether their preoperative planning would be similar to those who are experienced FAI surgeons.

2. Methods and Materials

Upon approval by the Marymount University Institutional Review Board, a total of 39 clinicians participated in the study. All of the participants were Board Certified orthopedic surgeons registered for the AANA Master's Experience in Hip Arthroscopy Course (Rosemont, IL). All of the subjects completed a survey describing their surgical history and level of experience (see the appendix).

In addition, the subjects were asked to evaluate the same digital radiographs of three patients with varying amounts of cam FAI. All 3 of the patients were seen at one center and were examined by the same highly experienced hip arthroscopist, with radiographs taken by one technician. High quality digital reproductions of A-P and Dunn lateral view radiographs were provided to the surgeons (Figure 1). Oral instructions were provided to all of the clinicians at the same time; they were asked to trace the area of optimal resection of the cam lesions in all images which were printed and distributed to them; investigators left the room during the tracing. These images were then scanned, converted to JPEG images, and digitally analyzed. The tracings (Figure 2) made by the study participants were retraced using image analysis software (Fiji/ImageJ software available at http://www.nih.gov/). This software also calculated area of resection for each image in pixels, which were compared between participants. Spatial calibration was accomplished by dividing pixels/mm and set for future images through Fiji/ImageJ software.

A single author performed all of the analyses to limit interrater error, who was blinded to all patient data. Results from the survey were used to describe surgeon characteristics and used in secondary analysis to determine correlations between survey responses and area indicated in the radiographs. Analysis of variance (ANOVA) was used as the primary analysis for subgroup characteristics. When significant differences were found, comparisons were made using a Bonferroni post hoc analysis. This analysis revealed differences only upon reaching 50 surgeries per year, allowing us to analyze the data by dividing surgeons into 2 groups, less than 50 surgeries and greater than 50, with no differences in greater than 50 or greater than 100 surgeries performed per year. For secondary data analysis, subjects were grouped according to the number of surgeries they performed. Secondary analysis employed the use of Student's t-tests and Pearson's correlations to assess differences in area of resection and the relationship between survey responses and calculated areas. A level of significance was set at $p < 0.05$. SPSS (version 17.0 Chicago, IL) was used for all statistical analyses.

Table 1: Surgeon characteristics as identified by survey.

Descriptor	Min	Max	Mode
Years performing surgery	1	25	1
Number of surgeries performed	0	>100	<5
% of surgeries including osteoplasty	<25%	>75%	>75%

3. Results

Study participants were grouped into instructors versus attendees. Of the 39 interviewees, 14 were instructors and 25 were attendees. Twenty-six of the participants had been performing surgeries for less than 5 years. The number of surgeries performed varied widely, with 26 surgeons performing <20 surgeries, 2 performing between 31 and 50, and 11 performing over 50. Minimum and maximum values and most frequently noted responses are outlined in Table 1 to illustrate the variance between participants.

Additional survey review revealed that instructors of the hip arthroscopy course were more likely to perform a cam osteoplasty compared to attendees ($r = 0.69$, $p < 0.01$). Among the attendees, the number of surgeries per year ($r = 0.72$, $p < 0.01$) shows a strong correlation with those who perform osteoplasty, while the number of years of experience ($r = 0.412$, $p < 0.05$) has a significant but moderate correlation. From survey data analysis, participants were grouped according to number of hip arthroscopies performed after finding a cut-off difference at 50 surgeries per year, as determined through post hoc analysis of our ANOVA (Table 1.) A positive correlation was found between number of years of surgical experience and number of surgeries performed per year ($r = 0.56$, $p < 0.01$). Pearson's test revealed a moderate but significant correlation of number of surgeries performed and area of resection for the 3 radiographs ($r = 0.39$, 0.47, and 0.39, $p < 0.05$).

Student's t-test detected significant differences in area of resection between groups. It is important to note that the radiographs all depicted obvious cam lesions. Surgeons performing greater than 50 cases per year traced a larger area of resection for the 3 patients' radiographs as compared to those performing less than 50 cases per year (117%, 143%, and 173%, $p < 0.05$) as illustrated in Table 2. No differences were seen between surgeons who performed > 50 versus > 100 surgeries per year.

4. Discussion

Because of the steep learning curve in the arthroscopic cam FAI osteoplasty and regional access to bony pathology arthroscopically, there is always a concern about the adequacy of resection of cam lesion [17–19]. Potential problems include inaccurate resection, underresection, and overresection, which may lead to suboptimal outcomes such as residual impingement or the creation of structural instability. One tool

TABLE 2: Average areas of resection for cam lesions.

Number of surgeries performed per year	Image 1 area (pixels)	Image 2 area (pixels)	Image 3 area (pixels)
Less than 50	10243.7 ± 1545.5*	17281.8 ± 6359.8*	6669.5 ± 4075.8*
More than 50	12413 ± 2796.8	23765.9 ± 8542.3	10184.8 ± 7208.4

Statistically significant differences denoted by * ($p < 0.05$) as compared to >50 surgeries performed per year.

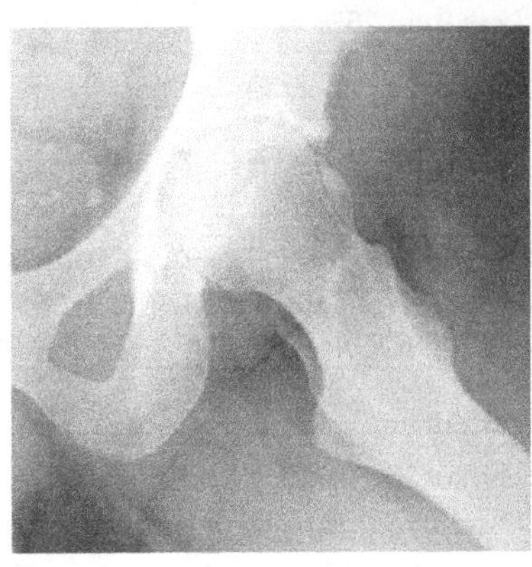

Image 1

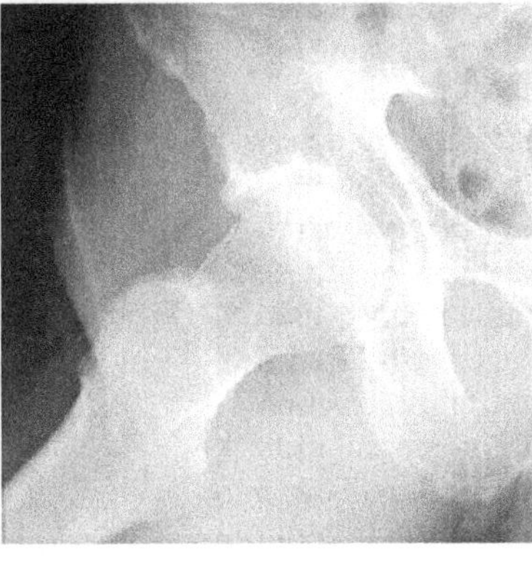

Image 2

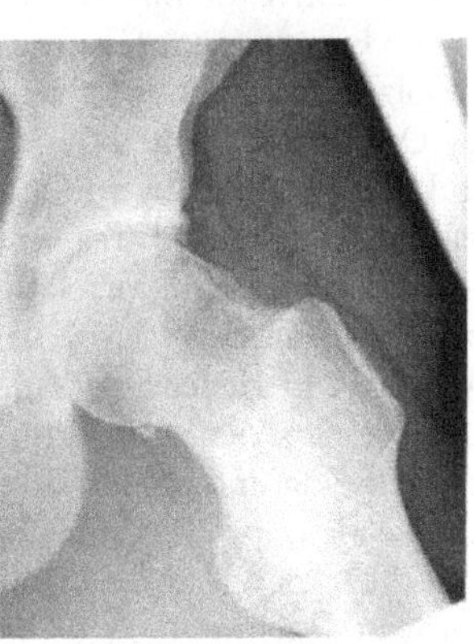

Image 3

FIGURE 1: Cam images presented to study participants.

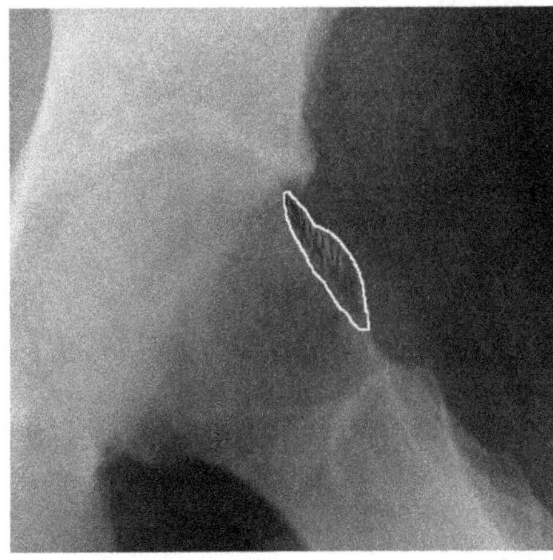

FIGURE 2: Scanned image of physician traced FAI lesion, with subsequent area determination using Fiji/ImageJ software.

to prevent these problems is preoperative planning. In our study, we provide an inexpensive tool [digitized radiographs and free software] to evaluate this skill level noninvasively. Our study supports that preoperative planning on X-ray is significantly different for those surgeons with greater than 50 surgeries per year compared to those with less than 50 per year ($p < 0.01$). There were significant differences in the area of resection between the 2 groups of surgeons, with those performing greater than 50 surgeries per year planning to resect more than the relatively inexperienced surgeons. Underresection by less experienced surgeons runs the risk of needing revision surgery or continued impingement. No difference was seen between surgeons who performed > 50 versus > 100 surgeries per year. Surgeons performing more than 50 hip arthroscopies per year planned surgical resection with similar variability as surgeons performing more than 100, and the variability was less than the surgeons performing <50 hip arthroscopies.

This study does not define the "correct" area of resection; it focuses on changes in variability of planned osteoplasty to experience. Likewise, the study did not focus on appropriateness of resection, the images used all had a moderate to severe cam lesion, and the participants were all in a course for arthroscopic management of this condition; thus each participant had a potential bias as to whether resection was necessary. Although this study identifies differences in planned resection, it does not speak to the capability of these surgeons' ability to accomplish a successful outcome.

5. Limitations

One of our limitations is the narrow population studied. Since our study group contained all course attendees, they all have vested interest in hip arthroscopy. Additionally, there were only 3 cases for each surgeon to examine; increasing this number may have shown more differences. Also, as a survey study, we chose to not use open-ended questions, but we rather assigned arbitrary cut-offs for the categories of number of surgeries per year. In doing so we felt we were eliminating recall bias: however, this study may slightly over- or underestimate the true number of surgeries related to the learning curve. For our analysis, we used post hoc results and identified 50 surgeries per year as a cut-off value; basing our results on this measurement has the potential to introduce error. We used a blinded review; however, we only used one reviewer, which could introduce bias to our study. Additionally, this study does not measure the actual surgical performance, which could potentially differ from a planned surgical resection. Lastly, this study is solely based on radiographs and did not explore other methods of evaluation which play a role in preoperative planning.

6. Conclusions

The primary objective of this study was to determine if surgeons of varying experience levels exhibited differences in preoperative planning methods for resection of FAI using hip arthroscopy. Our team evaluated characteristics between participants and grouped them by volume of surgeries to determine correlations to preferred area of surgical resection. This study demonstrates a positive correlation between number of surgeries performed and the area of planned resection. Those surgeons with less experience plan for less cam resection than those with more experience. In addition we introduced a method of evaluating and quantifying amount of resection for preoperative planning. This study can act as a foundation for future studies wishing to determine surgical skills and may help provide teaching tools or benchmarks that could be achieved during the learning curve and to facilitate studies based on surgical experience, surgical outcomes, and amount of resection. Our preoperative planning method might be a helpful tool to determine the amount of cam osteoplasty.

Appendix

Complete Hip Arthroscopy Survey: Hip FAI Surgeon Questionnaire

Please Answer All Questions. Indicate answer choice by checking the appropriate box or responding on line provided

(1) In what capacity are you attending this course?

□ Instructor
□ Attendee

(2) How many years have you performed hip arthroscopy as an attending?

□ 0–12 mos
□ if >12 mos, please provide # of years —

(3) Approximately how many hip arthroscopies do you perform per year?

□ Less than five
□ 5–10
□ 11–20
□ 21–30
□ 31–50
□ 51–100
□ Greater than 100

(4) Please estimate the percentage of hip arthroscopies that you perform that involve osteochondroplasty?

□ Less than 25%
□ 26–50%
□ 51–75%
□ Greater than 75%

(5) Please estimate, in your opinion, what the overall average of all hip arthroscopies performed in the United States involve osteochondroplasty?

□ Less than 25%
□ 26–50%
□ 51–75%
□ Greater than 75%

(6) In your opinion, what is the most common reason that you would NOT address existing femoroacetabular impingement while performing a hip arthroscopy?

□ Patient age
□ Patient has osteoporosis
□ Osteochondroplasty is not necessary
□ Osteochondroplasty is not covered by insurance
□ Technically demanding procedure
□ I would always address FAI with an osteoplasty

Conflict of Interests

The authors declare that there is no conflict of interests regarding the publication of this paper.

Acknowledgments

Financial affiliations include Tenex Health, Smith & Nephew, Arthrex, and Breg. The authors would like to thank Dr. Megan Geiger for her preparation of the abstract and poster associated with this study.

References

[1] S. Nordeck, J. Flanagan, L. Tenorio, W. Robertson, and A. Chhabra, "3-D Isotropic MR imaging for planning bone reconstruction in patients with femoroacetabular impingement," *Radiologic Technology*, vol. 87, no. 1, pp. 21–28, 2015.

[2] A. H. Gomoll, G. Pappas, B. Forsythe, and J. J. P. Warner, "Individual skill progression on a virtual reality simulator for shoulder arthroscopy: a 3-year follow-up study," *American Journal of Sports Medicine*, vol. 36, no. 6, pp. 1139–1142, 2008.

[3] S. Murphy, M. Tannast, Y.-J. Kim, R. Buly, and M. B. Millis, "Debridement of the adult hip for femoroacetabular impingement: indications and preliminary clinical results," *Clinical Orthopaedics and Related Research*, no. 429, pp. 178–181, 2004.

[4] D. Guttmann, R. D. Graham, M. J. MacLennan, and J. H. Lubowitz, "Arthroscopic rotator cuff repair: the learning curve," *Arthroscopy*, vol. 21, no. 4, pp. 394–400, 2005.

[5] N. R. Howells, M. D. Brinsden, R. S. Gill, A. J. Carr, and J. L. Rees, "Motion analysis: a validated method for showing skill levels in arthroscopy," *Arthroscopy*, vol. 24, no. 3, pp. 335–342, 2008.

[6] A. Insel, B. Carofino, R. Leger, R. Arciero, and A. D. Mazzocca, "The development of an objective model to assess arthroscopic performance," *The Journal of Bone & Joint Surgery—American Volume*, vol. 91, no. 9, pp. 2287–2295, 2009.

[7] P. J. O'Neill, A. J. Cosgarea, J. A. Freedman, W. S. Queale, and E. G. McFarland, "Arthroscopic proficiency: a survey of orthopaedic sports medicine fellowship directors and orthopaedic surgery department chairs," *Arthroscopy*, vol. 18, no. 7, pp. 795–800, 2002.

[8] R. Ganz, J. Parvizi, M. Beck, M. Leunig, H. Nötzli, and K. A. Siebenrock, "Femoroacetabular impingement: a cause for osteoarthritis of the hip," *Clinical Orthopaedics and Related Research*, no. 417, pp. 112–120, 2003.

[9] H. D. Martin, B. T. Kelly, M. Leunig et al., "The pattern and technique in the clinical evaluation of the adult hip: the common physical examination tests of hip specialists," *Arthroscopy*, vol. 26, no. 2, pp. 161–172, 2010.

[10] C. M. Larson, C. A. Guanche, B. T. Kelly, J. C. Clohisy, and A. S. Ranawat, "Advanced techniques in hip arthroscopy," *Instructional Course Lectures*, vol. 58, pp. 423–436, 2009.

[11] C. M. Larson and M. R. Giveans, "Arthroscopic debridement versus refixation of the acetabular labrum associated with femoroacetabular impingement," *Arthroscopy*, vol. 25, no. 4, pp. 369–376, 2009.

[12] M. J. Philippon, K. K. Briggs, Y.-M. Yen, and D. A. Kuppersmith, "Outcomes following hip arthroscopy for femoroacetabular impingement with associated chondrolabral dysfunction: minimum two-year follow-up," *The Journal of Bone & Joint Surgery—British Volume*, vol. 91, no. 1, pp. 16–23, 2009.

[13] L. Bogunovic, M. Gottlieb, G. Pashos, G. Baca, and J. C. Clohisy, "Why do hip arthroscopy procedures fail?" *Clinical Orthopaedics and Related Research*, vol. 471, no. 8, pp. 2523–2529, 2013.

[14] W. C. Brunner, J. R. Korndorffer Jr., R. Sierra et al., "Determining standards for laparoscopic proficiency using virtual reality," *American Surgeon*, vol. 71, no. 1, pp. 29–35, 2005.

[15] A. Brunner, M. Horisberger, and R. F. Herzog, "Evaluation of a computed tomography-based navigation system prototype for hip arthroscopy in the treatment of femoroacetabular cam impingement," *Arthroscopy*, vol. 25, no. 4, pp. 382–391, 2009.

[16] A. H. Gomoll, R. V. O'Toole, J. Czarnecki, and J. J. P. Warner, "Surgical experience correlates with performance on a virtual reality simulator for shoulder arthroscopy," *The American Journal of Sports Medicine*, vol. 35, no. 6, pp. 883–888, 2007.

[17] J. W. T. Byrd and K. S. Jones, "Arthroscopic Femoroplasty in the management of cam-type femoroacetabular impingement," *Clinical Orthopaedics and Related Research*, vol. 467, no. 3, pp. 739–746, 2009.

[18] A. Kassarjian, L. S. Yoon, E. Belzile, S. A. Connolly, M. B. Millis, and W. E. Palmer, "Triad of MR arthrographic findings in patients with cam-type femoroacetabular impingement," *Radiology*, vol. 236, no. 2, pp. 588–592, 2005.

[19] C. W. A. Pfirrmann, S. R. Duc, M. Zanetti, C. Dora, and J. Hodler, "MR arthrography of acetabular cartilage delamination in femoroacetabular cam impingement," *Radiology*, vol. 249, no. 1, pp. 236–241, 2008.

2

Treatment of Aseptic Hypertrophic Nonunion of the Lower Extremity with Less Invasive Stabilization System (New Approach to Hypertrophic Nonunion Treatment)

Metin Uzun,[1] Murat Çakar,[2] Ahmet Murat Bülbül,[3] and Adnan Kara[3]

[1] *Maslak Hospital, Orthopaedic Department, Acibadem University, Darüşşafaka Street, Büyükdere Street No. 40, Maslak, Sarıyer, İstanbul, Turkey*
[2] *Okmeydani Education and Training Hospital, Okmeydani, İstanbul, Turkey*
[3] *Orthopaedic Department, Medipol University, İstanbul, Turkey*

Correspondence should be addressed to Metin Uzun; drmetinuzun@gmail.com

Academic Editor: Werner Kolb

Aim. To evaluate whether aseptic hypertrophic nonunion in the long bones of the lower extremity can be treated successfully with LISS applied with closed methods without grafting. *Materials and Methods.* The study included 7 tibias and 9 femurs of 16 patients. All cases had hypertrophic nonunion. Initial surgical treatment was with intramedullary nailing in 14 cases, 6 of which had required an exchange of intramedullary nail. All the patients were treated with LISS plate with closed methods. *Results.* Union was obtained at mean 7 months in all patients. No implant loosening or breakage of the implant was observed and there was no requirement for secondary surgery. *Conclusion.* Cases of hypertrophic nonunion have excellent blood supply and biological potential. Therefore, there is no need for bone grafting and the addition of fracture stability is enough to achieve full union. Using a limited approach and percutaneous screw insertion, LISS provides fracture stabilization with soft tissue protection.

1. Introduction

Although good outcomes have been reported from the surgical treatment of tibia and femur diaphysis fractures, nonunion can always be a troubling complication. Nonunion may be seen as oligotrophic, hypertrophic, or atrophic. Hypertrophic nonunion differs from other forms of nonunion, as there is still the biological capacity for union. This nonunion type occurs as a result of mechanical instability. Many methods have been reported to enhance stability in the treatment of nonunion, such as plate, intramedullary (IM) nail, or external fixator. The standard treatment is to exchange the IM nail for a larger size, with or without applying graft.

The aim of this study was to evaluate the treatment of hypertrophic nonunion with closed reduction and fracture stability with LISS and to assess if this method was sufficient to achieve union without the necessity of grafting.

2. Materials and Methods

A retrospective evaluation was made of 16 patients with aseptic hypertrophic nonunion of the lower extremity treated with LISS between 2006 and 2009.

The diagnosis of nonunion was made clinically and radiologically. Clinical nonunion was defined as patients with pain and motion at the fracture site and radiological nonunion as no bone bridging observed 6 months after the initial treatment. The cases of hypertrophic nonunion included in the study met the criteria of the Weber and Cech classification. Patients were excluded if they had draining fistulas or infection determined by erythrocyte sedimentation rate, serum C-reactive protein, and white blood cell levels or if the nonunion was septic.

The patients comprised 9 males and 7 females with a mean age of 24 years (range, 15–48 years). The bones involved were

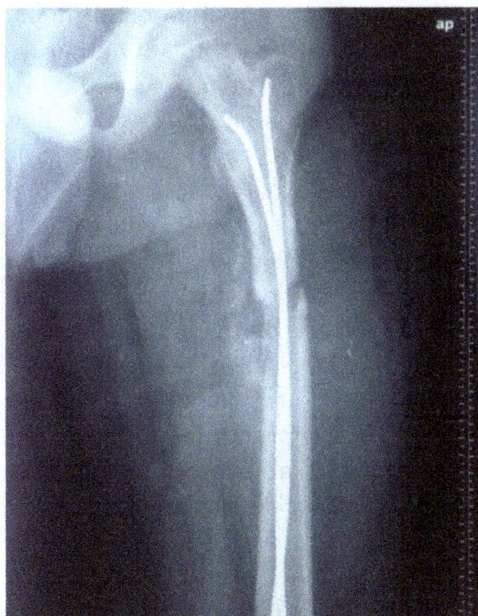

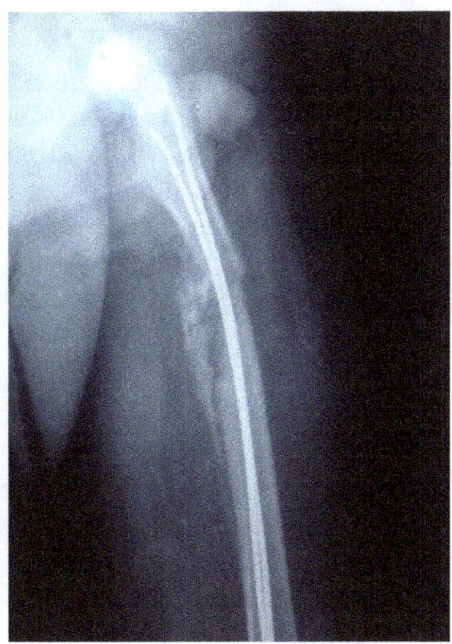

Figure 1: A 14-year-old boy 8 months after a traffic accident. Titanium intramedullary nail was initially applied and hypertrophic nonunion can be seen in the left femur.

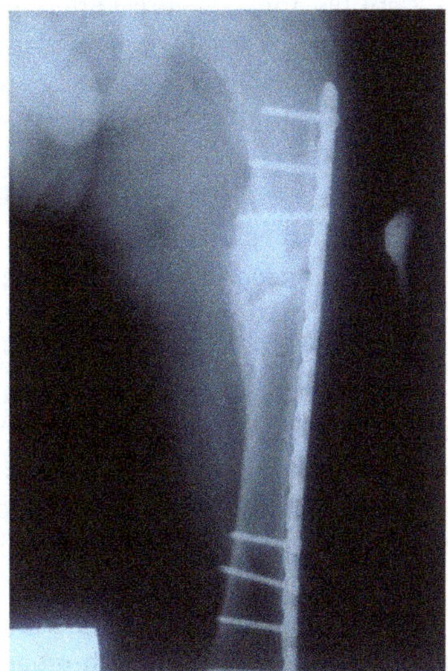

Figure 2: The same patient 3 months after the removal of nails and the application of LISS without grafting.

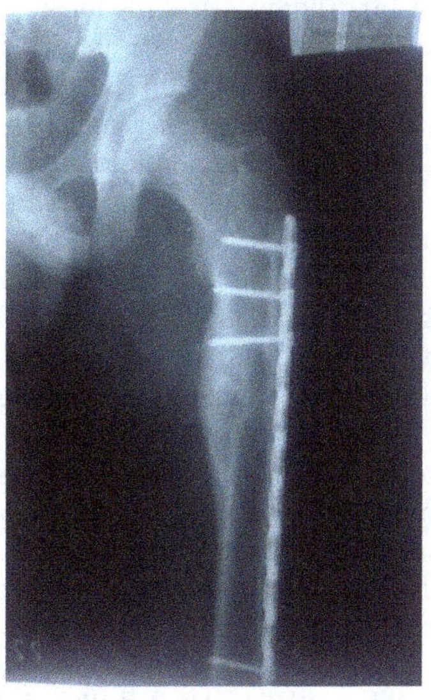

Figure 3: Postoperative 6 months.

7 tibias and 9 femurs with time of nonunion ranging from 7 to 18 months. Two patients were previously managed by cast immobilization only, and the remaining 14 patients were initially treated surgically with intramedullary nailing, 6 of whom had undergone intramedullary nail exchange.

Antibiotic prophylaxis was administered 30 minutes before surgery. The patients were positioned supine on a radiolucent operating table. After the necessary draping and preparation, the previous implants in 14 patients were removed from the previous skin incision (Figure 1). Reduction, alignment, and rotation were corrected under fluoroscopy; then tibial and femoral LISS implants were inserted without opening the fracture site (Figure 2). Postoperative active and passive range of motion exercises were started as soon as could be tolerated. All patients were mobilized on 2 crutches with partial weight-bearing. Antibiotic prophylaxis was continued for 2 days postoperatively. The mean duration of hospitalization was 5.6 days (range, 3–10 days). The patients were followed up clinically and radiologically on postoperative day 1 and then at 3, 6, and 12 weeks and 6, 9, 12, and 18 months. Radiological evaluation was made from standing anteroposterior and lateral radiographs. Clinical evaluation was based on pain, motion in the fracture site, infection, and function. A visual scale was used to evaluate the pain. Union was defined radiologically when there was bridging callus in at least three cortices (Figure 3).

3. Results

In this study, union was achieved in all patients at mean 7 months (range, 4–12 months). Superficial infection was determined in 3 cases (2 femurs and 1 tibia) which was successfully treated with oral antibiotics. Shortening of the limb of <2 cm was seen in 3 (13%) of the patients (1 femur and 2 tibias). No implant loosening or breakage of implants was determined. All patients achieved functional extremities without instability or pain.

4. Discussion

Bone fracture initiates a cascade of events to heal the bone [1, 2]. Any disruption to this cascade from biological or mechanical factors such as poor bone quality, comminution, bone loss, soft tissue damage, infection, insufficient mechanical stabilization, multiple surgery history, or smoking may result in delayed union or nonunion [1, 2].

Nonunion can be classified on the basis of anatomy, the presence and absence of infection, healing potential, or stiffness. The Weber and Cech classification is used for hypertrophic or atrophic nonunion based on the capability of biological reaction [3]. The hypertrophic form is characterized by abundant callus formation and a persistent radiolucent line at the fracture site. This form especially occurs due to lack of mechanical stability, but there is a sufficient blood supply and new bone formation. This nonunion type has biological potential and often only requires the addition of fracture stability to be able to achieve union.

Treatment of hypertrophic nonunion can be achieved through enhancement of stability. Therefore, many surgical techniques have been applied, including screw and plate fixation, external fixation, intramedullary nailing, bone transport, and free fibula grafting with or without bone grafting [2, 4–8]. However, if there is a history of surgery, the most popular treatment is to exchange the nail for a larger size with or without debridement at the nonunion site. If there is no surgical history or deformity, then open reduction and stabilization by plating with bone graft has been a standard treatment for diaphyseal nonunion of long bones [6, 9–11]. Some authors such as Bellabarbo and Weresh have reported difficulties and failure of exchange reamed intramedullary nails in nonunited femoral shaft fractures [6, 10, 11]. In the light of this, new techniques have been developed using LISS to enhance mechanical stability in lower extremity long bone hypertrophic nonunion, as was used in the current study [12–14].

When literature is examined, LCP was introduced for four reasons: (1) osteoporotic bone fracture, (2) comminution at the fracture site, (3) intra-articular fracture, and (4) short segment periarticular fracture [15–17]. The advantage of LCP is that stability does not depend on compression between the plate and bone and the periosteal blood supply to the fracture fragments is better preserved compared to DCP [16, 17]. Although many authors have tried to use this advantage for nonunion treatment, because of the prolonged immobilization periods and repeated operations required in severely osteopenic bones, good screw hold can not be achieved. Therefore, as a new treatment modality, LCP augmentation has been used with retaining hardware in cases previously treated with IM nail [5, 9, 10, 13, 14]. The advantages of the retaining nail are as follows: (1) alignment of the fracture is maintained and could help to maintain stability, (2) sometimes removal of the broken screw or nail may not be possible, and (3) there is no additional operating time entailing more blood loss and more soft tissue damage [15–17]. Chen et al. treated 55 patients with aseptic nonunion of femoral shaft fractures by retaining previous implants, open reduction, and internal fixation with DCP and supplementation with cancellous bone graft [12]. All nonunions united at 24 weeks and superficial wound infection developed in 1 case. Nadkarni et al. evaluated 11 patients who had previously undergone locked intramedullary nailing for fractures of long bones [13]. In all cases, the fracture site was exposed and LCP was applied over the intramedullary nail with autologous bone graft. Radiological union was achieved in all cases at 6.2 months and no complications developed. Kumar evaluated the role of locking plate with graft in difficult nonunion fractures. Roetman et al. analyzed augmentive plate fixation in 32 femoral nonunions after intramedullary nailing and it was concluded that augmentive plate fixation while leaving the nail in situ is simple and safe [14]. Different studies have found a union rate from 94% to 100% with plating [13, 14].

Although some authors have reported excellent results from the open method using LCP, there may be problems in the application of the plate due to bone surface deformation associated with hypertrophy at the fracture site. However, Wagner reported excellent results and showed that plate can be applied easily with no need to mould the plate [17].

In light of this information in literature, we considered that, with enhanced stability, union could be achieved without debridement and grafting. Therefore, all the patients in this study were treated with LISS applied with closed reduction and without any bone graft. Using the closed method resulted in a shorter operating time, less blood loss, no donor site problems for a bone graft area, and, consequently, less pain and less analgesia requirement. In this study, 16 patients with nonunion of the long bones were treated with LISS applied with the closed method without any bone graft. Union was achieved in all patients in mean 7 months (range, 4–12 months).

In conclusion, hypertrophic bone nonunion has an excellent blood supply and biological potential, so there is no need for bone grafting and just the addition of fracture stability will be enough to provide full osseous union. LISS provides fracture stabilization with soft tissue protection through the use of a limited approach and percutaneous screw insertion.

Disclosure

This is an original paper and its level of evidence is level 4 case series.

Conflict of Interests

The authors declare that there is no conflict of interests regarding the publication of this paper.

Acknowledgments

This paper was developed at the two centers of Acibadem University, Maslak Hospital, and Medipol University.

References

[1] K. J. Pugh and S. R. Rozbruch, "Nonunions and malunions," in *Orthopaedic Knowledge Update, Trauma*, M. R. Baumgaertner and P. Tornetta, Eds., pp. 117–118, American Acadamy of Orthopaedic Surgeons, Rosemont, Ill, USA, 2005.

[2] E. C. Rodriguez-Merchan and F. Forriol, "Nonunion: general principles and experimental data," *Clinical Orthopaedics and Related Research*, no. 419, pp. 4–12, 2004.

[3] B. G. Weber and O. Cech, *Pseudoarthrosis: Pathology, Biomechanics, Therapy, Results*, Hans Huber Medical Publisher, Berne, Switzerland, 1976.

[4] K.-D. Gao, J.-H. Huang, F. Li et al., "Treatment of aseptic diaphyseal nonunion of the lower extremities with exchange intramedullary nailing and blocking screws without open bone graft," *Orthopaedic Surgery*, vol. 1, no. 4, pp. 264–268, 2009.

[5] K.-D. Gao, J.-H. Huang, J. Tao et al., "Management of femoral diaphyseal nonunion after nailing with augmentative locked plating and bone graft," *Orthopaedic Surgery*, vol. 3, no. 2, pp. 83–87, 2011.

[6] D. J. Hak, "Management of aseptic tibial nonunion," *The Journal of the American Academy of Orthopaedic Surgeons*, vol. 19, no. 9, pp. 563–573, 2011.

[7] M. Kocaoğlu, L. Eralp, C. Sen, M. Cakmak, H. Dincyürek, and S. B. Göksan, "Management of stiff hypertrophic nonunions by distraction osteogenesis: a report of 16 cases," *Journal of Orthopaedic Trauma*, vol. 17, no. 8, pp. 543–548, 2003.

[8] L. X. Webb, "Bone defect nonunion of the lower extremity," *Techniques in Orthopaedics*, vol. 16, no. 4, pp. 387–397, 2001.

[9] C. Bellabarba, W. M. Ricci, and B. R. Bolhofner, "Results of indirect reduction and plating of femoral shaft nonunions after intramedullary nailing," *Journal of Orthopaedic Trauma*, vol. 15, no. 4, pp. 254–263, 2001.

[10] M. J. Weresh, R. Hakanson, M. D. Stover, S. H. Sims, J. F. Kellam, and M. J. Bosse, "Failure of exchange reamed intramedullary nails for ununited femoral shaft fractures," *Journal of Orthopaedic Trauma*, vol. 14, no. 5, pp. 335–338, 2000.

[11] A. J. Furlong, P. V. Giannoudis, P. DeBoer, S. J. Matthews, D. A. MacDonald, and R. M. Smith, "Exchange nailing for femoral shaft aseptic non-union," *Injury*, vol. 30, no. 4, pp. 245–249, 1999.

[12] C.-M. Chen, Y.-P. Su, S.-H. Hung, C.-L. Lin, and F.-Y. Chiu, "Dynamic compression plate and cancellous bone graft for aseptic nonunion after intramedullary nailing of femoral fracture," *Orthopedics*, vol. 33, article 393, 2010.

[13] B. Nadkarni, S. Srivastav, V. Mittal, and S. Agarwal, "Use of locking compression plates for long bone nonunions without removing existing intramedullary nail: review of literature and our experience," *The Journal of Trauma*, vol. 65, no. 2, pp. 482–486, 2008.

[14] B. Roetman, N. Scholz, G. Muhr, and G. Möllenhoff, "Augmentive plate fixation in femoral non-unions after intramedullary nailing. Strategy after unsuccessful intramedullary nailing of the femur," *Zeitschrift fur Orthopadie und Unfallchirurgie*, vol. 146, no. 5, pp. 586–590, 2008.

[15] K. A. Egol, E. N. Kubiak, E. Fulkerson, F. J. Kummer, and K. J. Koval, "Biomechanics of locked plates and screws," *Journal of Orthopaedic Trauma*, vol. 18, no. 8, pp. 488–493, 2004.

[16] W. R. Smith, B. H. Ziran, J. O. Anglen, and P. F. Stahel, "Locking plates: tips and tricks," *The Journal of Bone & Joint Surgery—American Volume*, vol. 89, no. 10, pp. 2298–2307, 2007.

[17] M. Wagner, "General principles for the clinical use of the LCP," *Injury*, vol. 34, supplement 2, pp. 31–42, 2003.

3

The Effect of a Femoral Fracture Sustained before Skeletal Maturity on Bone Mineral Density: A Long-Term Follow-Up Study

J. A. Kettunen,[1] S. Palmu,[2,3] K. Tallroth,[4] Y. Nietosvaara,[2] and M. Lohman[5]

[1] *Arcada University of Applied Sciences, Jan-Magnus Janssonin Aukio 1, 00550 Helsinki, Finland*
[2] *Children's Hospital, Helsinki University Central Hospital, P.O. Box 281, 00029 Helsinki, Finland*
[3] *Tampere Center for Child Health Research (TACC), University of Tampere and Tampere University Hospital, Lääkärinkatu 1, 33014 Tampere, Finland*
[4] *Orton Orthopaedic Hospital, Orton Foundation, P.O. Box 29, 00281 Helsinki, Finland*
[5] *Department of Radiology, HUS Medical Imaging Center, Helsinki University Central Hospital and University of Helsinki, P.O. Box 340, 00029 Helsinki, Finland*

Correspondence should be addressed to J. A. Kettunen; jyrki.kettunen@arcada.fi

Academic Editor: Werner Kolb

Background and Purpose. The possible effect of pediatric femoral fractures on the bone mineral density (BMD) is largely unknown. We conducted a study to investigate BMD in adults who had sustained a femoral shaft fracture in childhood treated with skeletal traction. *Materials and Methods.* Forty-four adults, who had had a femoral fracture before skeletal maturity, were reexamined on average 21 (range 11.4) years after treatment. Our follow-up study included a questionnaire, a clinical examination, length and angle measurements of the lower extremities from follow-up radiographs, and a DEXA examination with regional BMD values obtained for both legs separately. *Results.* At follow-up femoral varus-valgus ($P = 0.001$) and ante-/recurvatum ($P = 0.001$) angles were slightly larger in the injured lower-limb compared to the contralateral limb. The mean BMD of the entire injured lower-limb was lower than that of the noninjured (1.323 g/cm^2 versus 1.346 g/cm^2, $P = 0.003$). Duration of traction was the only factor in multiple linear regression analysis that was positively correlated with the BMD discrepancy between the injured and noninjured lower-limb explaining about 17% of its variation. *Conclusion.* The effect of a femoral fracture sustained during growth is small even in patients treated with traction.

1. Introduction

Decreased bone mineral density (BMD) has been diagnosed in adults as sequel of immobilisation and reduced weight bearing in the injured limb [1]. Henderson et al. [2] have reported a decreased BMD in proximal femur two years after tibial and femoral fractures in children that were immobilised for eight weeks or longer. Ferrari et al. [3] have found an association between a childhood fracture and low BMD in adulthood suggesting low peak bone mass and persistent bone fragility.

We studied long-term effects of pediatric femoral shaft fractures treated with skeletal traction on BMD.

2. Materials and Methods

Sixty-two pediatric patients (<16 years old, all Scandinavian Caucasian) that had sustained a femoral fracture were treated with skeletal traction (in a hospital bed) in Aurora Hospital, Helsinki, during 1980–1989. The most common injury type was a motor-vehicle accident.

Patient files and primary radiographs of these patients were analysed. A questionnaire about subjective treatment results as well as an invitation to participate in a follow-up examination (mean 21, range 11.4, standard deviation (SD) 2.8 years) was mailed to all patients [4]. Fifty-two of the patients agreed to participate. They all gave written informed consent

TABLE 1: Characteristics of patients at baseline and at follow-up.

Characteristics	At baseline (N = 44)	At follow-up (N = 44)
Age		
Years; mean (SD)[1]	8.0 (3.2)	29.1 (3.9)
Minimum–maximum	3–15	23–39
Height		
m; mean (SD)		1.76 (0.1)
Minimum–maximum		1.53–1.95
Weight		
kg; mean (SD)		74.8 (15.7)
Minimum–maximum		45–105
BMI[2]		
kg/m^2; mean (SD)		24.1 (3.9)
Minimum–maximum		16–31
Fracture location		
Proximal	13	
Distal	11	
Mid-shaft	28	
Treatment method		
Traction	44	
Tibial traction	34	
Femoral traction	10	

[1]SD: standard deviation.
[2]BMI: Body Mass Index.

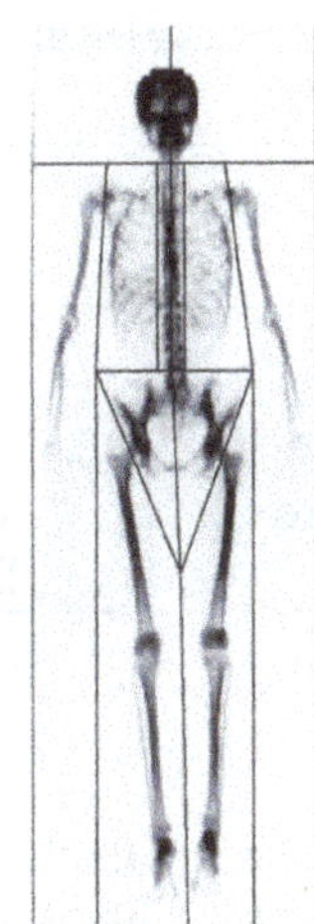

FIGURE 1: Whole body DEXA measurement, demonstrating measurement areas separately for each lower extremity.

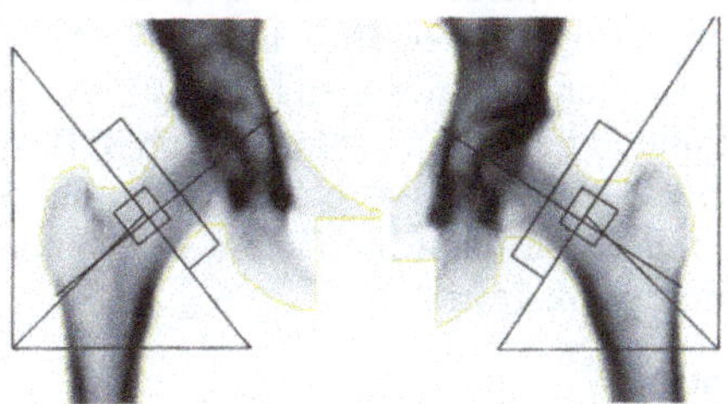

FIGURE 2: The areas for bone mass measurement for the right and left femoral neck.

approved by the local Ethics Committee of the Helsinki University Central Hospital (approval identification number 68/E7/2002).

Forty-four patients (15 females, 29 males, mean age 29 years) attended the follow-up study including clinical examination, lower-limb radiographs, and DEXA examination. None of our patients was known to have any metabolic or other disease, neither as child nor as adult. Demographics data of the patients are seen in Table 1.

The radiographic examinations were conducted at the time of the follow-up and consisted of standing anteroposterior radiographs of both legs and standing lateral views of the femurs. The anteroposterior hip-to-ankle radiographs were obtained separately of both extremities. They were taken in fluoroscopy control at a distance of 1.5 m on analog films. For length measurements a long radio-opaque ruler was fixed to the leg. The images were evaluated for the length of the lower-limbs and femurs in millimetres.

The mechanical axis of the entire leg was measured according to the method described by Hagstedt et al. [5]. In addition to the mechanical axis both femurs were analysed for angular deformity in two planes, that is, varus/valgus in the frontal view and ante-/recurvatum in the lateral view. For these assessments of the coronal and lateral curves lines through the midsection of the proximal and distal femoral diaphyses were drawn and measured with a manual goniometer.

DEXA examinations were performed using a narrow fan-beam Lunar Prodigy densitometer (GE Lunar Corporation, Madison, WI, USA). To verify the stability of the DEXA system a control procedure of the scanner was performed weekly in addition to a daily calibration according to manufacturer's instructions.

The subjects were positioned in supine position on the scanning table with the body aligned with the midline of the scanning table. The legs were straight and strapped in slight internal rotation. The Lunar Prodigy software uses a series of complex algorithms to calculate BMD and bone mass in the total body and for different anatomical regions, in our study the legs and femoral necks (Figures 1 and 2). The results were measured and reported as kilograms for total body weight (BW) and BMD was measured in g/cm^2.

Bone density was separately measured in the lower legs (Figure 1) and in femoral neck (Figure 2). In previous studies from our institution with the same scanner the precision of total bone and extremity density measurements have shown excellent repeatability and are expressed as the coefficient of variation 1,0% for total body [6] and 1,6% for the lower extremity [7]. The precision is consistent with the literature [8, 9].

Two senior musculoskeletal radiologists made all the radiographic (M. Lohman) and DEXA measurements (K. Tallroth) independently of each other and blinded regarding previous readings.

The statistical analysis was done with Statistical Package for the Social Sciences 21.0 (Norusis/SPSS, Inc., Chicago, IL).

TABLE 2: Lower-limb length, femur length, and lower-limb angular deformities at follow-up radiographic evaluation among patients with a childhood femoral fracture.

Characteristics	Noninjured mean (SD)[1]	Injured mean (SD)[1]	Noninjured–injured mean (95% CI)[2]	P value
Lower-limb length, cm	84.8 (5.9)	84.5 (6.2)	0.3 (−0.2 to 0.8)	0.287
Femur length, cm	47.5 (4.9)	46.9 (3.7)	0.7 (−0.4 to 1.7)	0.224
Mechanical axis, degrees	2.1 (1.9)	3.5 (2.8)	−1.4 (−2.3 to −0.6)	0.001
Femoral angulation				
Ante-/recurvatum, degrees	8.3 (2.3)	11.6 (6.4)	−3.3 (−5.1 to −1.4)	0.001
Varus-valgus, degrees	1.2 (2.0)	3.4 (3.6)	−2.2 (−3.4 to −1.0)	0.001

[1]SD: standard deviation.
[2]CI: confidence interval.

Paired samples or independent samples t-test was used to test differences between the lower-limbs among variables with normal distribution. Correspondingly, Wilcoxon signed rank test or Mann-Whitney U test was used among not normally distributed variables. Pearson's product moment correlation coefficient or Spearman's rho was used to investigate the relationship between different factors and BMD. Multiple linear regression analysis was used to study the determinants of the noninjured minus injured lower-limb BMD difference.

To evaluate the factors associated with the lower-limb BMD difference, the following factors were entered into a stepwise multiple regression analysis:

(i) gender,

(ii) age at injury,

(iii) traction time,

(iv) height,

(v) weight,

(vi) BMI,

(vii) follow-up time,

(viii) noninjured minus injured lower-limb length difference,

(ix) noninjured minus injured femur length difference,

(x) noninjured minus injured thigh circumference difference noninjured minus injured lower-limbs mechanical axis difference,

(xi) noninjured minus injured lower-limbs femoral varus-valgus difference,

(xii) noninjured minus injured lower-limbs femoral ante-/recurvatum difference.

3. Results

Mean duration of skeletal traction was 39.6 days (range 74, SD 15.8). Significant differences in leg lengths were not found (Table 2). Mean mechanical axis in both frontal and sagittal planes was slightly larger in the injured lower-limb compared to the noninjured contralateral limb (Table 2).

Whole body BMD was within normal limits in all patients according to the manufacturer's reference values. Mean BMD of the entire injured lower-limb was lower than that of the noninjured lower-limb (1.323 g/cm^2 versus 1.347 g/cm^2, $P = 0.003$). BMD of the femoral neck of the injured lower-limb did not differ from the limb without an injury (mean 0.998 g/cm^2 versus 0.995 g/cm^2, $P = 0.806$). BMD difference between the injured and the noninjured limb was statistically significant in male patients (mean 1.403 g/cm^2 versus 1.380 g/cm^2, $P = 0.023$), but not in female patients (mean 1.245 g/cm^2 versus 1.227 g/cm^2, $P = 0.203$).

The only factor that was associated with the lower-limbs BMD difference was the duration of traction explaining about 17% of its variation.

4. Discussion

In the 1980s most pediatric femoral fractures in Finland were treated without internal fixation, which allowed us to perform DEXA measurements on these patients without disturbing fixation devices such as metal plates or nails. The BMD was not evaluated before the fracture took place, which is obviously a limitation of our study. However, the mean follow-up time after the fracture was longer than in most of the previous studies.

Femoral fractures sustained before skeletal maturity have been reported to reduce the injured femur's BMD distal to the fracture site [1, 10], lower BMD values than in the noninjured extremity have been registered in the injured extremity 11 years after tibial shaft fractures [11], and girls have been reported to have a decreased body bone mineral content four years after a distal forearm fracture [12]. Our findings are in line with these earlier studies although we found that BMD of the injured lower extremity was only slightly lower compared (mean 2%) to the noninjured lower extremity. Furthermore, we did not find a decreased BMD proximal to the fracture. Malignment of the femur in neither frontal nor sagittal plane correlated with BMD in this study. No correlation was found between the mechanical axis of the lower extremity and the BMD. This is most likely explained by the fact that only few patients in our study with malunion had permanent deformity that is regarded unsatisfactory according to clinical guidelines [13].

Nikander et al. [14] concluded that exercise can significantly enhance bone strength at loaded sites in children. Leppälä and coworkers [10] found a positive correlation between muscle strength and bone density of the tibia in patients that had been rehabilitated from a tibial fracture. We did not collect data of physical activity nor test muscle function of our patients. No difference was however found in femoral circumferences suggesting recovery of muscle function of the injured leg.

Pediatric femoral fractures treated with several weeks long skeletal traction in bed do not lead to clinically significant decrease of BMD of the lower extremity in adulthood.

Conflict of Interests

The authors declare that there is no conflict of interests regarding the publication of this paper.

References

[1] B. E. Nilsson and N. E. Westlin, "Restoration of bone mass after fracture of the lower limb in children," *Acta Orthopaedica Scandinavica*, vol. 42, no. 1, pp. 78–81, 1971.

[2] R. C. Henderson, G. J. Kemp, and E. R. Campion, "Residual bone-mineral density and muscle strength after fractures of the tibia or femur in children," *Journal of Bone and Joint Surgery—Series A*, vol. 74, no. 2, pp. 211–218, 1992.

[3] S. L. Ferrari, T. Chevalley, J.-P. Bonjour, and R. Rizzoli, "Childhood fractures are associated with decreased bone mass gain during puberty: an early marker of persistent bone fragility?" *Journal of Bone and Mineral Research*, vol. 21, no. 4, pp. 501–507, 2006.

[4] S. A. Palmu, M. Lohman, R. T. Paukku, J. I. Peltonen, and Y. Nietosvaara, "Childhood femoral fracture can lead to premature knee-joint arthritis," *Acta Orthopaedica*, vol. 84, pp. 71–75, 2013.

[5] B. Hagstedt, O. Norman, T. H. Olsson, and B. Tjornstrand, "Technical accuracy in high tibial osteotomy for gonarthrosis," *Acta Orthopaedica Scandinavica*, vol. 51, no. 6, pp. 963–970, 1980.

[6] V. M. Mattila, K. Tallroth, M. Marttinen, O. Ohrankammen, and H. Pihlajamaki, "DEXA body composition changes among 140 conscripts," *International Journal of Sports Medicine*, vol. 30, no. 5, pp. 348–353, 2009.

[7] M. Lohman, K. Tallroth, J. A. Kettunen, and M. T. Marttinen, "Reproducibility of dual-energy x-ray absorptiometry total and regional body composition measurements using different scanning positions and definitions of regions," *Metabolism: Clinical and Experimental*, vol. 58, no. 11, pp. 1663–1668, 2009.

[8] G. M. Kiebzak, L. J. Leamy, L. M. Pierson, R. H. Nord, and Z. Y. Zhang, "Measurement precision of body composition variables using the Lunar DPX-L densitometer," *Journal of Clinical Densitometry*, vol. 3, no. 1, pp. 35–41, 2000.

[9] G. M. Chan, "Performance of dual-energy x-ray absorptiometry in evaluating bone, lean body mass, and fat in pediatric subjects," *Journal of Bone and Mineral Research*, vol. 7, no. 4, pp. 369–374, 1992.

[10] J. Leppälä, P. Kannus, S. Niemi, H. Sievänen, I. Vuori, and M. Järvinen, "An early-life femoral shaft fracture and bone mineral density at adulthood," *Osteoporosis International*, vol. 10, no. 4, pp. 337–342, 1999.

[11] J. Leppälä, P. Kannus, H. Sievänen, I. Vuori, and M. Järvinen, "A tibial shaft fracture sustained in childhood or adolescence does not c to interfere with attainment of peak bone density," *Journal of Bone and Mineral Research*, vol. 14, no. 6, pp. 988–993, 1999.

[12] I. E. Jones, R. W. Taylor, S. M. Williams, P. J. Manning, and A. Goulding, "Four-year gain in bone mineral in girls with and without past forearm fractures: a DXA study," *Journal of Bone and Mineral Research*, vol. 17, no. 6, pp. 1065–1072, 2002.

[13] J. M. Flynn and D. L. Skaggs, "Femoral shaft fractures," in *Rockwood and Wilkins' Fractures in Children*, Beaty and Kasser, Eds., chapter 22, pp. 797–841, Lippincott Williams & Wilkins, Philadelphia, Pa, USA, 7th edition.

[14] R. Nikander, H. Sievänen, A. Heinonen, R. M. Daly, K. Uusi-Rasi, and P. Kannus, "Targeted exercise against osteoporosis: a systematic review and meta-analysis for optimising bone strength throughout life," *BMC Medicine*, vol. 8, article 47, 2010.

4

Implementation of an Accelerated Rehabilitation Protocol for Total Joint Arthroplasty in the Managed Care Setting: The Experience of One Institution

Nicholas B. Robertson,[1] Tibor Warganich,[1] John Ghazarossian,[2] and Monti Khatod[2]

[1]Harbor UCLA Medical Center, Department of Orthopaedics, 1000 W. Carson Street Box 422, Torrance, CA 90245, USA
[2]Kaiser West Los Angeles, Department of Orthopaedics, 6041 Cadillac Avenue, Los Angeles, CA 90034, USA

Correspondence should be addressed to Monti Khatod; monti.x.khatod@kp.org

Academic Editor: Guoxin Ni

Accelerated rehabilitation following total joint replacement (TJR) surgery has become more common in contemporary orthopaedic practice. Increased utilization demands improvements in resource allocation with continued improvement in patient outcomes. We describe an accelerated rehab protocol (AR) instituted at a community based hospital. All patients undergoing total knee arthroplasty (TKA) and total hip arthroplasty (THA) were included. The AR consisted of preoperative patient education, standardization of perioperative pain management, therapy, and next day in-home services consultation following discharge. Outcomes of interest include average length of stay (ALOS), discharge disposition, 42-day return to Urgent Care (UC), Emergency Department (ED), or readmission. A total of 4 surgeons performed TJR procedures on 1,268 patients in the study period (696 TKA, 572 THA). ALOS was reduced from 3.5 days at the start of the observation period to 2.4 days at the end. Discharge to skilled nursing reduced from 25% to 14%. A multifaceted and evidence based approach to standardization of care delivery has resulted in improved patient outcomes and a reduction in resource utilization. Adoption of an accelerated rehab protocol has proven to be effective as well as safe without increased utilization of UC, ER, or readmissions.

1. Introduction

Total joint arthroplasty has historically not been considered an outpatient surgery among the majority of orthopedic surgeons. Some estimate the average cost per hospital stay to be $24,170 for primary total hip arthroplasty. In 2005, in an academic US practice, ALOS for revision versus primary THA was 6.5 and 5.6 days, respectively [1]. A recent study utilizing the national registry in Denmark quoted an average length of stay (ALOS) of 7.4 days after total hip arthroplasty (THA) and 8.0 days after total knee arthroplasty (TKA) [2]. A United States based study in 2004 revealed that a rapid recovery protocol decreased the average length of stay from 3.9 to 2.8 days while also decreasing readmission rates [3]. More recently, an accelerated rehabilitation (AR) protocol reduced ALOS an average of 1.36 days following primary THA (3.38 days for standard rehabilitation and 2.06 days for the AR protocol) [4]. Previous studies have evaluated the use of mini-incision THA and ALOS. Mears et al. found no advantage to mini-incision arthroplasty surgery regarding early discharge [5]. Ogonda et al. found that mini-incision THA does not improve early postoperative outcomes [6]. More important than the size of the incision, an aggressive pain protocol and patient education and in-home care preparation are key components to accelerated rehabilitation protocols.

Parvataneni et al. previously demonstrated in a randomized control trial that multimodal pain therapy alongside a periarticular injection could safely and effectively be used as an alternative to conventional pain control modalities [7]. The purpose of this investigation is to report the reduction in ALOS following primary THA and TKA in a US community hospital utilizing an intraoperative periarticular injection and multimodal perioperative pain protocol in conjunction with patient and family preparation for rapid rehabilitation.

Table 1

Number of surgeries	572	696	1,268
Number of patients	522	621	1,130
Age			
Average	68.0	71.0	69.6
Min.	26.0	41.0	26.0
Max.	96.0	96.0	96.0
Gender			
Male	186	213	398
Female	336	408	732
Total	522	621	1,130
Gender %			
Male	35.6%	34.3%	35.2%
Female	64.4%	65.7%	64.8%
Total	100.0%	100.0%	100.0%

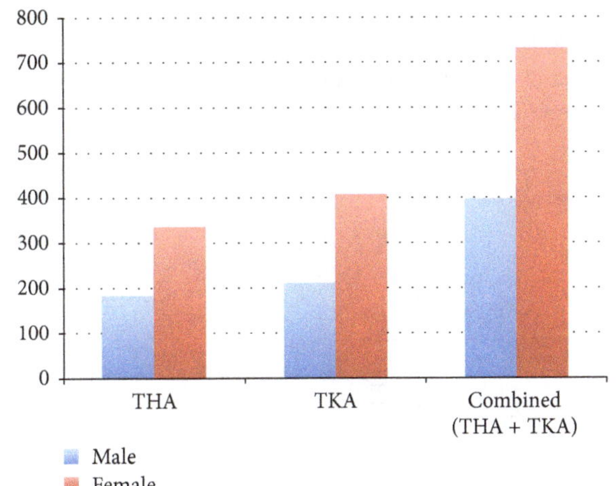

Figure 1: Gender demographics of patients receiving TJA.

At our institution in January 2011, we adopted a comprehensive, multidisciplinary approach to total joint replacement. Over a three-and-a-half-year period, we present the results of the implementation of an AR protocol and the effect of ALOS, placement in skilled nursing facilities (SNF), and decreased rehospitalizations, Emergency Department (ED), and Urgent Care (UC) visits within 42 days of the procedure. A secondary outcome is the rate of transfusion.

2. Materials and Methods

After obtaining approval by the institutional review board, a retrospective review was conducted on a total of 1,268 patients who received a total joint replacement from January 1, 2011, to July 31, 2014 (696 TKA and 572 THA). Demographic data including the age and gender of the patients can be seen in Appendix B, Table 1. The average age of the patients in the entire cohort is 69.6 (26–96). Of the patients in the cohort 35.2% were male and 64.8% were female. A graphical representation of gender can be seen in Appendix B, Figure 1. Utilizing the Kaiser Permanente West Los Angeles patient database, patients who had undergone "knee replacement" or "hip replacement" were utilized for the database query between January 2012 and July 2014. This was conducted using the data source system clarity optime. For the query, "knee replacement" included "Knee Replacement Total," "Knee Replacement Revision Total, Cemented," and "Knee Replacement Revision, All Component." "Hip replacement" consists of "Hip Replacement Total," "Hip Replacement Revision, Femoral Component," "Hip Replacement Revision, Both Acetabular And Femoral Component," "Hip Replacement Revision, Total," and "Hip Replacement Revision, Acetabular Liner And Femoral Head." For simplicity, the groups will be referred to as TKA and THA, respectively.

The patient information that was evaluated in this search included the ALOS, transfusion rates, readmission rates to the Urgent Care, Emergency Department, or inpatient hospitalization for the 42 days postoperatively. Secondary outcomes evaluated include discharge location (SNF, home ± home health), PE, DVT, mortality, and deep infection.

A total of four surgeons perform hip and knee arthroplasty surgery at this institution. All four surgeons adopted and implemented the accelerated rehabilitation protocol in January 2011. The advanced rehabilitation protocol involves a multidisciplinary approach to total joint replacement. This comprehensive program is standardized among the participating surgeons, physical therapists, nurses, anesthesiologists, and pharmacy. The key to the success of the program is an integrated system based approach and appropriate education of these multiple teams. Each member plays a crucial part in the success of the AR protocol. The rehabilitation protocol involves preoperative patient education (instruct patient on importance of ambulation on postoperative day 0 and prepare for next day hospital discharge), preoperative pain control administered in PACU, education to the ancillary staff (nursing and therapists) to anticipate a LOS of 24–48 hrs, intraoperative administration of local anesthesia, and physical therapy initiated on postoperative day 0 for transfer and gait training. Please see Appendix A for details.

A protocol to decrease the number of transfusions was also implemented by adopting a standardized protocol including the use of restrictive transfusion triggers. During the preoperative visit, if patients have a hemoglobin (Hb) > 13, no blood donation is required. For patients with a preoperative Hb of 10–13, patients are encouraged to donate 1 unit of blood. Patients with a preoperative Hb < 10 are referred to Internal Medicine for anemia work-up. All patients start iron supplementation (FeGluc 325 mg PO BID) at time of being scheduled for a total joint replacement. At time of surgery, patients without a contraindication are given one weight-based, preoperative dose of tranexamic acid prior to skin incision and one at the conclusion of the procedure in the PACU. Hb and hematocrit are drawn on the morning of POD#1, 2, and 3. Patients are transfused one unit of PRBC if Hb < 7. If Hb is between 7 and 9 and patient is symptomatic (tachycardia at rest or orthostatic hypotension), the patient is first resuscitated with fluids. If symptoms persist after fluid resuscitation, then the patient is transfused with 1 u PRBC. If Hb > 9, then patients are administered fluids only.

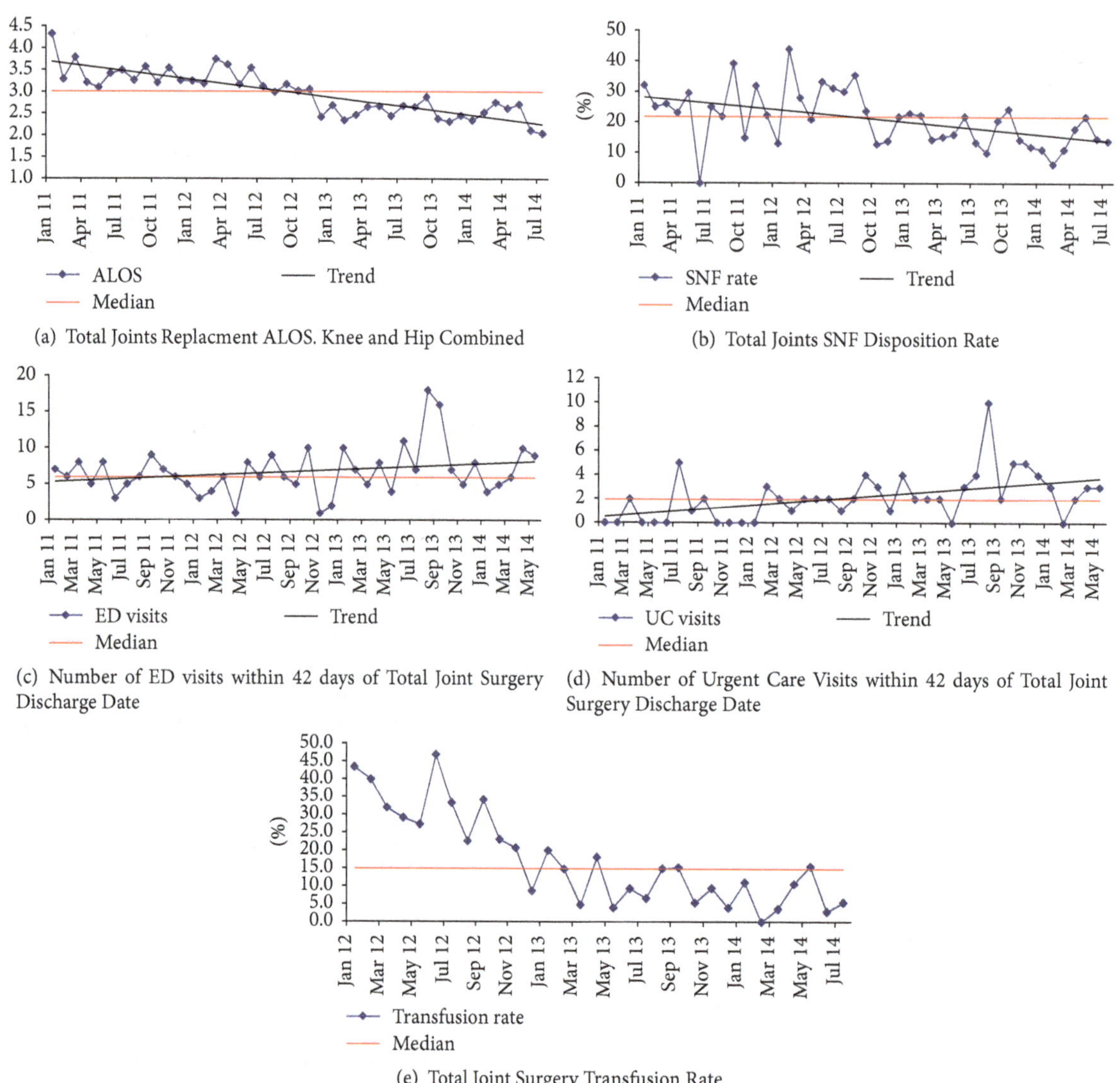

(a) Total Joints Replacment ALOS. Knee and Hip Combined

(b) Total Joints SNF Disposition Rate

(c) Number of ED visits within 42 days of Total Joint Surgery Discharge Date

(d) Number of Urgent Care Visits within 42 days of Total Joint Surgery Discharge Date

(e) Total Joint Surgery Transfusion Rate

FIGURE 2: (a) Total Joints ALOS. (b) Total Joints Disposition to SNF rate. (c) Emergency Department Visits within 42 days of total joint arthroplasty. (d) Emergency Department Visits within 42 days of total joint arthroplasty. (e) Total Joint Transfusion Rate.

3. Results

A total of 1,268 patients underwent hip or knee arthroplasty during the study period. There were 696 (54.9%) patients in the TKA group and 572 (45.1%) patients in the THA group.

In analyzing the entire group, the patients stayed a total of 3,725 hospital days with an ALOS of 2.9 days during the study period. With the implementation of the accelerated rehabilitation protocol, the ALOS was decreased from 3.5 in 2011 to 2.4 at the conclusion of the study period in 2014 (see Figure 2(a)). Postoperatively, 264 (20.8%) patients were discharged from the hospital to a SNF. The trend was for a decreased rate of SNF placement from 2011 to 2014, with 25% of patients discharged to SNF at start of study and 14% discharged at conclusion of the study (see Figure 2(b)). In total there were 276 (21.8%) visits to the ED, 87 (6.9%) visits to the UC, and 57 (4.5%) rehospitalizations within 42 days of surgery. In 2011, there were 75 visits (24%) to the ED and at the conclusion of the study there were 34 visits (16%) (see Figure 2(c)). In 2011, there were 10 UC visits (3%) and in 2014 there were 11 visits to UC (5%) (see Figure 2(d)). The number of IP admissions was 18 (6%) in 2011 and 7 (3%) in 2014.

During the study period, 696 patients underwent TKA, revision, or primary. These patients combined to a total of 2005 days hospitalized after surgery. The ALOS decreased each year from 2011 to 2014, 3.4, 3.2, 2.5, and 2.3, respectively. In 2011 and 2012 the rate of discharge to SNF was 26%. In 2013 and 2014 these numbers decreased to 16% and 13%, respectively. This group had a total of 165 ED visits, 45 UC visits, and 26 inpatient hospitalizations within 42 days of surgery during the study period. In 2011, there were 48 ED visits (25%) and 7 UC visits. In 2014 there were 19 ED visits (16%) and 7 UC visits (6%). The number of inpatient admissions decreased from 11 (6%) in 2011 to 6 (1%) in 2014.

Regarding the THA group, 572 surgeries were conducted during the study period for revision or primary. These patients had a sum of 1720 days hospitalized postoperatively. The rate of discharge to a SNF was 22% and 25% in 2011 and 2012, respectively. These rates decreased to 20% in 2013 and 14% in 2014. The ALOS also decreased from 3.6 in 2011 to 2.5 in 2014. In 2011 there were 27 (22%) ED visits and 3 (2%) UC visits. In 2014 there were 15 (4%) ED visits and 4 (4%) UC visits. There were 7 (6%) IP admissions in 2011 and 6 (6%) IP admission in 2014.

The transfusion rate was analyzed from 2012 to 2014, with 954 patients having undergone total joint replacement. In 2012, 106 (30.1%) patients were transfused. In 2013, 43 (11.1%) patients were transfused and in 2014, 15 (6.9%) patients were transfused (see Figure 2(e)).

4. Discussion

Primary total joint arthroplasty is an extremely successful operation with an inherently low risk for complications [8]. The epidemiologic data indicates that the demand for total joint arthroplasty will increase exponentially over time. Khatod et al. previously reported on the increased incidence of TKA from 1995 through 2004 at a rate of 5% per year [9]. Kurtz et al. project that by 2030 the demand for THA will grow by 174% and the demand for TKA will grow by 673% [10]. The increase in demand as well as the already extremely successful nature of the procedure requires that attention and effort be reallocated to the delivery of the perioperative care, including pain control, rehabilitation, and transfusion requirements. It has been shown in the critical care literature that protocols and standardization of medical practice lead to superior outcomes in the care of the critically ill patient [11]. The experience at our institution has been to persistently improve outcomes through the use of standardization in the delivery of care. The field of arthroplasty is particularly well positioned to benefit from standardization. A decrease in the ALOS in the hospital postarthroplasty is one area that can be improved as long as short-term outcomes are not compromised. This study is meant to present the early findings of the administration of a multidisciplinary action to improve the delivery of healthcare surrounding arthroplasty surgery at a single institution. Our findings indicate that the accelerated rehabilitation protocol alongside multimodal anesthesia therapy using an intraoperative periarticular injection can result in a decrease in the ALOS.

The ALOS in our study was reduced from 3.5 to 2.4 upon administration of the accelerated rehabilitation protocol. This required many system modifications to achieve. Some of these modifications include consensus among operating surgeons, anesthesia providers, in-hospital nursing, inpatient PT, home health nursing, and PT as well as preoperative patient education buy-in.

We also found a decrease in acute ED visits from 24% to 16% and a decrease in inpatient readmissions from 6% to 3%. There was no significant change in the number of UC visits. This provides evidence that the adoption of the accelerated rehabilitation program to decrease the ALOS did not shift the burden to the ED, nor did it result in readmissions. In fact, the number of visits had decreased throughout this study period. There also was a decrease in admission to SNF after surgery. This rate decreased from 25% in 2011 to 14% in 2014. This decrease in SNF admission was purposeful. Prior data revealed a reduction in perioperative complications when patients returned home versus a SNF after adjusting for patient comorbidities [12]. We utilized this information to guide our patients preoperatively to find adequate support for home discharge with the utilization of in home services provided by our institution. Further, the accelerated rehabilitation instilled confidence in the patients regarding their postoperative ambulation as well as performing activities of daily living. This resulted in many more patients feeling comfortable going home rather than to a SNF.

At the same time the accelerated rehabilitation protocol was administered and a transfusion protocol was also adopted. This was specifically to address the exceedingly high number of transfusions that were administered following arthroplasty procedures. Our results show a dramatic decrease in the rate of transfusion from 30.1% in 2012 to 6.9% in 2014. This dramatic decrease is likely due to the adoption of a transfusion protocol based on specific triggers as well as to the more widespread adoption of the use of tranexamic acid amongst all of the surgeons at the institution [13]. Transfusions have been shown to increase risk of prosthetic joint infection [14]. Adoption of an accelerated rehab protocol at our institution has proven to be safe, while the reduction in ALOS, transfusions, and reduction in SNF transfer translate into significant cost savings to the total joint program at our institution.

5. Conclusion

Standardization of care inclusive of perioperative patient education, aggressive pain management, blood management, and rapid discharge has led to improved patient outcomes as well as reduced length of stay. The standardization needs to be evidence based and a consensus must be reached by all participating surgeons at an individual facility to minimize variation.

Appendices

A. TKA and THA Rehab Protocol

A.1. Total Joint Clinical Pathway Optimization. At time of surgery scheduling one has the following:

(1) total joint education packet given to patient (including DVD of the shared decision making process),

(2) first date patient wishing to have surgery entered into the surgery request,

(3) adequate X-rays are completed for templating within 12 months,

(4) blood management protocol initiated:

  (a) males with Hb over 13 and females with Hb over 12, no predonation,

  (b) for males with Hb less than 13 and females with Hb less than 12, referral for anemia work-up,

- (c) all patients starting iron supplementation at time of surgery scheduling: FeGluc 325 mg PO BID,

(5) documenting the need/request for autologous blood in the progress note,

(6) patient geting a handout with the options for treatment, goals of treatment, risks of surgery which is also documented in the progress note at time of surgery scheduling (Informed Consent),

(7) patients with multiple medical problems (MI or stroke in the past, any cardiac disease, or over 60 years old) geting an Internal Medicine referral for preoperative risk stratification/optimization,

(8) all patients having the progress note forwarded to their PCP informing them that the patient will be undergoing total joint replacement and may be seen for medical optimization prior to surgery,

(9) patient signing up for kp.org with MA or confirming that account already exists,

(10) surgery scheduler ensuring the following:

- (a) patient having a ride home on POD#1 or 2,
  - (i) writing name of person in the chart,
  - (ii) writing phone number of person in the chart,
- (b) patient having assistance at home for 1 week following surgery,
- (c) having all financial questions answered:
  - (i) cost of procedure,
  - (ii) cost of hospital stay,
  - (iii) cost of potential rehab stay,
- (d) confirming that the patient has kp.org account active.

At time of preoperative visit one has the following:

(1) off work/activity form/caregiver forms given to patient and caregiver,

(2) placing orders for day of surgery in preoperative area, including preemptive analgesia:

- (a) Ancef 2 grams IV,
- (b) Mobic 15 mg po,
- (c) Percocet 1 or 2 tabs po,
- (d) Tramadol 50 mg po,
- (e) Pepcid 20 mg IV,

(3) placing outpatient PT referral with date of surgery,

(4) educating patient on importance of early gait and transfer training on day of surgery,

(5) education of the patient that the anticipated date of discharge will be postoperative day #1.

In the OR one has the following:

(1) pain protocol:

- (a) Total Hip Replacement:
  - (i) preemptive analgesia:
    - (1) Mobic 15 mg po on call to OR,
    - (2) Percocet 1 or 2 tabs po on call to OR,
    - (3) Tramadol 50 mg po on call to OR,
    - (4) Pepcid 20 mg IV on call to OR,
  - (ii) immediately prior to incision:
    - (1) tranexamic acid 1000 mg or 1500 mg IV to be ordered by MD prior to entering OR,
  - (iii) intraoperative periarticular injection with an 18-gauge spinal needle ordered prior to entering OR:
    - (1) Ropivacaine 250 mg,
    - (2) Epinephrine 0.5 mg,
    - (3) Ketorolac 30 mg,
    - (4) Clonidine 0.08 mg,
    - (5) total volume to 100 mL,
- (b) Total Knee Replacement:
  - (i) preemptive analgesia:
    - (1) Mobic 15 mg po on call to OR,
    - (2) Percocet 2 tabs po on call to OR,
    - (3) Tramadol 50 mg po on call to OR,
    - (4) Pepcid 20 mg IV on call to OR,
  - (ii) intraoperative:
    - (1) tranexamic acid 1000 mg or 1500 mg IV when tourniquet is taken down,
  - (iii) intraoperative periarticular injection with an 18-gauge spinal needle ordered prior to entering OR,
  - (iv) pericapsular/periarticular injection:
    - (1) Ropivacaine 250 mg,
    - (2) Epinephrine 0.5 mg,
    - (3) Ketorolac 30 mg,
    - (4) Clonidine 0.08 mg,
    - (5) total volume to 100 mL.

In PACU one has the following:

(1) postoperative check done by surgeon or assisting PA prior to leaving PACU,

(2) assessing patients mental status and pain control to ensure proper PT training.

On the floor one has the following:

(1) DVT and PE Prophylaxis:

- (a) Coumadin referral for Goal INR of 1.5 to 2.5 for 6 weeks in hips and knees,
- (b) selecting patients will get Aspirin 325 mg orally daily to start on day of surgery,

(2) All patients to be mobilized by the RN by getting them out of bed for meals (sitting up for dinner on the night of surgery),

(3) PT starting on POD#0:

(a) PT is not to be held due to blood transfusion,

(b) goal for 5 to 6 PT sessions by discharge,

(4) pain protocol:

(a) TKA:

(i) Oxycodone 5 mg PO every 4 hours for 24 hours (6 doses),
(ii) Zofran 5 mg IV every 4 hours with Oxycodone (6 doses), the prn,
(iii) Norco 1 tab prn q6h for moderate pain,
(iv) Norco 2 tabs prn q6h for severe pain,
(v) Meloxicam 15 mg PO daily (held for GFR < 30 which is equal to CKD 4 or 5),
(vi) Dilaudid 0.5 mg IV q2 hours prn breakthrough pain,

(b) THA:

(i) Oxycodone 5 mg PO every 4 hours for 24 hours (6 doses),
(ii) Zofran 5 mg IV every 4 hours with Oxycodone (6 doses), the prn,
(iii) Norco 1 tab prn q6h for moderate pain,
(iv) Norco 2 tabs prn q6h for severe pain,
(v) Meloxicam 15 mg PO daily (held for GFR < 30 which is equal to CKD 4 or 5),
(vi) Dilaudid 0.5 mg IV q2 hours prn breakthrough pain,

(5) GI Prophylaxis:

(a) Omeprazole 20 mg po q12 hours while inpatient,

(6) bowel protocol to be started the morning POD#1 and *not prn*:

(a) stool softener bid,

(b) MOM at night on POD#1, if no BM by then and holding for diarrhea,

(c) Dulcolax suppository on POD#2 morning, if no BM by then and holding for diarrhea,

(d) Enema to be given evening of POD#2 afternoon if no BM,

(7) labs:

(a) H/H drawn in AM of POD#1, 2, and 3:

(i) transfusion requirements:

(1) if Hb < 7, then transfuse 1 u PRBC,

(2) if Hb 7–9, then look for symptoms and fluid resuscitate, first:

(a) tachycardia (HR > 100) at rest,
(b) orthostatic symptoms,
(c) if positive symptoms then transfuse 1 u PRBC,

(3) if Hb > 9, then give fluids only.

Discharge instructions and discharge medication are as follows:

(1) discharge to be done by 4 pm on POD#1 on fast track patients and 9 am on POD#2 for all patients,

(2) deep breath and cough 2 times per hour for the next 2 days,

(a) patients should go home with their incentive spirometer,

(3) calling the office for persistent redness, increasing pain or fevers,

(4) coming to the office during working hours for wound drainage,

(5) home health referral for Home Health PT.

B. Demographic Data

See Table 1 and Figures 1 and 2.

Conflict of Interests

The authors declare that there is no conflict of interests regarding the publication of this paper.

Acknowledgment

This work is supported by Kaiser Permanente West Los Angeles, Department of Orthopaedics, Los Angeles, California.

References

[1] K. J. Bozic, P. Katz, M. Cisternas, L. Ono, M. D. Ries, and J. Showstack, "Hospital resource utilization for primary and revision total hip arthroplasty," *The Journal of Bone & Joint Surgery—American Volume*, vol. 87, no. 3, pp. 570–576, 2005.

[2] H. Husted, H. C. Hansen, G. Holm et al., "What determines length of stay after total hip and knee arthroplasty? A nationwide study in Denmark," *Archives of Orthopaedic and Trauma Surgery*, vol. 130, no. 2, pp. 263–268, 2010.

[3] K. R. Berend, A. V. Lombardi Jr., and T. H. Mallory, "Rapid recovery protocol for peri-operative care of total hip and total knee arthroplasty patients," *Surgical Technology International*, vol. 13, pp. 239–247, 2004.

[4] C. E. Robbins, D. Casey, J. V. Bono, S. B. Murphy, C. T. Talmo, and D. M. Ward, "A multidisciplinary total hip arthroplasty protocol with accelerated postoperative rehabilitation: does the patient benefit?" *The American Journal of Orthopedics*, vol. 43, no. 4, pp. 178–181, 2014.

[5] D. C. Mears, S. C. Mears, J. E. Chelly, F. Dai, and K. L. Vulakovich, "THA with a minimally invasive technique, multi-modal anesthesia, and home rehabilitation: factors associated with early discharge?" *Clinical Orthopaedics and Related Research*, vol. 467, no. 6, pp. 1412–1417, 2009, Erratum in *Clinical Orthopaedics and Related Research*, vol. 467, no. 7, p. 1928, 2009.

[6] L. Ogonda, R. Wilson, P. Archbold et al., "A minimal-incision technique in total hip arthroplasty does not improve early postoperative outcomes. A prospective, randomized, controlled trial," *The Journal of Bone & Joint Surgery—American Volume*, vol. 87, no. 4, pp. 701–710, 2005.

[7] H. K. Parvataneni, V. P. Shah, H. Howard, N. Cole, A. S. Ranawat, and C. S. Ranawat, "Controlling pain after total hip and knee arthroplasty using a multimodal protocol with local periarticular injections: a prospective randomized study," *Journal of Arthroplasty*, vol. 22, supplement 6, pp. 33–38, 2007.

[8] N. Nizar, N. N. Mahomed, J. A. Barrett et al., "Rates and outcomes of primary and revision total hip replacement in the united states medicare population," *Journal of Bone and Joint Surgery A*, vol. 85, no. 1, pp. 27–32, 2003.

[9] M. Khatod, M. Inacio, E. W. Paxton et al., "Knee replacement: Epidemiology, outcomes, and trends in Southern California: 17,080 replacements from 1995 through 2004," *Acta Orthopaedica*, vol. 79, no. 6, pp. 812–819, 2008.

[10] S. Kurtz, K. Ong, E. Lau, F. Mowat, and M. Halpern, "Projections of primary and revision hip and knee arthroplasty in the United States from 2005 to 2030," *The Journal of Bone & Joint Surgery—American Volume*, vol. 89, no. 4, pp. 780–785, 2007.

[11] B. W. Holcomb, A. P. Wheeler, and E. W. Ely, "New ways to reduce unnecessary variation and improve outcomes in the intensive care unit," *Current Opinion in Critical Care*, vol. 7, no. 4, pp. 304–311, 2001.

[12] S. A. Bini, D. C. Fithian, L. W. Paxton, M. X. Khatod, M. C. Inacio, and R. S. Namba, "Does discharge disposition after primary total joint arthroplasty affect readmission rates?" *Journal of Arthroplasty*, vol. 25, no. 1, pp. 114–117, 2010.

[13] G. M. March, S. Elfatori, and P. E. Beaulé, "Clinical experience with tranexamic acid during primary total hip arthroplasty," *HIP International*, vol. 23, no. 1, pp. 72–79, 2013.

[14] N. B. Frisch, N. M. Wessell, M. A. Charters, S. Yu, J. J. Jeffries, and C. D. Silverton, "Predictors and complications of blood transfusion in total hip and knee arthroplasty," *The Journal of Arthroplasty*, vol. 29, no. 9, supplement, pp. 189–192, 2014.

Incidence of Heterotopic Ossification in Patients Receiving Radiation Therapy following Total Hip Arthroplasty

Panagiotis Koulouvaris,[1] David Sherr,[2] and Thomas Sculco[3]

[1] *Orthopaedic Clinic, Attikon Hospital, University of Athens, Olympic Village Polyclinic, 36122 Athens, Greece*
[2] *New York Hospital, Cornell University, NY 10021, USA*
[3] *Hospital for Special Surgery, Cornell University, NY 10021, USA*

Correspondence should be addressed to Panagiotis Koulouvaris; info@drkoulouvaris.gr

Academic Editor: Guoxin Ni

Heterotopic ossification (HO) is a frequent complication of hip surgery. In this study the incidence of HO is analyzed in high risk patients who received radiation therapy (RT) after total hip replacement (THA) with regular and miniposterolateral hip approach. Two hundred and thirty five high risk patients received a single dose of 700 rad after THA. The incidence of HO was 15.7%. The incidence of HO in the high risk subgroup with the miniincision was lower (5.7%) but not significantly different ($P = 0.230$). Hypertrophic osteoarthritis was demonstrated to be the consistent predisposing factor for HO formation ($P = 0.005$).

1. Introduction

Heterotopic ossification (HO) is bone formation in the soft tissues which develops after hip replacement surgery without a well-defined precipitating event (Figure 1). HO represents one of the most frequent complications following THA with reported rates of HO after total hip arthroplasty (THA) ranging from 5% to 90% depending on the risk factors [1]. HO is approximately twice as prevalent in men as in women [2]. Patients with a history of HO after previous hip surgery are at increased risk for recurrent HO formation [3]. Men with hypertrophic osteoarthritis have markedly higher levels of HO after THA [4]. Hips with markedly diminished motion and hypertrophic ossification before surgery were statistically more likely to have HO [2, 4]. Surgical approach and trauma may be a risk factor for the development of HO after THA. In several studies anterior and lateral approaches increase the possibility of HO [5, 6]. The posterior approach for THA is associated with the lowest incidence of HO formation [5, 6]. HO has been found more after an epidural anesthesia than after general anesthesia [7]. Extraction of the femoral head in a fragmented state from the acetabulum has been linked with the occurrence of HO [8]. Patients who engaged in more physical activity before surgery developed HO more frequently than patients with minimal physical activity [7]. Bone formation has been found in patients with postoperative dislocations in the first week [9]. Also postoperative fever for more than five days, superficial wound infection, and postoperative hematoma have also been associated with HO [7, 8].

There has been no reported association between type of femoral fixation and HO [10, 11]. Severe ossification was more common in men than in women and in patients operated by relatively inexperienced surgeons [12]. Prophylactic measures include diphosphonates, indomethacin, and radiation therapy with most research studies supporting the radiation therapy as the most effective prophylaxis [13, 14].

The purpose of this study was to evaluate the incidence of HO in high risk patients with THR who received RT, to identify potential risk factors, and to compare the incidence of HO between patients with miniposterolateral approach (MIS) and a conventional posterolateral approach. The hypothesis in the surgical approach part of the study was that since MIS produced less soft tissue trauma, the occurrence of HO should be decreased.

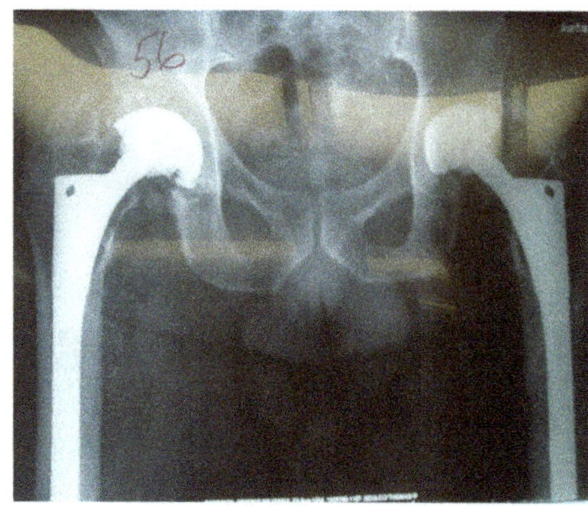

Figure 1: Bilateral HO formation 9 months after surgery.

2. Materials: Methods

In our hospital from January 1999 to March 2003 there were 12.325 THA. During this same period radiation therapy following THA was performed in 255 consecutive patients who were considered to be at risk for the development for HO. The high risk categories have been reported and include clinically severe hypertrophic osteoarthritis, ankylosing spondylitis, HO after previous surgery, and previous acetabulum fracture [15, 16]. Of these total patients 235 had complete radiographic follow-up.

There were 190 men and 45 women. Patient age at the time of operation was 63.7 (30–93) SD 14.7. Of the hips 185 had primary osteoarthritis, 7 rheumatoid arthritis, 8 ankylosing arthritis, 14 previous acetabulum fractures, 8 congenital dislocation, 2 previously slipped capital femoral epiphysis, and 4 avascular necrosis. There were 7 revision THR for aseptic loosening in the group. Thirty-five patients had THA with miniposterior incision with a skin incision of 5–8 cm. All patients were assessed for response to therapy with a mean follow-up 28.2 months (12–96) SD 18.2. Heterotopic bone formation was classified to one of four grades as described by Brooker et al. [17]

The posterolateral approach was used in all surgeries. All patients received a single 700 cGy fraction of RT to the affected hip within 24 to 72 hours following surgery. The RT treatments were delivered via equally weighted, parallelly opposed AP/PA portals with the RT dose prescribed to mid plane. The X-ray beam energies used ranged from 4 to 15 Mv, depending upon the AP diameter of the hip. The field sizes were usually 4 to 6 cm in width and 8 to 12 cm in length and included the hip abductor soft tissues.

The response to therapy was assessed by comparison of routine AP X-ray performed preoperatively, immediately postoperatively, and postoperatively during the last office visit. Possible risk factors like preoperative motion, diagnosis, date of radiation therapy, smoking, and severe osteoarthritis (large osteophytes) were recorded.

3. Statistical Analyses

All categorical are described with their absolute and relatives values, and all continuous variables are defined with their mean and median values, standard deviation, and range. Comparisons of frequencies will be tested using chi-square analysis. The calculations will be performed by using SPSS 12 for Windows.

4. Results

There were no revisions of any hips treated with radiation therapy. Of the 235 patients who received radiation therapy after THA, 15.7% developed heterotopic ossification (Table 1). In those developing HO after RT there were 27 male and 10 female patients. Twenty-two (59.5%) had Grade I, seven (18.9%) Grade II, and eight (21.6%) Grade III. A significant association was found between the rate of HO and primary OA in that 68.7% of the patients with HO had primary osteoarthritis (chi-square = 16.231^{a}; $P = 0.023$). A significant association was noted between hypertrophic osteoarthritis; 26 (70.2%) of the patients with HO had hypertrophic osteoarthritis (chi square = 7.795^{b}, $P = 0.005$). There was no statistical difference in the overall incidence of HO with transfusion rate (chi square = 2.237^{a}, $P = 0.505$), with bilateral THR (chi square = 0.470^{b}; $P = 0.493$), with preoperative diminished motion (chi square = 2.157^{a}; $P = 0.348$), with type of femoral fixation (chi square = 0.882^{b}; $P = 0.348$), with age (chi square = 0.844^{b}; $P = 0.348$), with type of thromboprophylaxis (chi square = 1.177^{a}; $P = 0.555$), and with smoking (chi square = 2.456^{a}; $P = 0.493$). In patients older than 65 years the total rate of HO was 56.2% compared to 43.5% in patients younger than 65 years old, and the older patients had a higher rate of Grade III HO but this was not statistically significant.

Of the 35 patients who had THR with MIS and received RT only two (5.7%) developed HO Grade I. No significant associations was determined between mini-incision and HO (chi-square = 1.444^{b}; $P = 0.230$).

5. Discussion

Heterotopic ossification is a serious complication after THA particularly when the amount of bone interferes with hip motion or produces pain. This has been reported in 3% to 10% of patients with HO after THA [18]. HO formation may become irritative as maturation occurs and warrant surgical excision if the symptoms cannot be controlled with NSAIDs and physical therapy modalities. Instability is a potential complication of HO after THA if the periarticular mass of bone contributes to impingement with limitation of hip excursion of the femur and initiation of dislocation. Maximal stimulus for the formation of HO has been reported to occur within 32 hours after surgery [15] and therefore optimal prophylactic regimens are instituted preoperatively or within the first 24 to 48 hours postoperatively. These measures can still be somewhat effective within four days after surgery [19]. Surgical removal of heterotopic ossification without prophylactic measures to prevent its recurrence is of little value since there is a high incidence of recurrence after excision [20]. Prophylactic measures have included systematic administration of diphosphonates, radiation therapy,

TABLE 1: The incidence of HO within primary diagnosis.

HO	OA	RA	AS	MA	AL	CDH	SCFH	AVN	Total
No	160	5	5	10	4	8	2	4	198
Yes	25 15 Grade I 5 Grade II 5 Grade III	2 Grade I	3 1 Grade I 2 Grade II	4 1 Grade I 3 Grade III	3 2 Grade I 1 Grade II	0	0	0	37
	10.6%	0.8%	1.2%	1.7%	1.2%	0.0%	0.0%	0.0%	15.7%
Total	185	7	8	14	7	8	2	4	235

Osteoarthritis OA, Rheumatoid Arthritis RA, Angylosing Spondylitis AS, Metatraumatic Arthritis MA, Aseptic Loosening AL, Congenital Dislocation of Hip CDH, Slipped Capital Femoral epiphysiolisthesis SCFH, Avascular Necrosis AVN.

and indomethacin; however, current research supports the effectiveness of radiation therapy [13, 14].

The present study was undertaken to report the incidence of HO formation in patients who received RT after THA and in patients who received RT and had THA with mini-posterolateral approach. A control group of patients without risk factors who had THA and no RT also were evaluated for HO.

The major limitation of this study is that it is retrospective and nonrandomized. However, follow-up of the patients in this study was quite high. Patients were evaluated for HO by three methods: (1) using the hospital and surgeon patient files, (2) checking all operative procedure likely to include subsequent excision of HO, and (3) radiographic evaluation at at least 1 year follow-up.

This study demonstrates an incidence of 15.7% HO formation in the RT group. Most of the patients were male and the diagnosis was primary osteoarthritis. This is consistent with the literature that reports a higher prevalence of HO in male patients [2]. This study also confirmed the consistent risk factor for HO of hypertrophic osteoarthritis reported in many studies [8, 15] he co. Also no association was determined between transfusion, bilateral THA, smoking, preoperative motion, type of thromboprophylaxis, and type of femoral fixation. Additionally the overall incidence of severe HO grade 2 was very small in this RT treated group; there was a higher rate of Grade III HO in patients older than 65 years. In the group of patients with the miniposterolateral approach the incidence of HO was lower than the conventional posterolateral approach (5.7% versus 23.2%); however, it was not significantly different.

Similarly other authors reported a lower rate of HO (7%) in a treated group with prophylaxsis compared to a control group (32%) with risk factors [13]. In another study, with high risk-patients receiving no preventive RT the rate of occurrence of HO was noted in 61.3% and in the patients who had no risk factors 60.9% which was not significantly different from that in the overall study population [12]. Our regimen was a single dose of 700 centigray delivered via equally weighted, parallelly opposed AP/PA portals. The efficacy of this regimen has been demonstrated by previous studies. Healy et al. [21] and Kennedy et al. [22] using a single dose of 700 centigray reported 10% and 11.9%, respectively. Many authors have reported the efficacy of a single dose of various regimens for preventive radiotherapy [16, 23, 24]. In addition, Pellegrini Jr. and Evarts [25] in a prospective randomized study reported 21% incidence of HO with a single dose 800 or 1000 centigray regimen.

In conclusion, the present study has shown that the incidence of HO (15.7%) is within the range of percentages reported in the literature. Also this study has confirmed the hypertrophic osteoarthritis as the main risk factor for HO formation. In addition, THA in high risk patients treated prophylactically with RT with miniposterolateral have a lower rate of HO but not significantly different than in THA with a conventional posterolateral approach.

These data suggest that RT targeted to specific THA patients with risk factors is effective in reduction of postoperative HO. However, future prospective randomized studies are required to evaluate the most efficient regimen to reduce the incidence of HO.

Disclosure

Investigation performed at the Hospital for Special Surgery, New York. The authors verify that all coauthors have seen and agreed with the contents and final version of this paper. The corresponding author had full access to all of the data in the study and takes responsibility for the integrity of the data and the accuracy of the data analysis. The contents of this paper have not been published, and it is not being submitted for publication elsewhere.

Conflict of Interests

The authors have no financial conflict of interests to disclose in association with this paper.

References

[1] L. Ahrengart and U. Lindgren, "Heterotopic bone after hip arthroplasty. Defining the patient at risk," *Clinical Orthopaedics and Related Research*, no. 293, pp. 153–159, 1993.

[2] M. A. Ritter and R. B. Vaughan, "Ectopic ossification after total hip arthroplasty. Predisposing factors, frequency, and effect on results," *The Journal of Bone and Joint Surgery. American*, vol. 59, no. 3, pp. 345–351, 1977.

[3] J. DeLee, A. Ferrari, and J. Charnley, "Ectopic bone formation following low friction arthroplasty of the hip," *Clinical Orthopaedics and Related Research*, no. 121, pp. 53–59, 1976.

[4] M. G. Lazansky, "Complications revisited. The debit side of total hip replacement," *Clinical Orthopaedics and Related Research*, no. 95, pp. 96–103, 1973.

[5] B. R. Horwitz, N. L. Rockowitz, S. R. Goll et al., "A prospective randomized comparison of two surgical approaches to total hip arthroplasty," *Clinical Orthopaedics and Related Research*, no. 291, pp. 154–163, 1993.

[6] V. S. Pai, "Heterotopic ossification in total hip arthroplasty: the influence of the approach," *Journal of Arthroplasty*, vol. 9, no. 2, pp. 199–202, 1994.

[7] C. Hierton, G. Blomgren, and U. Lindgren, "Factors associated with heterotopic bone formation in cemented total hip prostheses," *Acta Orthopaedica Scandinavica*, vol. 54, no. 5, pp. 698–702, 1983.

[8] L. Ahrengart, "Periarticular heterotopic ossification after total hip arthroplasty. Risk factors and consequences," *Clinical Orthopaedics and Related Research*, no. 263, pp. 49–58, 1991.

[9] J. R. Azcarate, J. de Pablos, F. Cornejo, and J. Canadell, "Postoperative dislocation: a risk factor for periprosthetic ectopic ossifications after total hip replacement," *Acta Orthopaedica Belgica*, vol. 52, no. 2, pp. 145–150, 1986.

[10] J. J. Purtill, K. Eng, R. H. Rothman, and W. J. Hozack, "Heterotopic ossification: incidence in cemented versus cementless total hip arthroplasty," *Journal of Arthroplasty*, vol. 11, no. 1, pp. 58–63, 1996.

[11] R. L. Wixson, S. D. Stulberg, and M. Mehlhoff, "Total hip replacement with cemented, uncemented, and hybrid prostheses. A comparison of clinical and radiographic results at two to four years," *The Journal of Bone and Joint Surgery. American*, vol. 73, no. 2, pp. 257–270, 1991.

[12] L. Vastel, L. Kerboull, P. Anract, and M. Kerboull, "Heterotopic ossification after total hip arthroplasty: risk factors and prevention," *Revue du Rhumatisme*, vol. 65, no. 4, pp. 238–244, 1998.

[13] M. H. Seegenschmiedt, H.-B. Makoski, and O. Micke, "Radiation prophylaxis for heterotopic ossification about the hip joint—a multicenter study," *International Journal of Radiation Oncology Biology Physics*, vol. 51, no. 3, pp. 756–765, 2001.

[14] E. E. Pakos and J. P. Ioannidis, "Radiotherapy vs. nonsteroidal anti-inflammatory drugs for the prevention of heterotopic ossification after major hip procedures: a meta-analysis of randomized trials," *International Journal of Radiation Oncology Biology Physics*, vol. 60, no. 3, pp. 888–895, 2004.

[15] R. Iorio and W. L. Healy, "Heterotopic ossification after hip and knee arthroplasty: risk factors, prevention, and treatment," *The Journal of the American Academy of Orthopaedic Surgeons*, vol. 10, no. 6, pp. 409–416, 2002.

[16] W. L. Healy, T. C. M. Lo, D. J. Covall, B. A. Pfeifer, and S. A. Wasilewski, "Single-dose radiation therapy for prevention of heterotopic ossification after total hip arthroplasty," *Journal of Arthroplasty*, vol. 5, no. 4, pp. 369–375, 1990.

[17] A. F. Brooker, J. W. Bowerman, R. A. Robinson, and L. H. Riley Jr., "Ectopic ossification following total hip replacement. Incidence and a method of classification," *The Journal of Bone and Joint Surgery. American*, vol. 55, no. 8, pp. 1629–1632, 1973.

[18] L. Ahrengart and U. Lindgren, "Functional significance of heterotopic bone formation after total hip arthroplasty," *Journal of Arthroplasty*, vol. 4, no. 2, pp. 125–131, 1989.

[19] J. E. Puzas, M. D. Miller, and R. N. Rosier, "Pathologic bone formation," *Clinical Orthopaedics and Related Research*, no. 245, pp. 269–281, 1989.

[20] N. R. Fahmy and B. M. Wroblewski, "Recurrence of ectopic ossification after excision in Charnley low friction arthroplasty," *Acta Orthopaedica Scandinavica*, vol. 53, no. 5, pp. 799–802, 1982.

[21] W. L. Healy, T. C. M. Lo, A. A. DiSimone, B. Rask, and B. A. Pfeifer, "Single-dose irradiation for the prevention of heterotopic ossification after total hip arthroplasty. A comparison of doses of five hundred and fifty and seven hundred centigray," *The Journal of Bone and Joint Surgery. American*, vol. 77, no. 4, pp. 590–595, 1995.

[22] W. F. Kennedy, T. A. Gruen, H. Chessin, G. Gasparini, and W. Thompson, "Radiation therapy to prevent heterotopic ossification after cementless total hip arthroplasty," *Clinical Orthopaedics and Related Research*, no. 262, pp. 185–191, 1991.

[23] R. J. Fingeroth and A. Q. Ahmed, "Single dose 6 Gy prophylaxis for heterotopic ossification after total hip arthroplasty," *Clinical Orthopaedics and Related Research*, no. 317, pp. 131–140, 1995.

[24] A. Konski, V. Pellegrini, C. M. Poulter et al., "Randomized trial comparing single dose versus fractionated irradiation for prevention of heterotopic bone: a preliminary report," *International Journal of Radiation Oncology Biology Physics*, vol. 18, no. 5, pp. 1139–1142, 1990.

[25] V. D. Pellegrini Jr. and C. M. Evarts, "Radiation prophylaxis of heterotopic bone formation following total hip arthroplasty: current status," *Seminars in Arthroplasty*, vol. 3, no. 3, pp. 156–166, 1992.

6

Is Single Use Portable Incisional Negative Pressure Wound Therapy System Suitable for Revision Arthroplasty?

Thomas Hester,[1] Shoib Mahmood,[2] and Farid Moftah[2]

[1]*Guys and St Thomas' NHS Trust, Department of Orthopaedics, Westminster Bridge Road, London SE1 7EH, UK*
[2]*Department of Orthopaedics, Darent Valley Hospital, Dartford DA2 8DA, UK*

Correspondence should be addressed to Thomas Hester; thomashester@gmail.com

Academic Editor: Ely Steinberg

Incisional negative pressure wound therapy (INPWT) has been used for high-risk surgery across specialties but has yet to be utilised for revision hip and knee surgery. Between 2013 and 2014, patients who underwent revision arthroplasty by the senior author were identified. 36 (9 hips and 27 knees) operations in 36 patients identified 18 (8 male, median age 77 (61–86)) who received standard dressing and 18 (12 male, median age 67 (58–81)) who received single use portable INPWT dressings (4 hips, 14 knees). Wound complications were seen in 3 (2 knees) from the standard group and 1 (hip) in the INPWT group ($p = 0.14$). There was no statistical difference in age or gender between groups. Risk factors (BMI > 30, smoking, and diabetes) were identified in 9 patients, median ASA 3, in the standard group and 10 patients, median ASA 2, in the INPWT group. There were no dressing related complications. This is the first study of INPWT with a low pressure single use 80 mmHg dressing with revision arthroplasty. This initial study showed a threefold decrease in wound complication in the INPWT group and that INPWT is a safe alternative to standard dressings.

1. Introduction

The use of negative pressure wound therapy (NPWT) and incisional NPWT is growing. More evidence is available to support its use and the technology has evolved and become more user-friendly and easier to apply and not cumbersome for the patient. Many studies have looked at INPWT use in plastic, general, cardiothoracic, and neurosurgery and it has been shown to be effective at reducing wound complications [1–3].

Surgical Site Infections (SSI) and persistent wound drainage are well-recognised complications with a reported incidence of approximately 1–3% in the general orthopaedic population [4]. Of these there are certain operative and patient groups, for example, trauma and raised body mass index, that have an associated higher risk [5]. Tibial plateau, calcaneal, or pilon fractures are known to have a high incidence of wound complications estimated at 10–40%, with promising results with the use of INPWT [6]. Revision hip and knee arthroplasty surgery is also associated with a rate of wound complication, 2% and 5%, respectively [5]. Despite this there are no studies looking at the effect of INPWT on this group. Saleh et al. and Pulido et al. extensively described risk factors associated with higher rates of periprosthetic infection such as malnutrition, excess anticoagulation, obesity, diabetes, and a high American Society of Anesthesiologists (ASA) score [7, 8]. However Patel et al. and Weiss and Krackow identified persistent wound drainage lasting greater than 48 hours after hip arthroplasty as also a risk factor for periprosthetic joint infection [9, 10]. As patients are optimised preoperatively, the dressing optimises the wound healing potential postoperatively by removing the excess wound fluid.

There are currently no standard guidelines for managing surgical wounds. Incisional NPWT is a relatively new application of the technology, with only a few studies in the published literature and only three studies looking at primary hip and knee arthroplasty [11–13]. By minimising the seroma around the wound, increasing local tissue perfusion, and angiogenesis this may decrease the wound complication rates [14, 15].

The aim of our study was to determine the complication rate associated with a single use INPWT system and the rate of wound infection in revision hip and knee arthroplasty.

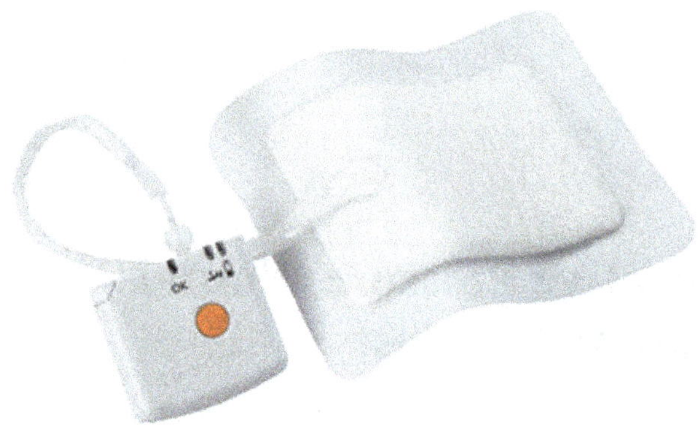

FIGURE 1: Smith & Nephew PICO dressing.

TABLE 1: Demographics of patients in both groups.

	Standard	INPWT
Total number of patients	18	18
Median age (years)	77	67
Median BMI (kg/m^2)	30	30.2
Median ASA	3	2
Surgical procedures		
Hip	5	4
Infection	1	1
Cup	4	2
Stem		1
Knee	13	14
Infection	1	1
Malalignment	2	1
Aseptic loosening	3	3
Anterior knee pain	7	6
UKR to TKR		2
Instability		1

2. Materials and Methods

Between January 2013 and January 2014, all patients who underwent revision arthroplasty surgery by the senior author were identified and case notes reviewed. 36 (9 hips and 27 knees) operations in 36 patients identified a control group of 18 (8 male, median age 77 (61–86)) who received standard dressing of blue gauze cotton wool and crepe bandaging for knees or pressure dressing for hips and 18 (12 male, median age 67 (58–81)) who received single use portable INPWT (PICO Smith & Nephew, Figure 1) dressings (4 hips, 14 knees).

Patients were allocated to the different dressing groups based on time of presentation. Prior to July 2013 all patients were in the standard dressing group and then all subsequent revisions that met the inclusion criteria were given the portable INPWT. Whilst not being prospective computer randomisation, this method does prevent allocation bias as at no point were patients deemed "more" or "less" at risk of wound complications and their dressing choice changed.

All patients had intraoperative cefuroxime or clarithromycin if penicillin allergic after appropriate microbiological samples were taken. Surgical approach to all revision knee patients was medial parapatella, under tourniquet with one drain placed. All revision hip arthroplasties were via an anterolateral approach. Wounds were closed with surgical clips and one drain was placed in all cases. All dressings were placed in theatre before the drapes were removed; then cotton wool and crepe bandage were applied to the knee replacements. Hip replacements received a surgical pad and pressure dressing.

Postoperatively, patients went to an elective orthopaedic ward; all drains were removed at 48 hours on the ward. All outer dressings were removed at 72 hours. As per the manufacturers guidelines, the INPWT dressing was changed at 7 days for a standard dressing. Clips were removed at 14 days by community arthroplasty nurse specialists. Antibiotics were continued for 6 weeks via a peripherally inserted central catheter if the revision was for infection. For all other revision arthroplasties 2 further doses were given. Patients were followed up 6 weeks postoperatively. Wound complications and dressing associated complications were recorded.

Inclusion criteria consisted of all revision knee and hip arthroplasty surgeries carried out by the senior author in the specified time frame. Exclusion criteria consisted of known allergy to the INPWT dressing or any adhesive dressing that was similar. The primary outcome measure was wound infection requiring further surgery or antibiotics in addition to those described above. Secondary outcome measures included any dressing related complications such as blistering. We obtained local research and development departmental approval before initiation of this study and patient medical records were used to collect data.

3. Results

In the standard dressing (control) group, 5 hips and 13 knees, the 5 hip revisions were as follows: 1, infection; 4, aseptic loosening of the cup. 13 knee revisions were as follows: 7, persistent anterior knee pain requiring patella resurfacing; 3, aseptic loosening; 2, malalignment; and one, infection. In the INPWT group, 4 hips and 14 knees, the 4 hip revisions were as follows: 1, second stage revision after infection; 2, aseptic loosening of the cup; and 1, aseptic loosening of the stem. The 14 knee revisions were as follows: 6, persistent anterior knee pain; 3, aseptic loosening; 2, revision unicompartmental knee replacements to total knee replacement; 1, malalignment; 1, infection; and 1, instability (see Table 1).

The median was ASA 3 in the standard group and ASA 2 in the INPWT group. There were 9 patients with identifiable risk factors in the standard group and 10 in the INPWT group (see Table 2).

TABLE 2: Medical comorbidities.

	Standard	INPWT
Patients with risk factors	9	11
None	9	7
BMI	9	9
Diabetes	1	1
Smoking		1
Antiplatelet drugs	2	2

There was no significant difference between the groups regarding age or gender. Neither group experienced any dressing related complications, such as blistering, maceration, or skin tearing.

Wound complications were seen in 3 (2 knees) from the standard group and 1 in the INPWT group ($p = 0.14$). In the standard group, wound complications were seen in 1 hip, which was being revised for infection where the patient had a BMI of 44 and type 2 diabetes. Two knees had wound complications, both for anterior knee pain, where one of the patients had a BMI of 48 and the other had no risk factors other than revision surgery. In the INPWT group the wound complication was seen in a revision hip arthroplasty for aseptic loosening of the femoral stem with only identifiable risk factor of BMI 37.

4. Discussion

NPWT has been widely accepted in the treatment of open wounds by secondary intention; however the role of INPWT is less clear. Although emerging criteria are starting to be defined such as high-risk lower extremity fractures, for example, tibial plateau, pilon, and calcaneal fractures as described by [1, 3], Stannard et al. reported both a decreased dehiscence rate in patients with high-risk lower extremity wounds with INPWT, 8.6% versus 16.5% with standard dressings, and decreased infection rate of 9% in the INPWT group versus 16.5% in the standard group with the relative risk of developing an infection being 1.9 times higher in control patients than in patients treated with INPWT [6].

Certain subgroups of elective orthopaedic surgery have a higher rate of wound complications, seen with 30-day and 90-day readmissions, such as that with revision total hip arthroplasty, with Schairer et al. showing at 90 days that primary THA (5%) had a lower unplanned readmission rate than revision THA (10%, $p < 0.001$) [16, 17]. Wound discharge has been considered as an important risk factor for wound complications with Patel et al. estimate that each day of persistent wound drainage increases the risk of infection by 42%, as the path that allows fluid to egress is a potential conduit for retrograde bacterial contamination into the wound [9]. Thus, one goal in managing persistent postoperative wound drainage is to minimise the time to achieve a dry, healed wound. Pachowsky et al. reported on decreased seroma formation with the use of INPWT in hip arthroplasty patients and concluded that this leads to improved wound healing [12].

Complications associated with INPWT have been reported. Howell et al. stopped their prospective randomised study early when 63% (15 of 24 knees) of those entered developed skin blisters compared to none in the standard group [13]. It is worth noting that the manufacturer has raised the possibility of incorrect dressing application as a contributing factor to these poor results and emphasises that those results have not been encountered elsewhere.

5. Conclusion

Our study is unique in that this is the first reported study to use a single use portable low pressure, 80 mmHg, INPWT dressing on high-risk revision knee and hip arthroplasty surgery. We showed a decrease in the number of wound complications when compared to standard dressings. Although not statistically significant, these results are encouraging. We also did not sustain any dressing related complications that have been previously published. There are of course limitations to this study such as the study size, retrospective nature, and the heterogeneous mix for causes of revision surgery, but the above points are important and should encourage further research into this new application of existing technology.

Conflict of Interests

The authors declare that there is no conflict of interests regarding the publication of this paper.

References

[1] M. H. Brem, H. J. Bail, and R. Biber, "Value of incisional negative pressure wound therapy in orthopaedic surgery," *International Wound Journal*, vol. 11, supplement 1, pp. 3–5, 2014.

[2] O. Adogwa, P. Fatemi, E. Perez et al., "Negative pressure wound therapy reduces incidence of postoperative wound infection and dehiscence after long-segment thoracolumbar spinal fusion: a single institutional experience," *Spine Journal*, vol. 14, no. 12, pp. 2911–2917, 2014.

[3] S. Karlakki, M. Brem, S. Giannini, V. Khanduja, J. Stannard, and R. Martin, "Negative pressure wound therapy for managementof the surgical incision in orthopaedic surgery: a review of evidence and mechanisms for an emerging indication," *Bone and Joint Research*, vol. 2, no. 12, pp. 276–284, 2013.

[4] F. A. Al-Mulhim, M. A. Baragbah, M. Sadat-Ali, A. S. Alomran, and M. Q. Azam, "Prevalence of surgical site infection in orthopedic surgery: a 5-year analysis," *International Surgery*, vol. 99, no. 3, pp. 264–268, 2014.

[5] M. R. Rasouli, C. Restrepo, M. G. Maltenfort, J. J. Purtill, and J. Parvizi, "Risk factors for surgical site infection following total joint arthroplasty," *The Journal of Bone & Joint Surgery—American Volume*, vol. 96, no. 18, article e158, 2014.

[6] J. P. Stannard, D. A. Volgas, G. McGwin III et al., "Incisional negative pressure wound therapy after high-risk lower extremity fractures," *Journal of Orthopaedic Trauma*, vol. 26, no. 1, pp. 37–42, 2012.

[7] L. Pulido, E. Ghanem, A. Joshi, J. J. Purtill, and J. Parvizi, "Periprosthetic joint infection: the incidence, timing, and predisposing factors," *Clinical Orthopaedics and Related Research*, vol. 466, no. 7, pp. 1710–1715, 2008.

[8] K. Saleh, M. Olson, S. Resig et al., "Predictors of wound infection in hip and knee joint replacement: results from a 20 year surveillance program," *Journal of Orthopaedic Research*, vol. 20, no. 3, pp. 506–515, 2002.

[9] V. P. Patel, M. Walsh, B. Sehgal, C. Preston, H. DeWal, and P. E. Di Cesare, "Factors associated with prolonged wound drainage after primary total hip and knee arthroplasty," *Journal of Bone and Joint Surgery A*, vol. 89, no. 1, pp. 33–38, 2007.

[10] A.-P. C. Weiss and K. A. Krackow, "Persistent wound drainage after primary total knee arthroplasty," *Journal of Arthroplasty*, vol. 8, no. 3, pp. 285–289, 1993.

[11] E. Hansen, J. B. Durinka, J. A. Costanzo, M. S. Austin, and G. K. Deirmengian, "Negative pressure wound therapy is associated with resolution of incisional drainage in most wounds after hip arthroplasty," *Clinical Orthopaedics and Related Research*, vol. 471, no. 10, pp. 3230–3236, 2013.

[12] M. Pachowsky, J. Gusinde, A. Klein et al., "Negative pressure wound therapy to prevent seromas and treat surgical incisions after total hip arthroplasty," *International Orthopaedics*, vol. 36, no. 4, pp. 719–722, 2012.

[13] R. D. Howell, S. Hadley, E. Strauss, and F. R. Pelham, "Blister formation with negative pressure dressings after total knee arthroplasty," *Current Orthopaedic Practice*, vol. 22, no. 2, pp. 176–179, 2011.

[14] P. Erba, R. Ogawa, M. Ackermann et al., "Angiogenesis in wounds treated by microdeformational wound therapy," *Annals of Surgery*, vol. 253, no. 2, pp. 402–409, 2011.

[15] S. Ichioka, H. Watanabe, N. Sekiya, M. Shibata, and T. Nakatsuka, "A technique to visualize wound bed microcirculation and the acute effect of negative pressure," *Wound Repair and Regeneration*, vol. 16, no. 3, pp. 460–465, 2008.

[16] W. W. Schairer, D. C. Sing, T. P. Vail, and K. J. Bozic, "Causes and frequency of unplanned hospital readmission after total hip arthroplasty," *Clinical Orthopaedics and Related Research*, vol. 472, no. 2, pp. 464–470, 2014.

[17] B. Zmistowski, C. Restrepo, J. Hess, D. Adibi, S. Cangoz, and J. Parvizi, "Unplanned readmission after total joint arthroplasty: rates, reasons, and risk factors," *Journal of Bone and Joint Surgery A*, vol. 95, no. 20, pp. 1869–1876, 2013.

7

A Brief History of Anterior Cruciate Ligament Reconstruction

Nikolaos Davarinos,[1] Barry James O'Neill,[2] and William Curtin[2]

[1] *Department of Trauma & Orthopaedics, The Adelaide & Meath Hospital, Tallaght, Dublin 24, Ireland*
[2] *Department of Trauma & Orthopaedics, Galway Regional Hospitals, Galway, Ireland*

Correspondence should be addressed to Nikolaos Davarinos; davarinn@me.com

Academic Editor: Palaniappan Lakshmanan

Reconstructions of the anterior cruciate ligament (ACL) are among the most frequently performed procedures in knee surgery nowadays. The history of ACL surgery can be traced as far back as the Egyptian times. The early years reflect the efforts to establish a viable, consistently successful reconstruction technique while, during the early 20th century, we witness an increasing awareness of, and interest in, the ligament and its lesions. Finally, we highlight the most important steps in the evolution of the ACL reconstruction surgery by discussing the various techniques spanning the years using not only autologous grafts (fascia lata, meniscal, hamstring, patella tendon, bone-patella tendon-bone, and double bundle grafts) but also synthetic ones and allografts.

1. Introduction

Rupture of the anterior cruciate ligament (ACL) is a common injury in active people, and one of the most common knee injuries in sports. It is estimated that the annual incidence of ACL injury is about 1 in 3,000 amongst the general population in the USA. That means more than 150,000 new ACL ruptures annually [1]. The healing response after ACL rupture is poor. Without surgical reconstruction the ACL deficient knee is limited. So are the patient's activities and such ACL deficiency can lead to future degenerative changes [2–5]. Nowadays, ACL reconstruction surgery is a major area of research worldwide. This is partly due to the large number of athletes being involved in professional sports where a fast recovery and rehab are essential to return quickly to the sport. It is also due to the greater awareness within the general public of their own healthcare matters and the higher expectations now evident in amateur sports-persons and non-sports-persons alike.

We present a brief history of ACL injury and the surgical measures taken to address it over the years as well as the modern ACL reconstruction techniques.

2. The Early Years

The cruciate ligaments have been known about since old Egyptian times and their anatomy was described in the famous Smith Papyrus (3000 BC). Hippocrates also (460–370 BC) mentioned the subluxation of the knee joint with ligament pathology, but Claudius Galen, a Greek physician in the Roman Empire, was the first to describe the true nature of the ACL [6].

Prior to Galen's description, it was believed that the cruciate ligaments were part of the nervous system, but Galen was the first to describe the ACL as being a structure that supports the joint and prevents abnormal knee motion. He called the cruciate ligaments genu cruciata but he did not describe in detail their function [6, 7].

In 1836, the Weber brothers from Goettingen in Germany noted an abnormal anterior-posterior movement of the tibia after transection of the ACL. They also described the roll and glide mechanism of the knee and the tension pattern of the different bundles of the cruciate ligaments and, to our knowledge, were the first to describe that each bundle of the ACL was tensioned in different degrees of flexion of the knee joint [6].

In 1845, Amade Bonnet (1809–1858) of Lyon, France, published his first cadaveric studies for the mechanism of knee ligament injuries in his treatise on the treatment of joint diseases [6]. The first recorded description of rupture of the ACL, however, was by Stark in 1850 [8].

In 1875, the Greek Georgios C. Noulis [6] described the technique of the Lachman test for the first time. He wrote: "fix the thigh with one hand, while with the other hand hold the lower leg just below the knee with the thumb in front and the fingers behind. Then, try to shift the tibia forward and backward. When only the anterior cruciate ligament is transected, this forward movement is seen when the knee is barely flexed, whereas a backward movement is noted in 110 degrees of flexion when the posterior cruciate ligament is transected." His 110 degrees of flexion would translate into 70 degrees of flexion today since at that time they used 180 degrees as full extension.

In 1879, Paul Segond described an avulsion fracture of the anterolateral margin of the tibial plateau. This is routinely associated with ACL disruption. This fracture is now known universally as a Segond fracture and is considered pathognomonic for ACL tears.

In 1900, Battle first reported an ACL repair. It was done two years earlier during treatment for dislocation of the knee. The results were satisfactory. No further description was made [7].

Battle published the first report and Mayo-Robson performed the first repair.

In 1903, he reported the repair of both cruciate ligaments of the knee in a 41-year-old miner. A diagnosis of rupture of the anterior and posterior cruciate ligaments was made. Further arthrotomy revealed that the ligaments had been avulsed from their femoral attachments and they were duly repaired with catgut sutures. After some weeks of cast immobilisation, the knee was allowed to move and six years postoperatively the patient reported the knee to be "perfectly strong" [9].

Mayo-Robson felt that this case should be published and that surgical repair was both "feasible and hopeful." Yet later in 1903, F Lange of Munich attempted to replace an ACL using braided silk attached to the semitendinosus as a ligament substitute. This ultimately failed. The importance of the anterior cruciate ligament (ACL) was recognised by Fick as early as 1911 [10].

In 1913, Goetjes produced a detailed study of ruptures of the cruciate ligaments [7]. He discussed ligament function and mechanisms of rupture, as determined by cadaver studies. He advocated repair for the acute injury and conservative treatment for chronic ruptures. By 1916 Jones [11] had remarked that stitching the ligaments is absolutely futile: "Natural cicatricial tissue... is the only reliable means of repair." Jones' early observation was confirmed 60 years later by Feagin and Curl [12] when they published their long-term follow-up of West Point cadets who had had ACL repair during their college years.

They concluded: "long-term follow-up evaluations do not justify the hope... that anatomic repositioning of the residual ligament would result in healing." Such views led to a trend away from primary ACL repair (without augmentation) and instead towards the concept of immediate reconstruction of the ACL.

3. Autologous Fascia Lata and Meniscal Grafts

In 1912, KH Giertz operated on a 13-year-old girl with a totally unstable knee. She had septic arthritis of her knee when she was one year old. First, he corrected the fixed flexion deformity of 45 degrees by an osteotomy. Two weeks later, he stabilised the knee with free transplanted strips of fascia lata, sutured on the medial side to the medial femoral epicondyle and to the tibial tubercle, and on the lateral side from the lateral epicondyle to the fibular head. Postoperatively the girl was asymptomatic and did not attend for follow-up for 6 months. For all practical purposes the knee was stable [13].

In 1917, Hey Groves published a short case report on reconstruction of the ACL [14]. He detached a strip of fascia lata from its insertion and directed it through a tunnel in the tibia. In the following year in 1918, Smith published a paper reporting on nine cases he had treated with Hey Groves' technique. Smith was critical of the incomplete nature of the construct, which failed to strengthen the medial collateral ligament. One year later, Hey Groves presented fourteen further cases in which he modified his technique by leaving the graft attached to the tibia and detaching it superiorly, following the same route as in the previous cases. Hey Groves in 1920 was the first to state clearly that flexion and extension of the knee affect tension within the ACL [14].

4. The Hamstring Graft

In 1934 the Italian orthopaedic surgeon Riccardo Galeazzi described a technique for ACL reconstruction using the semitendinosus tendon. The tendon was released from its musculotendinous junction and placed intra-articularly through a 5 mm diameter bone tunnel drilled in the tibial epiphysis and a tunnel drilled through the lateral femoral condyle, where it was fixed to the periosteum. Galeazzi used three incisions: one for harvesting of the semitendinosus tendon, another for arthrotomy, and a third laterally for fixation. He used a cast for 4 weeks and partially weight bearing for 6 weeks. He reported on three cases. One operated in 1932 had a follow-up of 18 months, and the final outcome was a stable knee with full extension and only a mild reduction of flexion. Galeazzi was the first that ever published the usage of hamstrings tendon autograft in ACL reconstruction [15].

In 1939 Macey reported on using the semitendinosus tendon for the reconstruction of the ACL [16]. Only the tendinous portion of the semitendinosus muscle was harvested. During harvesting Macey stopped short of the musculotendinous junction and attached the graft with the knee held in full extension. For many years it was believed that Macey was the first one to ever use hamstrings in ACL reconstruction. The Orthopaedic community had failed to take into consideration Galeazzi's publication 5 years earlier.

In 1950, Lindemann used the semitendinosus tendon as dynamic stabilizer of ACL deficient knees [17]. Augustine reported a similar procedure [18]. McMaster et al. in 1974 used the gracilis tendon alone [19]. It was left attached distally, pulled through the tibial and femoral tunnels, and fixed to the lateral condyle using a staple.

5. Patellar Tendon Grafts

In 1935, Campbell reported the first use of a tibia-based graft of the medial one- third of the patellar tendon, the prepatellar retinaculum, and a portion of the quadriceps tendon [20].

Campbell's technique involved the drilling of two tunnels, one in the tibia and one in the femur. The graft was sutured to the periosteum at the proximal end of the femoral tunnel. The procedure did not achieve widespread approval immediately. It was reintroduced by MacIntosh a few years later.

In 1944, Abbott noted that, in the absence of a fracture, examination of the knee joint was all too often superficial and cursory, with many ligamentous injury patterns grouped together as "internal derangements of the knee" and treated inadequately [21]. He advised that to avoid the later development of a painful, unstable joint with recurrent effusions, subsequent arthritic changes, and the attendant permanent disability, "a far greater precision in diagnosis and therapy is a necessity in a joint of such manifold complexity" [21].

6. Bone-Patellar Tendon-Bone Grafts

In 1963 Jones published a new surgical technique for the reconstruction of an irreparably damaged ACL [22]. Jones commented that while the need for surgical reconstruction of an irreparably torn ACL had long been appreciated, there was a need for a satisfactory technique to address the problem. The technique described was considered simpler and more "nearly physiological" than previous techniques. Jones described his technique as having the greatest application to old injuries, whilst suggesting that surgical repair was still the procedure of choice for acute injuries. The Jones procedure uses a medial parapatellar incision extending from one inch distal to the patella to just distal to the tibial tubercle. After drilling of a femoral tunnel, the middle third of the patellar tendon is then incised throughout its length, with the incisions continuing proximally across the patella and into the quadriceps tendon. A saw is then used to cut a triangular block of bone from the superficial cortex of the patella in line with the longitudinal incisions. The articular surface of the patella is not breached. In this manner, a graft consisting of a bone block from the patella and the central one-third of the patellar tendon is created, which is still in continuity with the tibia through the tibial insertion of the patellar tendon. This graft is then passed through the femoral tunnel, embedding the patellar component of the graft within the femoral tunnel, when pulled taut patellar tendon and the skin incision are then closed. Jones reported on 11 patients who underwent this procedure with excellent clinical outcomes.

Criticism of the technique centered around the fact that because the graft was so short, the femoral tunnel had to be drilled at the anterior margin of the notch and not at the insertion of the native ACL. The technique was simple, however, and caused minimal surgical trauma and so gained widespread acceptance.

Brückner described a similar technique in 1966, using the medial one-third of the patellar tendon [23]. The graft, harvested with a patellar bone block, was left attached to the tibia and then passed through a tibial tunnel, giving the graft more working length than in Jones' technique. After being passed through the joint, the graft was then placed in a socket in the femur and secured to the lateral aspect of the lateral femoral condyle of the femur with sutures passing through a button.

By 1969, Franke had further developed the techniques described by Jones and Bruckner. Franke pioneered the use of free bone-patellar tendon-bone graft consisting of one-quarter of the patellar tendon with blocks of bone derived from the patella and proximal tibia at opposite ends of the graft [24]. His graft was fixed with a wedge-like piece of bone anchored in the tibial plateau and a shell-like piece of bone implanted into the femoral condyle. Although very similar to the Jones and Bruckner techniques, this was the first description of a free graft used in this manner.

Marshall et al. in 1979 also used the central third of the patellar tendon but left it distally attached, and they added for length a strip of the quadriceps tendon, which was secured in the over-the-top position to the lateral condyle [25].

By the 1990s the technique of using a free bone-patellar tendon-bone graft harvested from the central one-third of the patella became the "Gold Standard" of treatment. This technique was broadly termed the Jones Procedure in reference to the pioneering work done by Kenneth Jones in the 1960s [22]. It was popular because it was relatively simple and because it yielded consistently good results. During this period researchers devised the metal interference screw as a form of tibial and femoral graft fixation. Bioabsorbable interference screws soon followed.

7. Synthetic Grafts

Benson suggested the potential biological and biomechanical significance of pure carbon in 1971 [26]. During the 1970s and early 1980s, a group from Cardiff experimented extensively with the use of carbon implants as an agent for the induction of new tendon synthesis in animal models [27–30]. Jenkins argued that "since a high proportion of the tissues of living organisms is composed of carbon compounds it would not perhaps be surprising that implants of the pure element should be well tolerated by these tissues" [29]. Initial results were promising with new tendon being formed around the carbon grafts at three months after implantation and no obvious clinical dysfunction in an ovine model [29]. Jenkins et al. concluded that filamentous carbon is accepted in living tissues with virtually no adverse reaction and that it can be used to induce the formation of new tendon or ligament with a physical strength equal to that of the normal structure [29]. The implants were extremely well tolerated in the ovine model with regard to foreign body response, and this encouraged the Cardiff group to progress to clinical trials in the human lower limb [31]. This study included two ACL reconstructions in isolation and thirty-one combined knee ligament procedures. The two ACL reconstructions were reviewed yearly postoperatively (maximum three years) and both reported a significant improvement in the function of their knees. The only complication documented in this preliminary report was of sinus formation overlying graft material in 2 ankles where the graft was considered too superficial. No complications were reported in the knee group.

In 1983 Rushton et al. reported the clinical, arthroscopic, and histological findings in ten knees that had undergone ACL reconstruction using a carbon-fibre graft [32]. Carbon-fibre ACL grafts had been implanted into thirty-nine patients and the ten reported cases had experienced pain and discomfort postoperatively. All ten patients had synovitis with evidence of carbon-fibre in the joint. Occasionally, the fibre stained the articular surface and menisci. The femoral notch of some patients contained inflamed synovium. Such synovium was stained black. In some patients a "new ligament" appeared to have formed but gentle probing with a blunt hook revealed this to be a thin, fibrous sheath covering unchanged carbon-fibre graft. Histologically two patients demonstrated a fibroblastic response to the carbon-fibre. Five patients showed evidence of chronic synovial inflammation and papillary proliferation of the synovium was present in all ten knees. A mild foreign-body giant-cell reaction to the carbon-fibre filaments and haemosiderin was seen in surface cells of the synovium, in macrophages, and around some fragments of carbon-fibre. Other complications included ulceration of the skin over subcutaneous carbon-fibre knots used to secure the graft, similar to the findings of the Jenkins study three years earlier [31].

8. The Use of Allograft

During the 1980s a remarkable interest developed in the use of allograft tissue for ACL reconstruction. The first experimental published studies concerning the mechanical, biological, and functional properties [33–37] were compensatory and this led sports medicine surgeons to adopt allografts in ACL reconstruction in humans.

Webster and Werner in 1983 conducted a study on dogs where they harvested flexor tendons from the forepaws and hind-paws of mongrel dogs [33]. These tendons were freeze-dried and then thawed, rehydrated, and implanted in recipient dogs as an ACL substitute graft. The purpose of the study was to ascertain whether or not freeze-dried grafts functioned as well as autografts over time. The use of allografts in theory would decrease the surgical morbidity associated with autograft harvest and would also allow for more precise graft size, shape, and quantity to be implanted than would autograft. Webster and Werner reported preliminary results similar to those for patellar tendon graft for graft strength and similar to normal ACL for mode of failure.

In 1985 Curtis et al. reported on a similar study, where freeze-dried fascia lata grafts were implanted in dogs as an ACL substitute graft [34]. All grafts were found to be intact at sacrifice with no overt evidence of biologic incompatibility. The knees displayed only mild instability to clinical testing without evidence of arthrosis. Histologically, the grafts appeared to function as collagenous scaffolding for revascularization and fibrovascular creeping substitution. Shino et al. echoed these findings. They found no significant differences between the mechanical properties of allografts and autografts and also reported no evidence of implant rejection [35].

Nikolaou et al. in 1986 seemed so sure of the future of freeze-dried allografts that they attempted to design and implement an experimental model for testing the feasibility of cryopreserved ACL allotransplantation [36]. Groups of dogs were used to evaluate the effect of cryopreservation on ligament strength and to compare the relative performance of both autograft and allograft ACL transplants up to 18 months after implantation. The ligaments were examined mechanically, histologically, and microangiographically. They reported that the cryopreservation process and duration of storage had no effect on the biomechanical or structural properties of the ligament. The mechanical integrity of the allografts was similar to that of the autografts, with both achieving nearly 90% of control ligament strength by 36 weeks. Revascularization approached normal by 24 weeks in both autograft and allograft. No evidence of structural degradation or immunological reaction was seen. Based on these results, Nikolaou et al. believed that a cryopreserved ACL allograft could provide the ideal material for ACL reconstruction and so outlined a surgical technique for harvesting and implanting this graft clinically.

In 1987 Jackson et al. reported disappointing results of implanted freeze-dried bone-ACL-bone graft in goats [37].

By 1991, however, the same group reported much better results in a similar trial whereby the graft material was frozen in situ and then subjected to a freeze-thaw process whereby the graft material was devitalised and devascularised prior to harvesting [38]. This resulted in a significant increase in graft strength and a decrease in knee laxity at six weeks and six months. The authors deduced that the loss of strength seen in allografts postoperatively was not a result of the freezing and revascularisation process, but rather the consequence of improper orientation and tensioning of the graft. They concluded that techniques of implantation that precisely provide proper orientation and tensioning of the graft might minimise the loss of strength.

During the 1980s, techniques for arthroscopic ACL reconstruction were becoming increasingly popular. There were two distinct schools of thought with regard to this. Some surgeons preferred the outside-in method, where the ligament is routed into the joint through a femoral tunnel [39, 40]. Yet other surgeons preferred the inside-out technique, where the ligament is routed from inside the joint into a femoral socket [41]. Despite the differing techniques, the 1980s were a time when arthroscopic ACL reconstruction became popularised, leading to a much better understanding of the ligament and its sites of attachment.

9. The Double-Bundle graft

The Jones procedure did of course have its drawbacks, including pain at the graft donor site and stiffness within the extensor apparatus of the knee. This led to further experimentation with the use of hamstring grafts.

In 2003 Marcacci et al. described a double-bundle gracilis and semitendinosus graft that they claimed guaranteed a more anatomic ACL reconstruction and avoided the use of hardware for graft fixation [42].

The technique is designed to reproduce the kinematic effect of both anteromedial and posterolateral bundles of the ACL with a 4-bundle reconstruction. Modifications of this technique have been described by a number of authors [43–48]. Research into this area continues, and although many surgeons now practice variations of this technique, many ACL reconstruction procedures are still done using bone-patellar tendon-bone graft.

10. Conclusion

The history of ACL reconstruction can be traced as far back as the Egyptians times. Research and innovation abound in this area, with improvements in clinical outcomes being achieved constantly. Knowledge of the evolution of ACL reconstruction is invaluable to those who continue to try to improve the outcomes of the procedure, in order to further the advances already made, but also to reduce the risk of repeating the mistakes of the past.

Conflict of Interests

The authors declare that they have no conflict of interests, financial or otherwise, with regard to this paper. It has not been submitted to any other journal for consideration for publication.

References

[1] K. Miyasaka, D. Daniel, M. Stone, and P. Hirshman, "The incidence of knee ligament injuries in the general population," *The American Journal of Knee Surgery*, vol. 4, pp. 3–8, 1991.

[2] D. L. Butler, "Anterior cruciate ligament: its normal response and replacement," *Journal of Orthopaedic Research*, vol. 7, no. 6, pp. 910–921, 1989.

[3] C. Frank, D. Amiel, S. L.-Y. Woo, and W. Akeson, "Normal ligament properties and ligament healing," *Clinical Orthopaedics and Related Research*, vol. 196, pp. 15–25, 1985.

[4] F. R. Noyes, L. A. Mooar, C. T. Moorman III, and G. H. McGinniss, "Partial tears of the anterior cruciate ligament. Progression to complete ligament deficiency," *Journal of Bone and Joint Surgery. British*, vol. 71, no. 5, pp. 825–833, 1989.

[5] S. M. Strickland, J. D. MacGillivray, and R. F. Warren, "Anterior cruciate ligament reconstruction with allograft tendons," *Orthopedic Clinics of North America*, vol. 34, no. 1, pp. 41–47, 2003.

[6] V. Chouliaras and H. H. Passler, "The history of the anterior cruciate ligament from Galen to double-bundle acl reconstruction," *Acta Orthopaedica et Traumatologica Hellenica*.

[7] G. A. Snook, "A short history of the anterior cruciate ligament and the treatment of tears," *Clinical Orthopaedics and Related Research*, vol. 172, pp. 11–13, 1983.

[8] J. Stark, "Two cases of ruptured crucial ligaments of the knee-joint," *The Edinburgh Medical and Surgical*, vol. 5, pp. 267–271, 1850.

[9] A. W. M. Robson, "Ruptured crucial ligaments and their repair by operation," *Annals of Surgery*, vol. 37, pp. 716–718, 1903.

[10] H. E. Cabaud, "Biomechanics of the anterior cruciate ligament," *Clinical Orthopaedics and Related Research*, vol. 172, pp. 26–31, 1983.

[11] R. Jones, "Disabilities of the knee joint," *British Medical Journal*, vol. 2, pp. 169–173, 1916.

[12] J. A. Feagin Jr. and W. W. Curl, "Isolated tear of the anterior cruciate ligament: 5 year follow up study," *American Journal of Sports Medicine*, vol. 4, no. 3, pp. 95–100, 1976.

[13] K. H. Giertz, "Über freie Transplantation der Fascia lata als Ersatz für Sehnen und Bänder," *Deutsche Zeitschrift für Chirurgie*, vol. 125, no. 5-6, pp. 480–496, 1913.

[14] "The classic. Operation for repair of the crucial ligaments Ernest W. Hey Groves, MD., F.R.C.S.," *Clinical Orthopaedics and Related Research*, vol. 147, pp. 4–6, 1980.

[15] R. Galleazzi, "La ricostituzione dei ligamenti cociati del ginocchio," *Atti e Memorie della Società Lombarda di Chirurgia*, vol. 13, pp. 302–317, 1924.

[16] H. Macey, "A new operative procedure for the repair of ruptured cruciate ligaments of the knee joint," *Surgery, Gynecology & Obstetrics*, vol. 69, pp. 108–109, 1939.

[17] K. Lindemann, "Plastic surgery in substitution of the cruciate ligaments of the knee-joint by means of pedunculated tendon transplants," *Zeitschrift für Orthopädie und ihre Grenzgebiete*, vol. 79, no. 2, pp. 316–334, 1950.

[18] R. W. Augustine, "The unstable knee," *The American Journal of Surgery*, vol. 92, no. 3, pp. 380–388, 1956.

[19] J. H. McMaster, C. R. Weinert Jr., and P. Scranton Jr., "Diagnosis and management of isolated anterior cruciate ligament tears: a preliminary report on reconstruction with the gracilis tendon," *Journal of Trauma*, vol. 14, no. 3, pp. 230–235, 1974.

[20] W. Campbell, "Repair of the ligaments of the knee: report of a new operation for the repair of the anterior cruciate ligament," *Surgery, Gynecology & Obstetrics*, vol. 62, pp. 964–968, 1936.

[21] L. C. Abbott, J. B. M. Saunders, F. C. Bost, and C. E. Anderson, "Injuries to the ligaments of the knee joints," *The Journal of Bone and Joint Surgery. American*, vol. 26, pp. 503–521, 1944.

[22] K. G. Jones, "Reconstruction of the anterior cruciate ligament using the central one-third of the patellar ligament," *Journal of Bone and Joint Surgery. American*, vol. 52, no. 4, pp. 838–839, 1970.

[23] H. Brückner, "A new method for plastic surgery of cruciate ligaments," *Chirurg*, vol. 37, no. 9, pp. 413–414, 1966.

[24] K. Franke, "Clinical experience in 130 cruciate ligament reconstructions," *Orthopedic Clinics of North America*, vol. 7, no. 1, pp. 191–193, 1976.

[25] J. L. Marshall, R. F. Warren, T. L. Wickiewicz, and B. Reider, "The anterior cruciate ligament: a technique of repair and reconstruction," *Clinical Orthopaedics and Related Research*, vol. 143, pp. 97–106, 1979.

[26] B. J. Benson, "Elemental carbon as a biomaterial," *Journal of Biomedical Materials Research*, vol. 5, no. 6, pp. 41–47, 1972.

[27] I. W. Forster, Z. A. Ralis, B. McKibbin, and D. H. R. Jenkins, "Biological reaction to carbon fiber implants: the formation and structure of a carbon-induced 'neotendon," *Clinical Orthopaedics and Related Research*, vol. 131, pp. 299–307, 1978.

[28] D. H. R. Jenkins, "The repair of cruciate ligaments with flexible carbon fibre. A longer term study of the induction of new ligaments and of the fate of the implanted carbon," *Journal of Bone and Joint Surgery. British*, vol. 60, no. 4, pp. 520–522, 1978.

[29] D. H. R. Jenkins, I. W. Forster, B. McKibbin, and Z. A. Ralis, "Induction of tendon and ligament formation by carbon implants," *Journal of Bone and Joint Surgery. British*, vol. 59, no. 1, pp. 53–57, 1977.

[30] R. N. Tandogan, Ö. Taşer, A. Kayaalp et al., "Analysis of meniscal and chondral lesions accompanying anterior cruciate ligament tears: relationship with age, time from injury, and level of sport," *Knee Surgery, Sports Traumatology, Arthroscopy*, vol. 12, no. 4, pp. 262–270, 2004.

[31] D. H. R. Jenkins and B. McKibbin, "The role of flexible carbon-fibre implants as tendon and ligament substitutes in clinical practice. A preliminary report," *Journal of Bone and Joint Surgery. British*, vol. 62, no. 4, pp. 497–499, 1980.

[32] N. Rushton, D. J. Dandy, and C. P. E. Naylor, "The clinical, arthroscopic and histological findings after replacement of the anterior cruciate ligament with carbon-fibre," *Journal of Bone and Joint Surgery. British*, vol. 65, no. 3, pp. 308–309, 1983.

[33] D. A. Webster and F. W. Werner, "Freeze-dried flexor tendons in anterior cruciate ligament reconstruction," *Clinical Orthopaedics and Related Research*, vol. 181, pp. 238–243, 1983.

[34] R. J. Curtis, J. C. Delee, and D. J. Drez Jr., "Reconstruction of the anterior cruciate ligament with freeze dried fascia lata allografts in dogs. A preliminary report," *American Journal of Sports Medicine*, vol. 13, no. 6, pp. 408–414, 1985.

[35] K. Shino, T. Kawasaki, and H. Hirose, "Replacement of the anterior cruciate ligament by an allogeneic tendon graft. An experimental study in the dog," *Journal of Bone and Joint Surgery. British*, vol. 66, no. 5, pp. 672–681, 1984.

[36] P. K. Nikolaou, A. V. Seaber, and R. R. Glisson, "Anterior cruciate ligament allograft transplantation. Long-term function, histology, revascularization, and operative technique," *American Journal of Sports Medicine*, vol. 14, no. 5, pp. 348–360, 1986.

[37] D. W. Jackson, E. S. Grood, B. T. Cohn, S. P. Arnoczky, T. M. Simon, and J. F. Cummings, "The effects of in situ freezing on the anterior cruciate ligament: an experimental study in goats," *Journal of Bone and Joint Surgery. American*, vol. 73, no. 2, pp. 201–213, 1991.

[38] S. M. Howell, M. P. Wallace, M. L. Hull, and M. L. Deutsch, "Evaluation of the single-incision arthroscopic technique for anterior cruciate ligament replacement: a study of tibial tunnel placement, intraoperative graft tension, and stability," *American Journal of Sports Medicine*, vol. 27, no. 3, pp. 284–293, 1999.

[39] W. G. Clancy Jr., R. G. Narechania, and T. D. Rosenberg, "Anterior and posterior cruciate ligament reconstruction in rhesus monkeys. A histological, microangiographic, and biomechanical analysis," *Journal of Bone and Joint Surgery. American*, vol. 63, no. 8, pp. 1270–1284, 1981.

[40] F. R. Noyes, D. S. Matthews, P. A. Mooar, and E. S. Grood, "The symptomatic anterior cruciate-deficient knee. Part II. The results of rehabilitation, activity modification, and counseling on functional disability," *Journal of Bone and Joint Surgery. American*, vol. 65, no. 2, pp. 163–174, 1983.

[41] J. Gillquist and M. Odensten, "Arthroscopic reconstruction of the anterior cruciate ligament," *Arthroscopy*, vol. 4, no. 1, pp. 5–9, 1988.

[42] M. Marcacci, A. P. Molgora, S. Zaffagnini, A. Vascellari, F. Iacono, and M. Lo Presti, "Anatomic double-bundle anterior cruciate ligament reconstruction with hamstrings," *Arthroscopy*, vol. 19, no. 5, pp. 540–546, 2003.

[43] H. Asagumo, M. Kimura, Y. Kobayashi, M. Taki, and K. Takagishi, "Anatomic reconstruction of the anterior cruciate ligament using double-bundle hamstring tendons: surgical techniques, clinical outcomes, and complications," *Arthroscopy*, vol. 23, no. 6, pp. 602–609, 2007.

[44] G. Bellier, P. Christel, P. Colombet, P. Djian, J. P. Franceschi, and A. Sbihi, "Double-stranded hamstring graft for anterior cruciate ligament reconstruction," *Arthroscopy*, vol. 20, no. 8, pp. 890–894, 2004.

[45] K. Yasuda, E. Kondo, H. Ichiyama, Y. Tanabe, and H. Tohyama, "Clinical evaluation of anatomic double-bundle anterior cruciate ligament reconstruction procedure using hamstring tendon grafts: comparisons among 3 different procedures," *Arthroscopy*, vol. 22, no. 3, pp. 240–251, 2006.

[46] S.-J. Kim, K.-A. Jung, and D.-H. Song, "Arthroscopic double-bundle anterior cruciate ligament reconstruction using autogenous quadriceps tendon," *Arthroscopy*, vol. 22, no. 7, pp. 797.el–797.e5, 2006.

[47] P. U. Brucker, S. Lorenz, and A. B. Imhoff, "Aperture fixation in arthroscopic anterior cruciate ligament double-bundle reconstruction," *Arthroscopy*, vol. 22, no. 11, pp. 1250.el–1250.e6, 2006.

[48] J. H. Ahn and S. H. Lee, "Anterior cruciate ligament double-bundle reconstruction with hamstring tendon autografts," *Arthroscopy*, vol. 23, no. 1, pp. 109.el–109.e4, 2007.

8

A Simplified Approach for Arthroscopic Repair of Rotator Cuff Tear with Dermal Patch Augmentation

Anthony C. Levenda and Natalie R. Sanders

Lakeshore Bone and Joint Institute, 601 Gateway Boulevard, Chesterton, IN 46304, USA

Correspondence should be addressed to Anthony C. Levenda; alevenda@yahoo.com

Academic Editor: Padhraig O'Loughlin

Here, we describe an arthroscopic method specifically developed to augment rotator cuff repair using a flexible acellular dermal patch (ADP). In this method, an apparently complex technique is simplified by utilizing specific steps to augment a rotator cuff repair. In this method, using a revised arthroscopic technique, rotator cuff repair was performed. This technique allowed easy passage of the graft, excellent visualization, minimal soft tissue trauma, and full four-corner fixation of an ADP. Twelve patients underwent rotator cuff repair with augmentation using the combination of this method and ADP. Due to the technique and biomechanical characteristics of the material, the repairs have been stable and with high patient satisfaction.

1. Introduction

Rotator cuff tears primarily affect the older segment of the population which is increasingly growing in size and activity level [1]. It is estimated that more than 40% of those over 60 years of age suffer from a rotator cuff tear [2]. In treating this condition, it is estimated that, for 2010 in the United States alone, there were a total of 81,000 major (≥3 cm tear) rotator cuff repairs performed and 24,600 of these used some kind of augmentation [1]. By 2014, the number of major procedures is expected to rise to 109,100 [1]. For treatment, many patients with partial-thickness tears look first to noninvasive treatment options which can include icing the affected area and anti-inflammatory injections such as cortisone and physical therapy. If the injury does not heal, is painful, or is too severe (full-thickness, large, or massive tear), for those patients who wish to proceed with surgery and are willing to accept the risks and the demands of postoperative physical therapy, arthroscopic surgery can be advantageous. Since no two rotator cuff tears are alike, the way the tears are addressed is different for each case. Primary rotator cuff repair using standard arthroscopic technique is often not optimal in patients with large to massive tears [1]. In addition to the tear type, there are differences in tissue quality, patients' comorbidities (diabetic, smoker, etc.), revision tears, and chronic tears. All of these factors must be taken into consideration when evaluating a patient for possible arthroscopic rotator cuff repair.

When surgery is indicated, large to massive rotator cuff tears may be augmented using a material with biomechanical integrity. Failed rotator cuff repairs can sometimes occur due to knot tying or anchor fixation; however, this should not be a concern for a skilled arthroscopist. Even for a skilled surgeon, challenges remain in repairing rotator cuffs arthroscopically. Several studies have shown high imaging test (MRI, ultrasound) failure rates for nonaugmented repairs with failure defined by a nonintact rotator cuff [3–5]. Recognizing this, surgeons choosing augmented repair with either an allograft, a xenograft, or a synthetic graft, over just sutures, made up about 30% of all major rotator cuff repairs in 2010 [1]. This percentage is estimated to increase to as much as 37% by 2014 [1]. One option for difficult repairs is augmentation with biological scaffolds.

Biological scaffolds commonly used to augment rotator cuff repair include xenografts and allografts. Common xenograft tissues are typically collagen-based sheets such as equine pericardium, bovine dermis, or porcine small intestinal submucosa. Repairs using xenografts counted for slightly less than half of all augmented repairs in 2010 [1]. The other major category of biological scaffold augment material is decellularized human skin allografts which made up slightly more than half of the augmented repair market in 2010 and this number is expected to increase [1] as surgeons choose allografts over both xenografts and nonaugmented repairs. Decellularized human skin allografts have been used for a variety of medical procedures, primarily wound healing, soft tissue reconstruction, and sports medicine applications [6–24]. In theory, decellularization serves to remove potentially immunogenic material and also provides a clean scaffold for host cellular and vascular ingrowth [25]. Augmentation in repair of rotator cuff tears is among reported clinical applications for decellularized human dermis [9, 11, 13, 21, 24, 26]. During these procedures, the dermal matrix is typically used to augment a repair procedure in order to provide biomechanical strength and support directed healing.

Here, we describe arthroscopic rotator cuff augmentation using a method specifically tailored to the use of flexible of a human ADP.

2. Technique

The criteria used for selecting patients included patients with large to massive rotator cuff tears and those who needed revision repairs. Tears with poor tissue quality or having poor mobilization of tissue were prime candidates for augmented repair. Finally, patients who exhibited comorbidities such as smoking or diabetes could greatly benefit from ADP.

Patients consented to participation in the study and the surgical extremity was marked. Most patients received interscalene block in the preoperative area by an anesthesiologist. General anesthesia was induced and the patient was placed in the lateral decubitus position on a bean bag using an axillary roll and padding all bony prominences. The extremity was prepped and draped and the arm was placed in traction at 15 degrees of forward flexion and 60 degrees of abduction. A rolled towel was placed in the axillary pouch. Bony landmarks were outlined. A standard posterior portal was made and arthroscope was introduced. Intra-articular exam was performed and an anterior portal was made from an outside-in technique using a spinal needle. Any intra-articular pathology was addressed. The camera was then redirected to the subacromial space.

Once in the subacromial space, a spinal needle was introduced laterally for proper positioning of the lateral portal. Once in proper position, a stab incision was made and a complete bursectomy was performed using a shaver and electrocautery. If a subacromial decompression or distal clavicle extension was to be performed this was done at this time. Next, the rotator cuff was inspected by evaluating mobilization, size of tear, and tendon quality (Figure 1). If repairable, the footprint was prepared. Soft tissue releases (anterior and posterior slides) were performed if necessary. Next, Arthrex BioCorkscrews, double loaded (Arthrex, Naples, FL), were implanted at the edge of the articular surface (Figure 2). Visualization was from the lateral portal. Using Arthrex Lassos, Arthrex FiberWire (Arthrex, Naples, FL) was passed from the corkscrew through the rotator cuff tear in a mattress type fashion carefully not to over-tension the repair (Figure 3). The sutures were tied arthroscopically and excess material was cut (Figure 4).

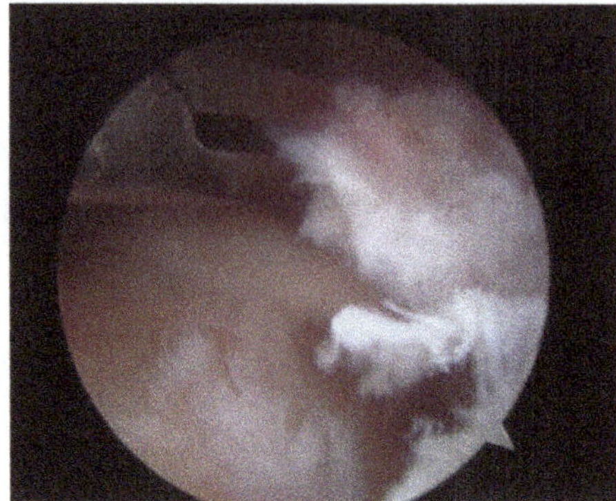

Figure 1: Identify rotator cuff tear pattern.

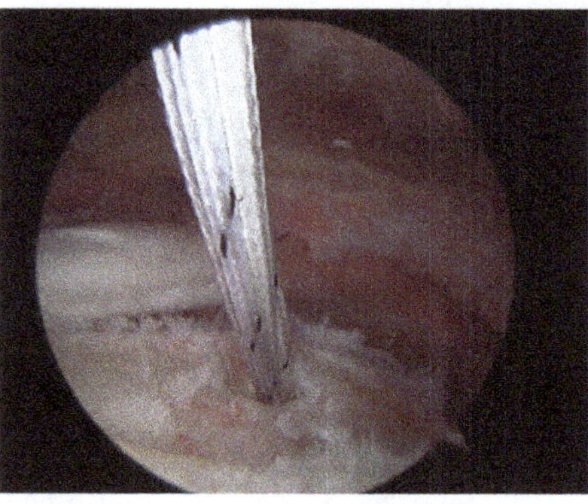

Figure 2: 5.5 BioCorkscrew anchor loaded with double FiberWire.

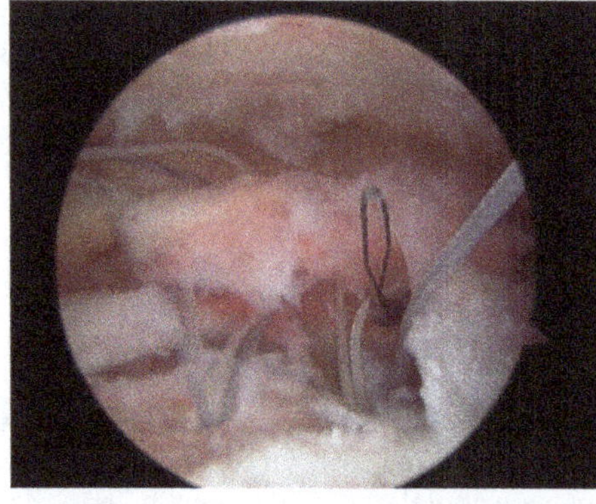

Figure 3: Pass sutures in mattress fashion through cuff utilizing Arthrex Lasso.

In patients with poor tissue quality, revision surgery, or combination of both, an allograft was used. Using a calibrated probe, the area that needs augmentation was measured. It is important to measure the area from anterior to posterior and from medial to lateral. A lateral cannula was placed at this point for suture management. Three FiberWires were placed medially to the sutures tied in the cuff repair. These should be placed in the anterior position, the midline position, and posterior position. This was done with an Arthrex Lasso.

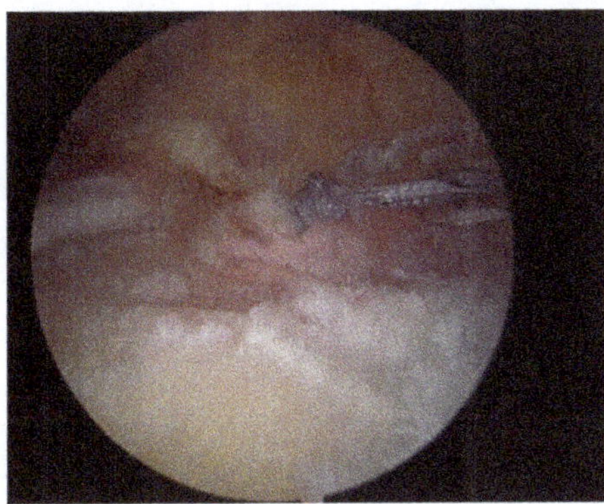

Figure 4: Repaired cuff to medial edge of footprint. As noted, entire footprint is prepared for placement of the ArthroFlex dermal patch.

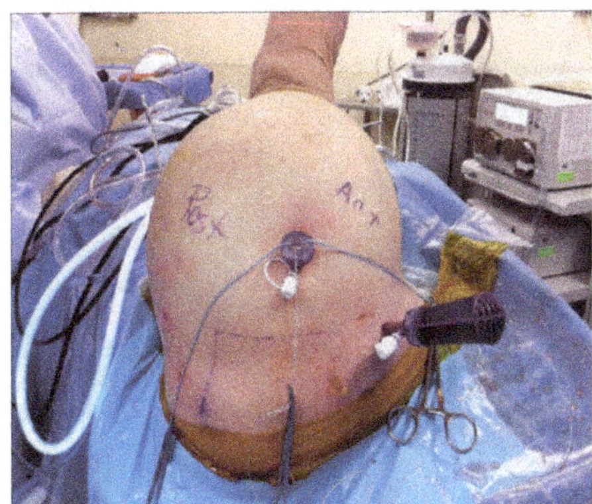

Figure 5: Three medial FiberWires for the ADP are passed through lateral cannula. Cannula is used to keep sutures from crossing.

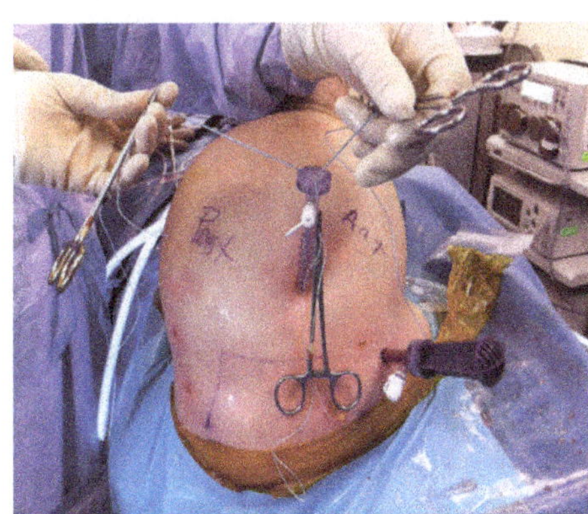

Figure 6: With assistance, the sutures are kept separate as the cannula is removed.

The sutures were not tied. It is advisable to use alternating colored FiberWire to assist in suture management. The camera was placed in the posterior portal and the sutures were grasped individually through the lateral cannula using caution not to cross sutures. Then, they were tagged with hemostats (Figure 5). With assistance, the cannula was carefully removed while keeping the sutures separated (Figure 6). The graft passed easier through skin incision versus a cannula.

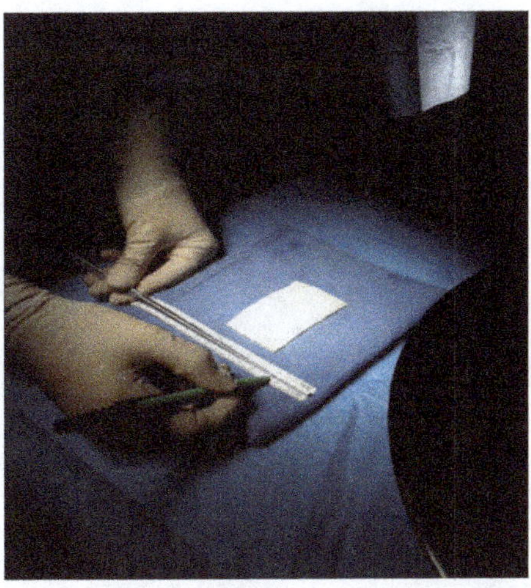

Figure 7: Arthroscopically the defect to be filled is measured with a probe. The measurements taken are anterior to posterior and medial to lateral.

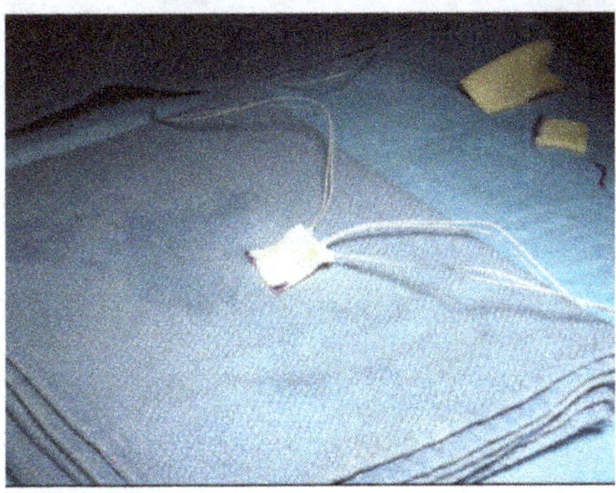

Figure 8: Two to three fiber cinches are placed on the lateral side for lateral fixation and stabilization.

Once the cannula was removed and the sutures were kept separated and tagged, attention was turned to the graft. Using the measurements obtained, the ADP (ArthroFlex, LifeNet Health, Virginia Beach, VA) was prepared (Figure 7). The graft was slightly undersized due to the need to place tension on the graft during the augmentation. Next, three Arthrex FiberLinks (Arthrex, Naples, FL) were passed through the lateral edge of the graft (Figure 8). These were used for ease of graft passage and for double row fixation.

The graft was then placed on the arm laterally to the lateral portal with the correct side up. One arm of each suture previously passed through the cuff was then passed through the anterior, midline, and posterior sides of the graft (Figures 9 and 10).

The graft was carefully passed through the lateral incision alternating a knot pusher over each anterior and posterior suture as they were passed. A mulberry knot can be used on the medial midline suture to help advance the graft into position. During this step, an assistant held slight tension on the lateral Cinch sutures to aid in passing the graft (Figure 11). Once the graft was in position, the sutures were each tied medially (Figure 12). After the medial edge was down,

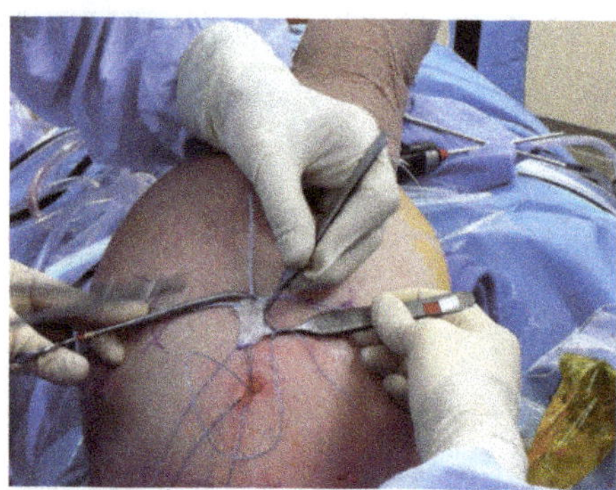

Figure 9: The three medial FiberWires are passed through the medial side of the ADP in a simple fashion.

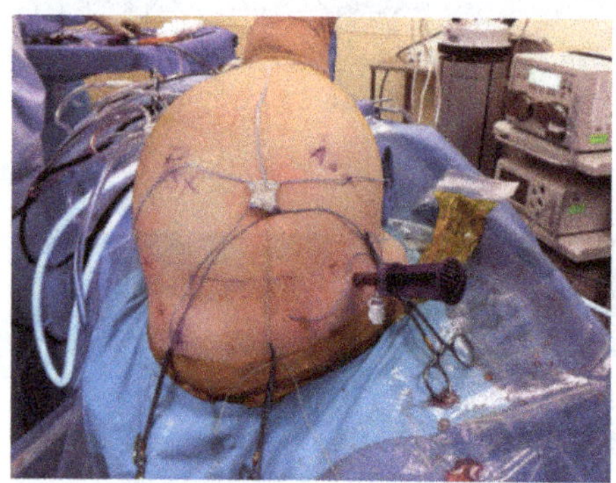

Figure 10: All medial and lateral sutures were passed through ADP.

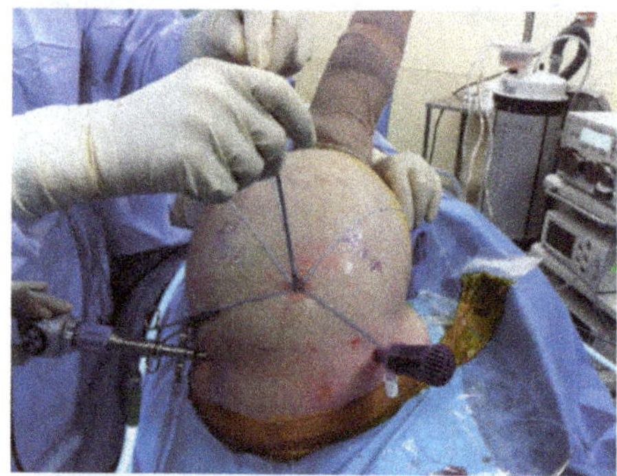

Figure 11: Utilizing a knot pusher and viewing arthroscopically the graft is passed into the subacromial space. Note the tension placed by the assistant on the lateral sutures. The knot pusher is alternated on the medial fiberwire sutures passing through the graft.

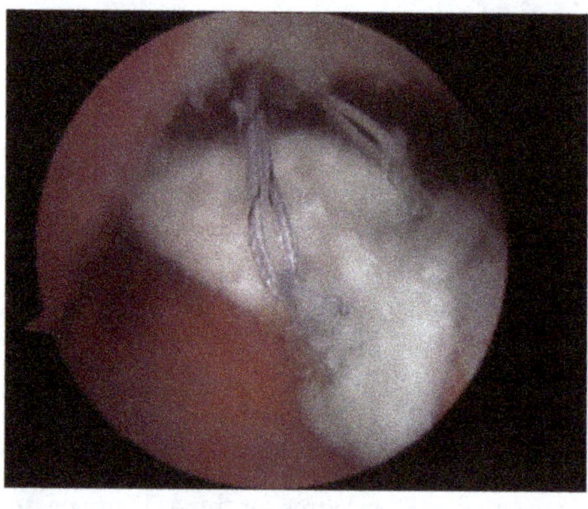

Figure 12: The three medial FiberWire sutures are tied arthroscopically to stabilize the graft.

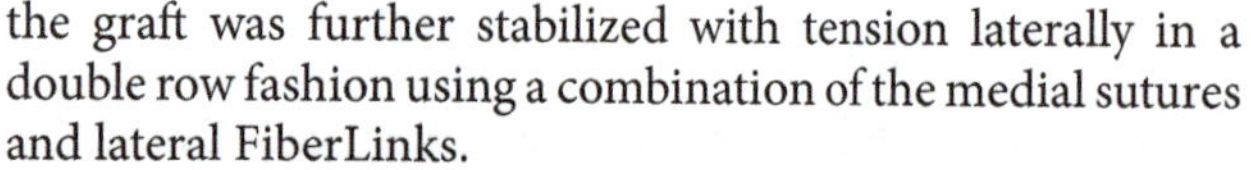

the graft was further stabilized with tension laterally in a double row fashion using a combination of the medial sutures and lateral FiberLinks.

Additional small stab incisions can be made laterally to obtain optimal points of fixation for the double row (Figures 13(a) and 13(b)). A spinal needle can be used to obtain these positions. It is easier to stabilize the midline lateral FiberLink first. The repair was then evaluated and additional fixation was performed as needed on the anterior and posterior edges using a lasso and additional free FiberWires to allow further tensioning (Figure 14).

The technique described allowed ease of passage of the graft, excellent visualization, and minimal soft tissue trauma. Generally, the only cannula utilized was the small orange cannula from Arthrex and only during suture management of the ADP.

Postoperative protocol was patient dependent but began with true protected passive ROM for the first 6–8 weeks. An abductor sling was worn for the first 6–8 weeks except for hygiene and therapy. At 6–8 weeks, general active motion was started. Resistance or strengthening was not begun until the fourth month.

3. Results

Thus far, ADP has been used in 12 patients with 2–4 cm tears using the technique described here (Table 1). The patients ranged in age from 52 to 71 years with a mean age of 61.8 years and had an equal male to female ratio. Two patients had type II diabetes and one patient had type I diabetes. Three of the patients presented with revision tears, unrelated to the augment patch.

Patients were evaluated at 2 weeks, 6 weeks, 12 weeks, 16 weeks, 6 months, and 1 year following the procedure. Patients showed both an increased range of motion and increased strength. They also experienced a significant decrease in pain when graded on the VAS Numeric Pain Distress Scale. The preoperative average score of 9 was greatly reduced to a postoperative average of 3 following surgery using this technique. The results of several studies [13, 21, 26] have suggested the clinical outcomes of rotator cuff repairs might not be dependent or even correlated with cuff integrity determined by MRI. In light of these findings, the additional expense of MRI scanning was deemed unnecessary if the patient demonstrated clinical success, pain relief, and satisfaction with the repair.

As a case example, a 66-year-old female underwent primary arthroscopic rotator cuff repair without ADP augmentation in June, 2011. She had an uneventful postoperative course for 6 weeks and then she sustained a fall. She then began to have increased pain in her shoulder. A repeated MRI without contrast revealed retear of rotator cuff

Table 1: Patient demographics and outcomes.

Patient	Age y.o.	Gender	Present w/revision	Tear size (cm)	Pre-op VAS*	Post-op VAS	Increase in strength	Successful repair
1	58	M	No	4 × 4	7	0	Yes	Yes
2	66	F	Yes	3 × 2	10	2	Yes	Yes
3	52	F	Yes	2.5 × 3	10	5	Yes	Yes
4	59	F	No	2 × 2	8	2	Yes	Yes
5	71	F	No	3 × 3	8	4	Yes	Yes
6	55	M	No	3 × 3	10	4	Yes	Yes
7	67	M	No	2.7 × 2.7	10	5	Yes	Yes
8	67	F	No	2 × 2	9	1	Yes	Yes
9	57	M	Yes	3 × 3	7	0	Yes	Yes
10	67	M	No	2 × 2	10	2	Yes	Yes
11	62	F	No	2.5 × 2.5	10	0	Yes	Yes
12	62	M	No	2 × 3	9	2	Yes	Yes

*Visual Analog Numeric Pain Distress Scale.

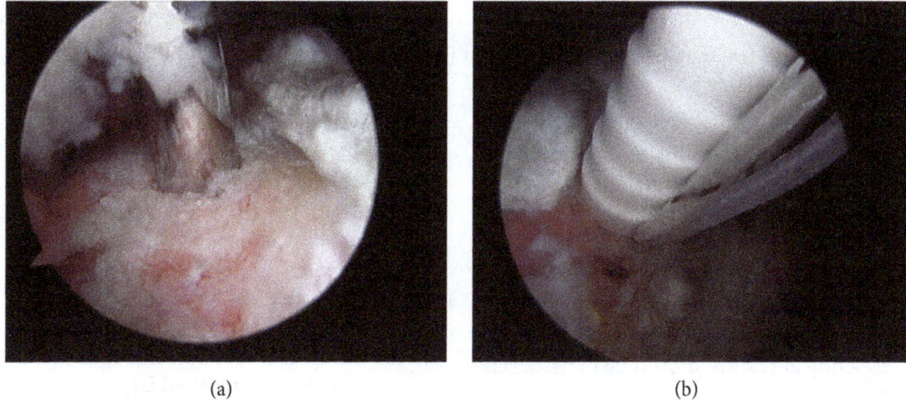

(a) (b)

Figure 13: (a) Push locks are used laterally to perform a double row repair and stabilize the graft laterally. (b) Push lock is used laterally for double row fixation.

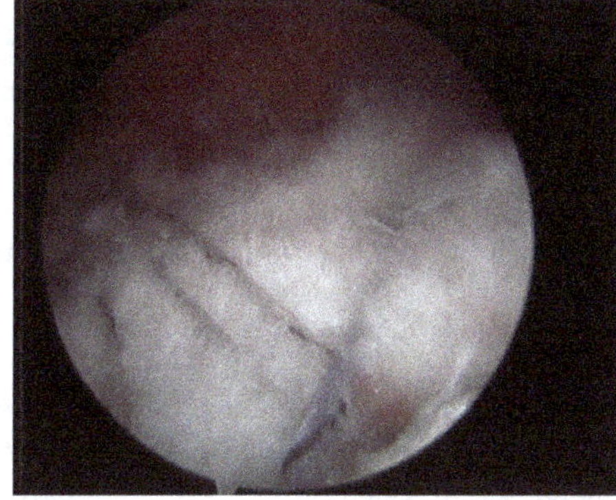

Figure 14: Final repair viewed from lateral portal.

(Figure 15(a)). She went on to have an arthroscopic revision rotator cuff repair augmented with the allograft. Another MRI was ordered seven months after operation which demonstrated healed rotator cuff repair with ADP augmentation (Figure 15(b)).

There were no complications due to infection, adhesions, or neurological injuries. However, two failures of ADP augmentation occurred due to postoperative falls resulting in retear of their rotator cuff. Both patients went on to have reverse total shoulder arthroplasty. Of note, during reverse total shoulder arthroplasty the graft and tissue were evaluated. The retear had occurred medial to the graft. The graft and the footprint were intact.

4. Discussion

Using this simplified approach to graft augmentation of arthroscopic rotator cuff repair has resulted in high quality surgical fixation. This is in large part due to the improved visualization for graft augmentation, when compared to a mini-open technique, as well as the ease of ADP handling and the favorable biomechanical characteristics of the graft. The advantage of improved visualization from using an arthroscopic technique may be offset by the benefit of a potentially stronger fixation at the suture-tendon interface provided by a mini-open or open repair [3, 26]. However, the use of an allograft to augment the arthroscopic repair can increase the strength of the suture-tendon interface, thus minimizing the advantage of an open repair, while also benefitting

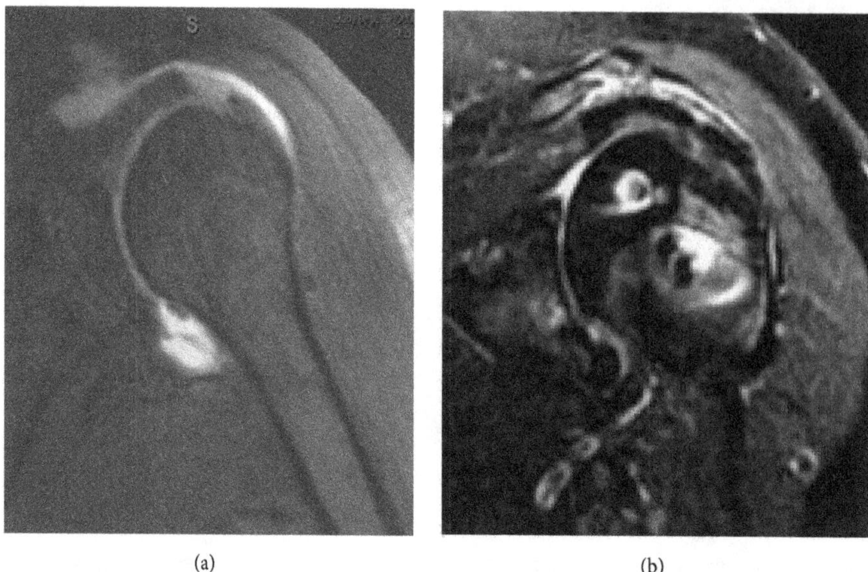

(a) (b)

Figure 15: Retear rotator cuff two months after original repair (a) and seven months after RCR with ADP augmentation (b).

the patient with decreased wound morbidity and pain. Using our arthroscopic method, follow-up through one year after operation has demonstrated high patient satisfaction. The ADP was very manageable to use in performing arthroscopic graft augmentation despite the average graft size being 3 cm by 3 cm. In addition, the graft exhibited superior strength since it did not tear and resisted pull out with tension of the sutures. However, these clinical results should be considered with the limitations of an informal case series. Our intent was to focus on this innovative augmentation technique and we only provided the initial clinical results as an interest of note.

5. Conclusion

This surgical technique demonstrates a new method to arthroscopically augment a standard rotator cuff repair with a graft which is provided ready to use. Patients exhibited a significant decrease in postoperative pain. While further long-term study and the larger patient base are necessary to have significance, these short-term results demonstrate favorable outcomes especially in patients with an increased risk of failure.

Conflict of Interests

The authors declare that there is no conflict of interests regarding the publication of this paper.

References

[1] The Millennium Research Group, "Rotator cuff reinforcement graft market," US markets for soft tissue repair devices, 2010, pp. 93-109.

[2] K. A. Derwin, S. F. Badylak, S. P. Steinmann, and J. P. Iannotti, "Extracellular matrix scaffold devices for rotator cuff repair," *Journal of Shoulder and Elbow Surgery*, vol. 19, no. 3, pp. 467–476, 2010.

[3] J. Bishop, S. Klepps, I. K. Lo, J. Bird, J. N. Gladstone, and E. L. Flatow, "Cuff integrity after arthroscopic versus open rotator cuff repair: a prospective study," *Journal of Shoulder and Elbow Surgery*, vol. 15, no. 3, pp. 290–299, 2006.

[4] L. M. Galatz, C. M. Ball, S. A. Teefey, W. D. Middleton, and K. Yamaguchi, "The outcome and repair integrity of completely arthroscopically repaired large and massive rotator cuff tears," *The Journal of Bone & Joint Surgery A*, vol. 86, no. 2, pp. 219–224, 2004.

[5] S. J. Nho, M. K. Shindle, R. S. Adler, R. F. Warren, D. W. Altchek, and J. D. MacGillivray, "Prospective analysis of arthroscopic rotator cuff repair: subgroup analysis," *Journal of Shoulder and Elbow Surgery*, vol. 18, no. 5, pp. 697–704, 2009.

[6] D. Albo, S. S. Awad, D. H. Berger, and C. F. Bellows, "Decellularized human cadaveric dermis provides a safe alternative for primary inguinal hernia repair in contaminated surgical fields," *American Journal of Surgery*, vol. 192, no. 5, pp. e12–e17, 2006.

[7] F. A. Barber, M. A. Herbert, and M. H. Boothby, "Ultimate tensile failure loads of a human dermal allograft rotator cuff augmentation," *Arthroscopy: The Journal of Arthroscopic and Related Surgery*, vol. 24, no. 1, pp. 20–24, 2008.

[8] F. A. Barber, M. A. Herbert, and D. A. Coons, "Tendon augmentation grafts: biomechanical failure loads and failure patterns," *Arthroscopy*, vol. 22, no. 5, pp. 534-538, 2006.

[9] J. L. Bond, R. M. Dopirak, J. Higgins, J. Burns, and S. J. Snyder, "Arthroscopic replacement of massive, irreparable rotator cuff tears using a GraftJacket allograft: technique and preliminary results," *Arthroscopy: Journal of Arthroscopic and Related Surgery*, vol. 24, no. 4, pp. 403–409, 2008.

[10] S. A. Brigido, S. F. Boc, and R. C. Lopez, "Effective management of major lower extremity wounds using an acellular regenerative tissue matrix: a pilot study," *Orthopedics*, vol. 27, no. 1, supplement, pp. s145–s149, 2004.

[11] W. Z. Burkhead Jr., S. C. Schiffern, and S. G. Krishnan, "Use of Graft Jacket as an augmentation for massive rotator cuff tears," *Seminars in Arthroplasty*, vol. 18, no. 1, pp. 11–18, 2007.

[12] R. Candage, K. Jones, F. A. Luchette, J. M. Sinacore, D. Vandevender, and R. L. Reed II, "Use of human acellular dermal matrix for hernia repair: friend or foe?" *Surgery*, vol. 144, no. 4, pp. 703–711, 2008.

[13] R. Dopirak, J. L. Bond, and S. J. Snyder, "Arthroscopic total rotator cuff replacement with an acellular human dermal allograft matrix," *International Journal of Shoulder Surgery*, vol. 1, no. 1, pp. 7–15, 2007.

[14] S. A. Kapfer and T. H. Keshen, "The use of human acellular dermis in the operative management of giant omphalocele," *Journal of Pediatric Surgery*, vol. 41, no. 1, pp. 216–220, 2006.

[15] D. K. Lee, "Achilles tendon repair with acellular tissue graft augmentation in neglected ruptures," *Journal of Foot and Ankle Surgery*, vol. 46, no. 6, pp. 451–455, 2007.

[16] D. K. Lee, "A preliminary study on the effects of acellular tissue graft augmentation in acute Achilles tendon ruptures," *The Journal of Foot & Ankle Surgery*, vol. 47, no. 1, pp. 8–12, 2008.

[17] C. R. Mitchell and R. R. Cima, "A novel technique for the repair of urostomal hernias using human acellular dermal matrix," *Urology*, vol. 77, no. 3, pp. 746–750, 2011.

[18] M. Y. Nahabedian, "AlloDerm performance in the setting of prosthetic breast surgery, infection, and irradiation," *Plastic and Reconstructive Surgery*, vol. 124, no. 6, pp. 1743–1753, 2009.

[19] K. L. Randall, B. A. Booth, A. J. Miller, C. B. Russell, and R. T. Laughlin, "Use of an acellular regenerative tissue matrix in combination with vacuum-assisted closure therapy for treatment of a diabetic foot wound," *The Journal of Foot and Ankle Surgery*, vol. 47, no. 5, pp. 430–433, 2008.

[20] C. A. Salzberg, "Nonexpansive immediate breast reconstruction using human acellular tissue matrix graft (AlloDerm)," *Annals of Plastic Surgery*, vol. 57, no. 1, pp. 1–5, 2006.

[21] S. J. Snyder and J. L. Bond, "Technique for arthroscopic replacement of severely damaged rotator cuff using 'GraftJacket' allograft," *Operative Techniques in Sports Medicine*, vol. 15, no. 2, pp. 86–94, 2007.

[22] R. M. Wilkins, "Acellular dermal graft augmentation in quadriceps tendon rupture repair," *Current Orthopaedic Practice*, vol. 21, no. 3, pp. 315–319, 2010.

[23] C. L. Winters, S. A. Brigido, B. A. Liden, M. Simmons, J. F. Hartman, and M. L. Wright, "A multicenter study involving the use of a human acellular dermal regenerative tissue matrix for the treatment of diabetic lower extremity wounds," *Advances in skin & wound care*, vol. 21, no. 8, pp. 375–381, 2008.

[24] I. Wong, J. Burns, and S. Snyder, "Arthroscopic GraftJacket repair of rotator cuff tears," *Journal of Shoulder and Elbow Surgery*, vol. 19, no. 2, pp. 104–109, 2010.

[25] L. W. Norton and J. E. Babensee, "Innate and adaptive immune responses in tissue engineering," in *Fundamentals of Tissue Engineering and Regenerative Medicine*, U. Meyer, T. Meyer, J. Handschel, and H. P. Weismann, Eds., pp. 721–747, Springer, Berlin, Germany, 2009.

[26] F. A. Barber, J. P. Burns, A. Deutsch, M. R. Labbé, and R. B. Litchfield, "A prospective, randomized evaluation of acellular human dermal matrix augmentation for arthroscopic rotator cuff repair," *Arthroscopy: The Journal of Arthroscopic and Related Surgery*, vol. 28, no. 1, pp. 8–15, 2012.

Management of Neglected Achilles Tendon Division: Assessment of Two Novel and Innovative Techniques

Pradeep Jain,[1] Parthapratim Dutta,[1] Prabal Goswami,[1] Amol Patel,[1] Shammi Purwar,[1] and Vaibhav Jain[2]

[1] *Department of Plastic Surgery, Institute of Medical Sciences, Banaras Hindu University, Varanasi 221005, India*
[2] *Department of Plastic Surgery, Institute of Postgraduate Medical Education & Research, Kolkata 700020, India*

Correspondence should be addressed to Pradeep Jain; drpmjain@rediffmail.com

Academic Editor: Mel S. Lee

Objective. Repair of injured Achilles tendon in neglected cases is one of the difficult and challenging procedures for surgeon. Here, we share our experience with the use of two innovative techniques for repair of chronic rupture of Achilles tendon. *Design.* Prospective Study. *Setting.* Tertiary care hospital. *Patients.* Twelve patients with chronic Tendo Achilles rupture were followed up over a period of three to five years. *Intervention.* Patients were divided in two groups, A and B. In Group A, the repair was done with Gastroc-soleus turndown flap and weaving with Plantaris tendon graft and in Group B, with modified Kessler's technique strengthened with the free plantaris tendon graft. *Outcome Assessment.* Clinically and by Modified Rupp Scoring system. *Results.* At an average follow-up of 4 years (Group A, 3.7 and Group B, 4.4 years), the majority of the patients had excellent to good results as assessed with Modified Rupp Scoring with few minor complications in both the groups. There was no significant difference in the baseline variables such as age and gender and also in the Rupp's score between the two groups. *Conclusion.* The two techniques are novel and simple and have been found to be useful for repair of chronically ruptured Achilles tendon.

1. Introduction

Achilles tendon repair in neglected cases is one of the difficult and challenging procedures for the treating surgeon. Several methods and moifications have been described in the literature to treat this complicated situation with rather simplified modifications [1–5]. Success of procedure selected in a given case is dependent upon surgeon's skills, nature of the defect, patients' compliance, adequacy of repair, availability of graft reenforcement, and proper rehabilitation.

Augmentation of surgically repaired fresh total Achilles tendon rupture has not been found to have any advantage over simple end-to-end repair [6]. There is no consensus on the technique of repair, type, and strength of suture and method of postoperative rehabilitation.

We hypothesized that the technique of Gastroc-soleus turndown flap augmented with plantaris tendon would be as efficacious as the simple end-to-end repair of divided Tendo Achilles augmented with plantaris. Since chronic Achilles tendon injuries are more difficult to manage due to surrounding tissue fibrosis, larger defect, and muscle wasting, augmentation of repaired tendon in one way or the other would perhaps be desirable.

2. Patients and Methods

A prospective study was carried out from the year 2004 to 2009 enrolling 29 patients in which a diagnosis of Tendo Achilles rupture was made by performing Thomson's test [7] and palpating a defect in continuity of Tendo Achilles. Ultrasonography was done to assess the defect and for presence or absence of plantaris tendon. The patients were subjected to repair by one of the two proposed techniques. Inclusion criteria were chronic rupture at least 6 weeks old, unilateral rupture, and skeletal maturity.

Patients with bilateral injury (1), fresh ruptures (11), avulsion of bone (1), and with absence of plantaris tendon (4, 13.8%) were excluded. Thus, a total of 12 patients were available for final follow-up. Of the available patients, 7

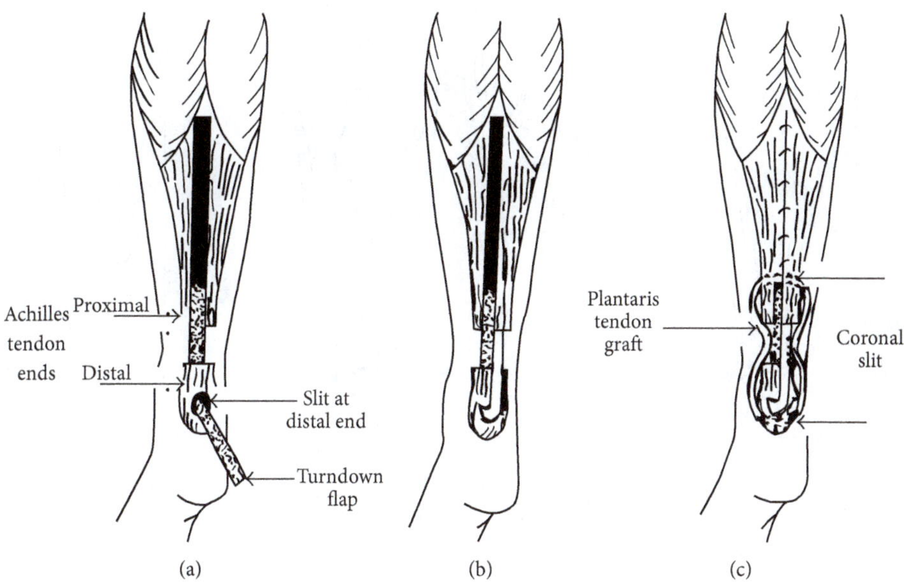

Figure 1: Diagrammatic illustration of gastroc-soleus turneddown flap ((a), (b)) and plantaris augmentation (c). Plantaris tendon graft passed through coronal slit and sutured with turndown flap.

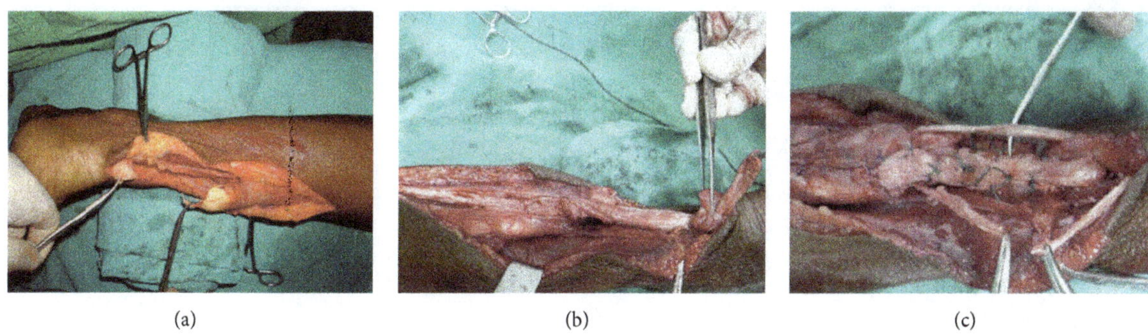

Figure 2: (a) 5 cm gap between two ends of Achilles tendon to be managed by GTPA. (b) Turndown flap passed through a slit made in distal end TA. (c) Plantaris tendon graft passed through coronal slit.

patients (5 males, 2 females) were treated with Gastroc-soleus turndown flap with plantaris augmentation (GTPA), and the remaining 5 (4 males, 1 female) were managed with primary repair with Kessler's suture technique and free plantaris autografting (KFPA). The age of Patients in the study ranged from 20 to 55 years. Average time between injury and surgery was approximately 3 months (range 2–4 months, Table 2).

2.1. Statistical Analysis. Mann Whitney U test was used to find the statistical significance of quantitative variables and Fisher's exact probability test for qualitative values.

2.1.1. Surgical Technique 1: Gastroc-Soleus Turndown Flap with Plantaris Augmentation (GTPA). Achilles tendon was explored by a lazy S incision under spinal anesthesia. The gap between two ends of ruptured/divided tendon was identified. Plantaris tendon graft around 18 cm in length was harvested from the same limb. A central turndown flap, of 14×2 cm size distally based from proximal end of Achilles tendon was raised. The base of the flap was placed 2.5 cm from the proximal cut end (Figure 1). This flap was passed through a slit made in distal end of tendon, turned up and both the raw surfaces of the turned down and turned up, flap were sutured together with nonabsorbable 3–0 polypropylene/No. 5 polyester suture. The plantaris tendon graft was passed spirally through coronal slit in distal and proximal ends, and both ends were sutured together (Figures 2(a) and 2(c)). Plantaris tendon and turned down flap were also sutured to each other with 4–0 polypropylene.

2.2. Postoperative Management. The patients were immobilized in above knee and below knee plaster splint for 2 weeks each with foot in planter flexion. Neutral position of ankle joint was achieved gradually over the next 2 weeks. Passive physiotherapy and partial weight bearing were allowed in further 3 weeks. This was followed by total weight bearing with restriction of strenuous exercise postoperatively.

2.3. Surgical Technique 2: Primary End-to-End Repair with Kessler's Suture and Free Plantaris Autografting (KFPA).

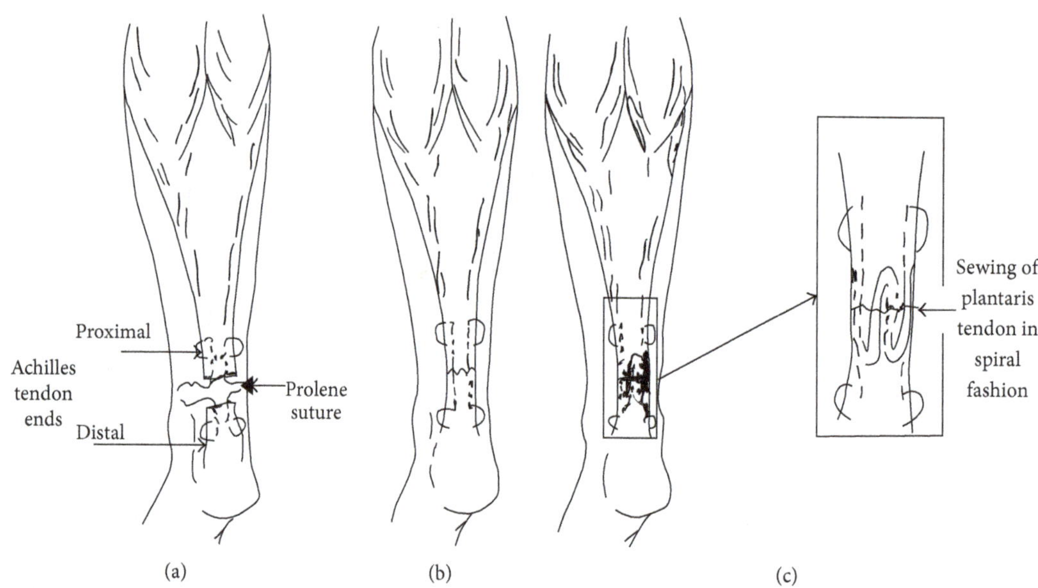

FIGURE 3: Diagrammatic illustration of primary repair with Kessler's suture ((a), (b)) and free plantaris autografting (KFPA) and sewing in spiral fashion (c).

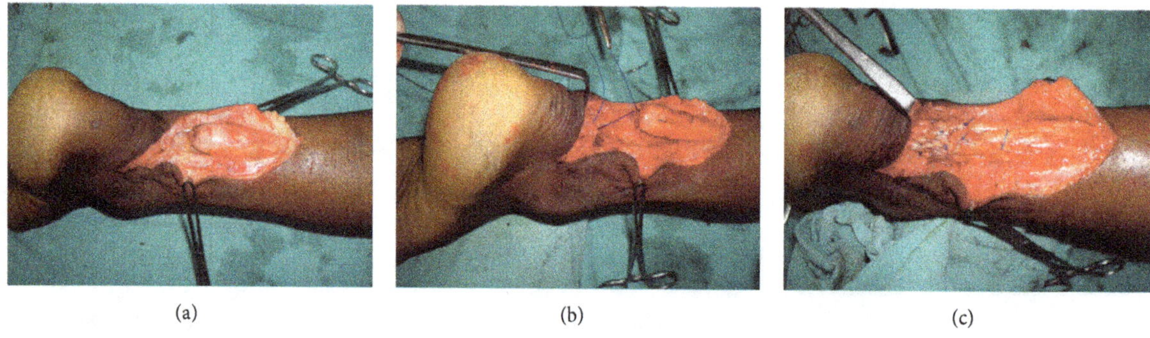

FIGURE 4: (a) 2 cm gap without soft tissue loss to be managed by KFPA. (b) Repair with Kessler's technique. (c) Sewing of plantaris tendon.

Achilles tendon was explored by a lazy S incision. Fibrous ends of the tendons were trimmed and mobilized. Plantaris tendon was harvested. Modified Kessler's stitch with number 1 prolene was applied between two divided ends of tendon and epitenon was repaired with 4–0 prolene with the foot in planter flexion. Sewing of plantaris tendon in spiral fashion away from the epitenon suture was additionally done (Figures 3, 4(a), 4(b), and 4(c)). Postoperative management was similar to previous technique.

All cases were operated by senior author (PJ). KFPA technique was initially advocated but, since 2007, majority of neglected cases with gaps ≥3 cm were managed by GTPA technique. Mean operative time was 72 minutes for GTPA and 58 minutes for KFPA technique.

2.4. Evaluation. All patients were followed up for assessment of integrity of repair and functional status. At each follow-up, ankle range of movements was measured by goniometer. The calf thickness was measured and compared with that of contralateral limb. The neurological status of foot, single limb hopping, strength of plantar flexors with heel raised standing, and ability to perform repeated heel raises were assessed. At the final follow-up, patients' satisfaction was assessed with Kerkhoffs' Modified Rupp Scoring system [8] (Table 1). Results of this scoring were rated as excellent (>30 points), good (15–30 points), fair (5–15 points), and poor (<5 points).

3. Results

As the GTPA technique was started later (since 2007), patients in this group had an average follow-up of approximately 3.7 years while patients with KFPA had a longer average follow-up of 4.4 years. Steroid injection (6 of 12 patients, 50%) in tendon was the most common cause of chronic rupture as these patients were having a tendinitis in the past. On an average, in both the groups, the injury was neglected for approximately a mean of 3 months (Table 2).

Ankle ROM and Calf diameter was found to be within 95th percentile of the operated and normal limb in both the groups. At final follow-up, all the patients could return to their daily activities and could perform single leg hopping

Table 1: Modified Rupp's Scoring system for subjective evaluation.

(1) Patient satisfaction	
Excellent	5
Good	1
Fair	−1
Poor	−5
(2) Do you experience pain during weight bearing?	
None	5
With extended weight bearing	1
With slight weight bearing	−2
Continuous	−5
(3) Do you experience pain independent of weight bearing?	
None	5
Pain a/w changes in weather	1
Pain sometimes a/w rest	−2
Continuous pain	−5
(4) Has your ankle function decreased since the operation?	
No	±2
Tendency to swelling	±2
Reduction of muscle strength	±2
Tendency to cramp	±2
(5) Do you fear rerupture?	
Yes	−1
No	1
(6) Do you have limitations of your work?	
Does not apply	0
None	5
Minor	−1
Major	−3
Changed profession due to TA problem	−5
(7) Do you have limitation of sports activity?	
Does not apply	0
None	5
Minor	−1
Major	−3
Stopped due to problems with Tendo Achilles	−5
Total score	
>30	Excellent
15–30	Good
5–15	Fair
<5	Poor

for 30 seconds, repeated heel raises, and heel standing. There was no significant difference between the two groups at the final follow-up with regard to pain, stiffness of ankle joint, calf muscle weakness, range of ankle motion, and overall outcome. There was no significant difference in the baseline variables such as age, gender, and so forth, and also in the Rupp's score between the two groups. Modified Rupp's score was excellent in 4, good in 2, and fair in 1 in GTPA, and excellent in 2, good in 2, and fair 1 in KFPA groups, thus making a total of 50% as excellent, 33.3% as good, and 16.6% as fair results with a satisfactory outcome (Table 3). There was no statistically significant difference in the overall Rupp's score between the two groups, thus proving our hypothesis.

3.1. Complications. No patient in these groups ever had sural nerve neuropraxia. Superficial marginal flap necrosis in one patient of Group A was managed conservatively. Superficial suture point infection (n = 3, 1 in Group A, 2 in B) was also managed conservatively (Group A) and by exploration and extracting the buried suture (Group B). At 6 months follow-up, these patients were having little discomfort at the heel but no limitation in ROM as they were followed up for long. Functional recovery was near complete at the time of final follow-up.

4. Discussion

Many methods have been described in the literature for Achilles tendon repair. Selection of particular method depends upon the type and size of the defect. When there is no major defect, the surgeon can have different options like percutaneous suture method, modified Kessler, Bunnel, and Krackow techniques. But in our patients, we found larger gaps (>2 cms) between two cut/ruptured ends of Achilles tendon. For management of neglected Achilles tendon rupture with significant gap, the basic requirement is to bridge the defect by tissue or synthetic materials which can unite the cut ends with satisfactory strength and allow full range of tendon excursion. The popular options are Lindholm technique [9], Bosworth technique [10], and V-Y repair [11]. In Group A, we raised an inferiorly based and centrally situated tendon flap attached for 2.5 cm at the distal part of proximal cut end of tendon like Bosworth but in our method, the harvested central strip was much broader and shorter in length (14 cm × 2 cm in our technique as compared to Bosworth in which tendon strip of 1.5 cm × 17.5 to 22.5 cm) assuming that broader and shorter tendon strip can provide more viability to the tendon strip and strength to repair and be superior in terms of graft stiffness, ease of handling and with lesser residual weakness of ankle dorsiflexion as demonstrated in our series of Group A patients. Our use of flap is totally different from Bosworth technique. We sutured raw surfaces together after passing it through the slit made in proximal healthy part of distal cut end of the tendon. Secondly, we further strengthened our repair by plantaris tendon graft (Figure 1) which was not described by Bosworth.

Maffulli has very rightly advised to individualize the treatment according to concern and health of the patient [12]. End-to-end repair is possible for gaps of <2.5 cm between the divided ends of the tendon [13]. Apart from Achilles tendon itself, Perez Teuffer [14] deployed peroneus brevis and Wapner et al. used flexor hallucis longus for Achilles tendon repair. Although these were good options, we avoided sacrificing another tendon in an already injured limb because

TABLE 2: Patients' characteristics: Group A (GTPA) and B (KFPA).

Pt name	Age	Sex	Side involved	Duration since injury (months)	Duration of follow-up (years)	Mode of injury	Complications	Rupp's score
Group A								
RS	32	M	L	3	4	Steroid injection	Superficial marginal necrosis	25
HP	20	M	R	2	3	Traumatic	—	31
KP	22	M	L	2	4	Cut injury	—	31
JK	54	F	R	3	5	Steroid injection	Superficial suture point infection	14
JD	45	M	R	4	3	Steroid injection	—	32
MR	48	M	L	3	3	Steroid injection	—	22
VK	25	F	L	3	4	Cut injury	—	33
Mean	**33**			**2.85**	**3.71**			
Group B								
ONS	33	F	L	2	5	Traumatic	—	31
RB	46	M	R	4	5	Steroid injection	Superficial suture point infection	23
JK	55	M	R	3	5	Cut injury	Superficial suture point infection	14
FR	29	M	L	2	4	Cut injury	—	32
IA	52	M	R	4	3	Steroid injection	—	30
Mean	**43**			**3**	**4.4**			
"*P*" value	**0.323**	**0.746**	**0.575**	**0.774**	**0.181**			**0.843**

TABLE 3: Rupp's score in both the groups at final follow-up.

Modified Rupp's Scoring	Group A (GTPA)	Group B (KFPA)	Overall total (%)
Excellent	4 (57.14%)	2 (40%)	50%
Good	2 (28.57%)	2 (40%)	33.3%
Fair	1 (14.28%)	1 (20%)	16.6%
Poor	0	0	0

in our opinion by doing so, there may be some functional loss related to transferred tendon. We reserved these tendon grafts in cases of rerupture of repair by our techniques in either of the group. Plantaris tendon is the most useful locally available tendon for further strengthening of Achilles tendon repair and has been advocated for use by surgeons in different ways. In Group B, we utilized the free plantaris tendon graft in a novel way to strengthen the repair. Lynn [1] advised the Achilles tendon repair using the plantaris tendon as a reinforcing membrane. They placed the previously harvested plantaris tendon in a fascial needle and passed it circumferentially, first through the posterior and then through anterior part of the tendon 2 cm from the rupture and fanned out and tucked over the repair after primary repair of tendon by Kessler's stitch. In White and Kraynic [15] modification of Perez Teuffer's technique, they also utilized the plantaris tendon strengthening after repairing the Achilles tendon by bridging the gap with peroneus brevis tendon. They placed the harvested plantaris tendon on a fascial needle and passed it in a figure of eight manner through the ruptured ends of the tendon. In our described method, we did the darning by previously harvested plantaris tendon-free graft by placing it on fascial needle and passing it spirally through the cut ends of the tendon and tucking it over the repair after applying modified Kessler's stitch, without sacrificing peroneus brevis.

Our technique (KFPA) offered advantage over other technique of Lynn [1] that fanning the tendon in membrane form might lose the tensile strength of repair and application of Bunnel's suture has the disadvantage of knots being left exposed on the tendon surface [10]. In contrast to Kraynick's modification of Perez Teuffer's technique, we did primary repair with modified Kessler's intratendinous suture to reduce intratendinous ischemia caused by classical Bunnell's suture and instead of increasing the bulk of repair by doing a figure of eight threading of plantaris tendon, we passed the graft spirally. We also repaired epitenon separately from the spiral graft in order to improve the vascularity of repair. Frequently, these neglected injuries present to us with more complex defects of soft tissues including loss of skin cover, either primarily or secondarily due to a previously failed operative intervention. Many methods like grafting to technically demanding free flap repair have been described in the literature for this purpose. The first and the foremost quality of the flap for providing skin cover over repaired tendon site is to allow adequate tendon excursion besides being easy to harvest, locally available, less morbid, and acceptable cosmetically. In our opinion, adipofascial flap described by Mohanty and Jain [16] and local fascial flap described by Fong et al. [17] fulfill all the criteria mentioned above for providing a suitable cover over tendon repair. The strength of our two techniques is that they are simple, surgeon friendly, less complex, and useful method of tendon repair in neglected cases with large interfragment gap as shown in their final outcome. Peroperative risk of sural nerve damage was minimal as we stayed posteromedially to the ruptured Tendo Achilles. An average follow-up of nearly four years in both the groups may be considered satisfactory in view of the opinion of Olsson et al. [18] that only minor improvements occur after the first year of repair. However, main disadvantage includes a small sample size in either of the group. Comparative analysis between both the groups could not yield significant difference as it required more number of patients. Biomechanical studies are also required to determine the tensile strength and vascularity at the repair site. Also, identification of factors leading to poor or successful outcome needs to be done with regression analysis. Hadi et al. in a review of management options for chronic rupture of Achilles tendon advocate that the surgery is the best option and emphasize on the need of randomized controlled trials with validated functional outcome measures [19].

In conclusion, the techniques described by us are newer and relatively easy ones based on present knowledge of tendon healing and its augmentation which seems to provide a reasonably good outcome.

Disclosure

Level of evidence is IV.

Conflict of Interests

None of the authors has any conflict of interests regarding the publication of this paper.

References

[1] T. A. Lynn, "Repair of the torn achilles tendon, using the plantaris tendon as a reinforcing membrane," *Journal of Bone and Joint Surgery A*, vol. 48, no. 2, pp. 268–272, 1966.

[2] K. L. Wapner, G. S. Pavlock, P. J. Hecht, F. Naselli, and R. Walther, "Repair of chronic Achilles tendon rupture with flexor hallucis longus tendon transfer," *Foot and Ankle*, vol. 14, no. 8, pp. 443–449, 1993.

[3] M. Takao, M. Ochi, K. Naito, Y. Uchio, M. Matsusaki, and K. Oae, "Repair of neglected Achilles tendon rupture using gastrocnemius fascial flaps," *Archives of Orthopaedic and Trauma Surgery*, vol. 123, no. 9, pp. 471–474, 2003.

[4] N. J. Bevilacqua, "Treatment of the neglected achilles tendon rupture," *Clinics in Podiatric Medicine and Surgery*, vol. 29, no. 2, pp. 291–299, 2012.

[5] S. Rahm, C. Spross, F. Gerber, M. Farshad, F. M. Buck, and N. Espinosa, "Operative treatment of chronic irreparable Achilles tendon ruptures with large flexor hallucis tendon transfers," *Foot & Ankle International*, vol. 34, pp. 1100–1110, 2013.

[6] T. C. Thompson and J. H. Doherty, "Spontaneous rupture of tendon of Achilles: a new clinical diagnostic test," *The Journal of Trauma*, vol. 2, pp. 126–129, 1962.

[7] A. Pajala, J. Kangas, P. Siira, P. Ohtonen, and J. Leppilahti, "Augmented compared with nonaugmented surgical repair of a fresh total achilles tendon rupture: a prospective randomized study," *Journal of Bone and Joint Surgery A*, vol. 91, no. 5, pp. 1092–1100, 2009.

[8] G. M. M. J. Kerkhoffs, P. A. A. Struijs, E. L. F. B. Raaymakers, and R. K. Marti, "Functional treatment after surgical repair of acute Achilles tendon rupture: wrap vs walking cast," *Archives of Orthopaedic and Trauma Surgery*, vol. 122, no. 2, pp. 102–105, 2002.

[9] A. Lindholm, "A new method of operation in subcutaneous rupture of the Achilles tendon," *Acta Chirurgica Scandinavica*, vol. 117, pp. 261–270, 1959.

[10] D. M. Bosworth, "Repair of defects in the tendoachilles," *The Journal of Bone & Joint Surgery*, vol. 38, pp. 111–114, 1956.

[11] E. Abraham and A. M. Pankovich, "Neglected rupture of the Achilles tendon: treatment by V-Y tendinous flap," *Journal of Bone and Joint Surgery A*, vol. 57, no. 2, pp. 253–255, 1975.

[12] N. Maffulli, "Rupture of the Achilles tendon," *Journal of Bone and Joint Surgery A*, vol. 81, no. 7, pp. 1019–1036, 1999.

[13] N. Maffulli and A. Ajis, "Management of chronic ruptures of the achilles tendon," *Journal of Bone and Joint Surgery A*, vol. 90, no. 6, pp. 1348–1360, 2008.

[14] A. Perez Teuffer, "Traumatic rupture of the Achilles tendon. Reconstruction by transplant and graft using the lateral peroneus brevis," *Orthopedic Clinics of North America*, vol. 5, no. 1, pp. 89–93, 1974.

[15] R. K. White and B. M. Kraynic, "Surgical uses of peroneous brevis tendon," *Surgery, Gynecology & Obstetrics*, vol. 108, pp. 117–121, 1959.

[16] A. Mohanty and P. Jain, "Reconstructing and resurfacing open neglected Achilles tendon injury by distal posterior tibial artery perforator based adipofascial flap," *European Journal of Plastic Surgery*, vol. 27, no. 4, pp. 196–199, 2004.

[17] E. P. Fong, R. P. G. Papini, M. V. McKiernan, and G. S. Rao, "Reconstruction of an Achilles tendon skin defect using a local fascial flap," *European Journal of Plastic Surgery*, vol. 20, no. 5, pp. 266–269, 1997.

[18] N. Olsson, K. Nilsson-Helander, J. Karlsson et al., "Major functional deficits persist 2 years after acute Achilles tendon rupture," *Knee Surgery, Sports Traumatology, Arthroscopy*, vol. 19, no. 8, pp. 1385–1393, 2011.

[19] M. Hadi, J. Young, L. Cooper, M. Costa, and N. Maffulli, "Surgical management of chronic ruptures of the Achilles tendon remains unclear: a systematic review of the management options," *British Medical Bulletin*, vol. 108, pp. 95–114, 2013.

10

Biomechanical Comparison of Different External Fixation Configurations for Posttraumatic Pelvic Ring Instability

Simon Tiziani,[1] Georg Osterhoff,[1] Stephen J. Ferguson,[2] Gregor Spreiter,[2] Max J. Scheyerer,[1] Gian-Leza Spinas,[1] Guido A. Wanner,[1] Hans-Peter Simmen,[1] and Clément M. L. Werner[1]

[1] *Department of Surgery, Division of Trauma Surgery, University Hospital Zurich, Raemistrasse 100, 8091 Zurich, Switzerland*
[2] *Institute for Biomechanics, ETH Zurich, HCI-E355.2 Wolfgang-Pauli-Strasse 10, 8093 Zurich, Switzerland*

Correspondence should be addressed to Simon Tiziani; simon.tiziani@uzh.ch

Academic Editor: Jörn Kircher

Background. External fixation is useful in the primary treatment of pelvic ring injuries. The present study compared the biomechanical stability of five different configurations of an external pelvic ring fixation system. *Methods.* Five configurations of an anterior external pelvic ring fixation system were tested using a universal testing machine. One single connecting rod was used in group "SINGLE," two parallel connecting rods in group "DOUBLE," two and four rods, respectively, in a tent-like configuration in groups "SINGLE TENT" and "DOUBLE TENT," and a rhomboid-like configuration in group "RHOMBOID." Each specimen was subjected to a total of 2000 consecutive cyclic loadings at 1 Hz lateral compression/distraction (±50 N) and torque (±0.5 Nm) loading alternating every 200 cycles. Translational and rotational stiffness were determined at 100, 300, 500, 700, and 900 cycles. *Results.* The "SINGLE TENT" and "RHOMBOID" configurations already failed with a preloading of 50 N compression force. The "DOUBLE" configuration had around twice the translational stability compared with the "SINGLE" and "DOUBLE TENT" configurations. Rotational stiffness observed for the "DOUBLE" and "DOUBLE TENT" configurations was about 50% higher compared to the SINGLE configuration. *Conclusion.* Using two parallel connecting rods provides the highest translational and rotational stability.

1. Background

Although unstable pelvic ring injuries are relatively rare [1], patients suffering from such injuries often show extensive haemorrhage [2]. Blood loss can occur from osseous structures at the fracture site, venous bleeding from the sacral plexus, or arterial bleeding [3]. Pelvic volume increases with pelvic ring disruption, which further hinders haemostasis. The primary objective in such situations is to reestablish pelvic ring integrity and stability, reducing pelvic volume in the process [3, 4]. Together with pelvic packing and clamping, external pelvic fixation has become an established adjunct for stabilizing unstable fractures and increasing chances of haemostasis [5–10]. External fixation may assist haemostasis in different ways, reducing fracture surfaces, ensuring blood clot stability, stopping venous bleeding, and achieving some tamponade by reducing pelvic volume [11, 12], though it has been shown that it may not induce pressure-induced tamponade [6]. There are numerous different external fixator constructs with each making different configurations possible. Furthermore there are different locations for pin anchoring in the pelvis. A supra-acetabular placement of the external fixator pins has been shown to be superior in stability compared to pins placed in the iliac crest [13, 14]. Continuing stability of the external fixation is crucial in ensuring optimal chance for haemostasis. Patients rarely present with isolated injuries to the pelvis. Concomitant abdominal injuries are frequent, making, for example, further abdominal surgery necessary [15]. This and the fact that some patients are obese, have made it necessary to come up with different configurations of the external fixation construct to fit the respective situations. The following configurations, tested in this study, were in use at

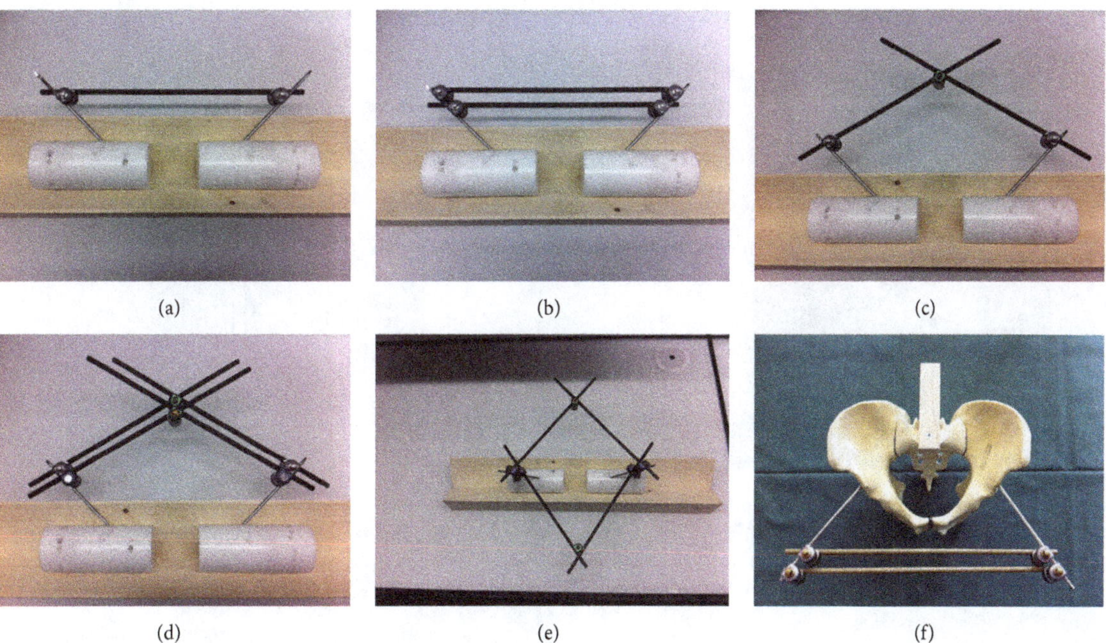

FIGURE 1: Configurations and pelvic instrumentation. (a) The "SINGLE" configuration. (b) The "DOUBLE" configuration. (c) The "SINGLE-TENT" configuration. (d) The "DOUBLE-TENT" configuration. (e) The "RHOMBOID" configuration. (f) A "DOUBLE" configuration mounted on a synthetic Synbone pelvis.

our University Hospital when treating unstable pelvic ring fractures. The "SINGLE" (Figure 1(a)) and "DOUBLE" (Figure 1(b)) configurations represent standard configurations. The "SINGLE TENT" (Figure 1(c)) and "DOUBLE TENT" (Figure 1(d)) configurations are used where the distance from the symphysis to the skin is increased in obese patients, making the application of the "SINGLE" and "DOUBLE" configurations impossible. Finally the "RHOMBOID" (Figure 1(e)) configuration is installed when further abdominal procedures (e.g., laparotomy) are to be expected.

The aim of the study was to compare the stability of five different configurations of the same external pelvic fixation construct. The hypothesis was that there would be no difference in stability between the different configurations.

2. Materials and Methods

2.1. Samples. The testing protocol included the testing of five different configurations of the same external fixation construct for the pelvis (Hoffmann II, Stryker, Kalamazoo, MI, USA). The groups to be tested included the following configurations: "SINGLE" (Figure 1(a)), "DOUBLE" (Figure 1(b)), "SINGLE TENT" (Figure 1(c)), "DOUBLE TENT" (Figure 1(d)), and "RHOMBOID" (Figure 1(e)). The fixator's pins (diameter 5 mm) were inserted into polyoxymethylene cylinders (diameter 70 mm) (Delrin, DuPont, Wilmington, DE, USA), one for each pin. Distance between the two polyoxymethylene cylinders and angle of pin insertion were measured at an external fixation device mounted in the supra-acetabular region of a synthetic model of the pelvis (Pelvis, Synbone, Malans, Switzerland) (Figure 1(f)). The pins were than screwed into the polyoxymethylene cylinders at a 45 degree angle and 7 cm from the later inward facing edge, making the distance from pin entry to pin entry site 21 cm. The couplings interfacing the pins and the rods were always placed with their upper edge on the first mark on the pins. In the "TENT" and "DOUBLE-TENT" configuration the distance between the pin-rod interface and the rod-rod interface was 24 cm (in the "DOUBLE-TENT" configuration this refers to the outer tent), resulting in a distance from rod-rod coupling to the surface of the cylinders of 25 cm in the plumb line. The distance from rod-pin interface to the rod-rod interface in the "RHOMBOID" configuration was 26 cm on all sides. The shapes of the different configurations were determined by an experienced orthopedic trauma surgeon (C.W). The five different configurations were attached to the pins via the rod-pin interface couplings, which all were tightened by the same person (S.T).

2.2. Biomechanical Testing. For the tests two different loading scenarios were selected. Firstly a translational loading scenario was applied, where the construct was loaded simulating compression and distraction in the pelvis. Secondly a rotational loading scenario was applied that would simulate, for example, hip bending. These two scenarios were chosen because they address the most common situations occurring in the postop phase: patients in supine position, leg movement, and patient transfer.

Thus all samples were tested using a universal testing machine (ElectroPulse E10000, Instron, Norwood, MA, USA) (Figure 2) according to the following protocol: alternating cycles of compression and distraction (along the cylindrical axis) and rotational loading (rotation around the cylindrical axis). Each sequence consisting of 200 cycles at 1 Hz was

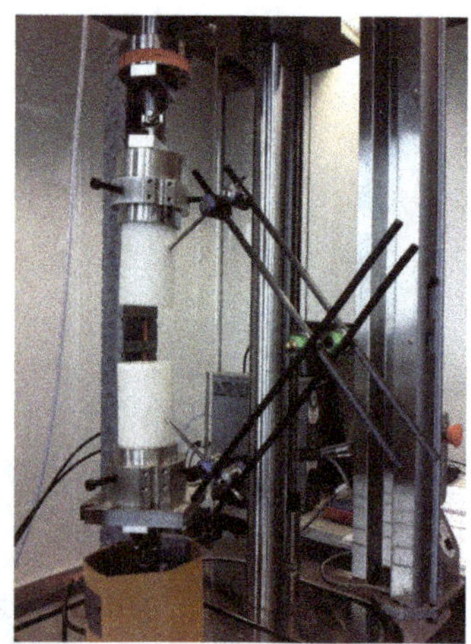

FIGURE 2: Experimental setup. Two polyoxymethylene cylinders instrumented with a Hoffmann II external fixator in the "DOUBLE-TENT" configuration mounted on the Intron testing machine. Testing included compression/distraction and rotational loading.

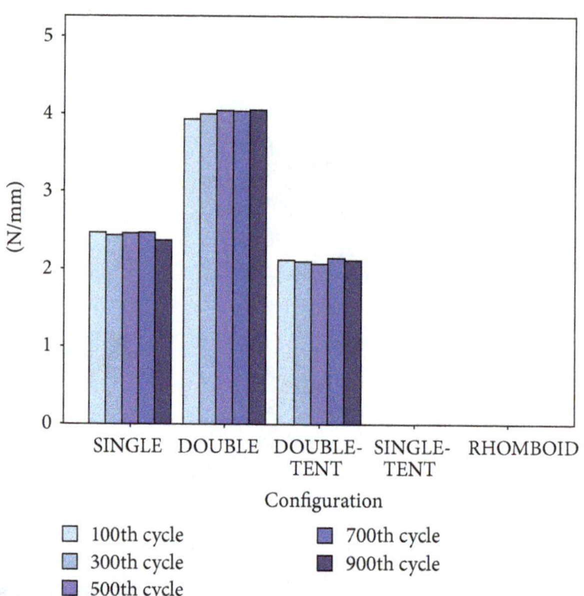

FIGURE 3: Translational stiffness. Results for translational stiffness of the five different configurations at 100, 300, 500, 700, and 900 cycles. The "SINGLE-TENT" and the "RHOMBOID" configurations failed and thus yielded no results.

run 5 times, making a total of 2000 cycles (1000 cycles each) per sample.

After slowly loading and observing a displacement of >25 mm with ±50 N translational load, 50 N was chosen for loading the cycles in translational loading. Rotational torque was set at ±5 Nm.

Measurements during testing were recorded by a ±1000 N (compression/distraction forces) and a 25 Nm (torque forces) loading cell and the computer programme calculated translational and rotational stiffness. Failure, as defined in the testing protocol, leading to abort of testing included: displacement overshooting the machine's range of motion (±30 mm translation and ±135 degrees rotation) and/or interface or construct failure.

2.2.1. Evaluation

Translational Stiffness [N/mm]. Translational stiffness readings were taken at 100, 300, 500, 700, and 900 cycles to be analysed statistically. This is a measure for resisting displacement when loaded simulating lateral compression and distraction.

Rotational Stiffness [Nm/degree]. Rotational stiffness readings were taken at 100, 300, 500, 700, and 900 cycles to be analysed statistically. This is a measure for resisting torque forces on the pelvis.

2.3. Statistical Analysis. After preliminary testing, a sample size calculation was performed using PS power and sample size calculations 3.0 (alpha error: 0.05) [16].

With an expected difference in means of 0.5 N/mm and a standard deviation of 0.15 N/mm for translational stiffness and an expected difference in means of 0.08 Nm/degree and a standard deviation of 0.025 Nm/degree for rotational stiffness the calculated number of samples to be able to reject the null hypothesis that the population means of the experimental and control groups are equal with a probability (power) of 0.8 was 3 per group.

Comparison of translational and rotational stiffness was done using a one-way ANOVA with a post hoc Bonferroni adjustment for multiple comparisons using SPSS for Windows V20.0 (SPSS, Chicago, Illinois, USA). Differences were considered significant for values of $P < 0.05$.

3. Results

The "SINGLE TENT" and the "RHOMBOID" configurations showed more than 30 mm displacement before reaching 50 N lateral compression-distraction loading, resulting in failure as defined by the testing protocol.

3.1. Translational Stiffness (Figure 3). The "DOUBLE" configuration was 59%–71% stiffer than the "SINGLE" configuration at 100, 300, 500, 700, and 900 cycles ($P = .002$, .003, .005, .001, and .001). Comparing it to the "DOUBLE TENT" configuration, the "DOUBLE" configuration was between 86% and 95% stiffer ($P = .001$, .001, .001, .001, and .001). There was no significant difference in translational stiffness between the "DOUBLE TENT" and the "SINGLE" configuration.

3.2. Rotational Stiffness (Figure 4). The "DOUBLE" configuration exceeded the "SINGLE" configuration in stiffness by 35% to 60% at 100, 300, 500, 700, and 900 cycles ($P = .025$, .019, .031, .003, and .004). The "DOUBLE TENT" configuration was stiffer than the SINGLE configuration at 100 cycles (41%, $P = .012$), 500 cycles (43%, $P = .011$), 700 cycles (57%, $P = .005$), and 900 cycles (55%, $P = .006$); there was no

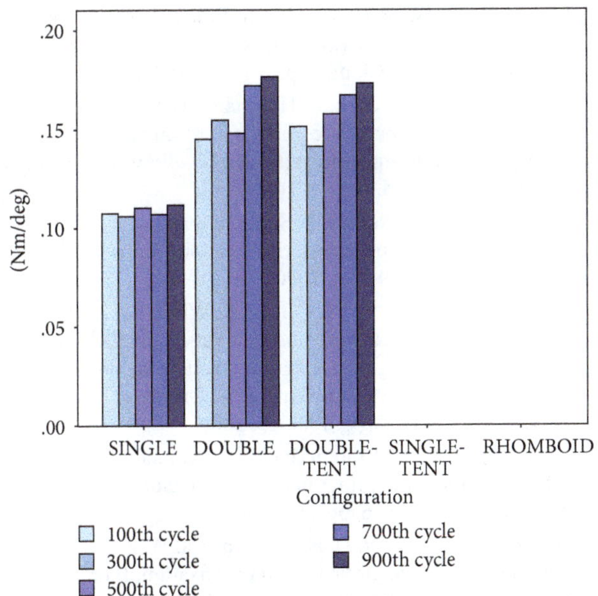

Figure 4: Rotational stiffness. Results for rotational stiffness of the five different configurations at 100, 300, 500, 700, and 900 cycles. The "SINGLE-TENT" and the "RHOMBOID" configurations failed and thus yielded no results.

significant difference at 300 cycles. Also, there was no significant difference between the "DOUBLE" and the "DOUBLE TENT" configurations.

No permanent deformation was observed in any of the tested implants. No interface failure occurred.

4. Discussion

The aim of the study was to compare different configurations of the same external pelvic fixation construct, testing them for translational and rotational stiffness. The "SINGLE" configuration showed two-third of the "DOUBLE" configuration's stiffness and the "DOUBLE" configuration was twice as stiff as the "DOUBLE TENT" configuration in terms of translational stiffness. There was no significant difference between the "DOUBLE" and the "DOUBLE TENT" configurations regarding rotational stiffness. Between the "DOUBLE TENT" and "SINGLE" configuration there was a significant difference in rotational stiffness and the "DOUBLE TENT" was twice as stiff. Both the "RHOMBOID" and the "SINGLE TENT" configurations failed.

In the beginning there were efforts to devise external fixator constructs that would by themselves stabilize vertically unstable pelvic fractures. This was demonstrated not to be possible [17, 18]. As soon as this was realized, complexity in external fixation construct decreased, seeing as multiple pins increase the chance for pin-tract infections [19]. Research has since been focused on finding the optimal pin placement site [13, 20] or determining difference in stability between different fixator constructs and configurations [21–24]. It was not clear how our fixation construct's stability would change when the configuration was adapted for obese patients or patients undergoing abdominal surgery.

There are a few limitations innate to the testing protocol. Failure within our test setup does not have to result in failure in the clinical setup. The testing setup was devised solely to analyse construct stiffness, ignoring additional factors like intact ligaments, soft tissue, or pelvic contents that might contribute to overall stability. The upside of focusing on the construct is that we isolate the effect of different configurations on stiffness. The influence of pin anchoring strength in the bone as a possible confounding factor was avoided in this experimental setup, as all tests were conducted with the same pins anchored in the same polyoxymethylene cylinders. Rod configuration by itself should not have an impact on pin anchoring strength. One limitation might be that the pin-rod interfaces were not tightened by use of a torque spanner, but the same person (S.T), applying maximal force. However we are confident that this did not influence the results as no interface failure occurred and difference in stiffness was due to elastic deformation within the rods and pins rather than interface loosening. It is possible that a bulkier configuration would be prone to screw loosening, being more difficult to handle in postop care. An additional limitation is that forces on the pelvis in real patients are not limited to those addressed in this study. It is possible that the construct and its configurations react differently to a combination of translational and rotational forces or a completely different force vector.

There might be other configurations with better biomechanical properties than those tested in our study. Based on the data of the five tested, however, it seems that where the rod was in parallel alignment with the applied force (for the compression/distraction part), the stiffness was greatest. Moreover where an additional rod could be applied, a significant increase in translational stiffness was recorded. Therefore, when the circumstances (patient size, concomitant injuries, etc.) allow it, one should always choose a configuration where the rod is aligned parallel to the expected force vector. If possible the configuration should be augmented with an extra rod, set up the same way as the first one. The study has shown that the "DOUBLE TENT" configuration is significantly less stiff than the "DOUBLE" one. It is not possible to tell from this study whether a "TENT" configuration provides sufficient stability in obese patients in the clinical environment as obesity is also associated with higher loads. An alternative might be a subcutaneous internal anterior fixator, with which the distance from pin entry sites to the connecting rods can be decreased [25, 26]. This method would also be an option where further abdominal surgeries are expected avoiding a potentially unstable "RHOMBOID" configuration. There is some evidence that such a device would be at least as stable as an external fixator [27].

Any future studies should look at failure of different constructs in the clinical setup and try to come up with quantifiable, maybe in vivo, results.

5. Conclusion

Using two parallel connecting rods for external pelvic ring fixation provides the highest translational (lateral compression/distraction) and rotational (bending of the hip) stability.

Conflict of Interests

The authors declare that there is no conflict of interests regarding the publication of this paper.

References

[1] Z. Balogh, K. L. King, P. Mackay et al., "The epidemiology of pelvic ring fractures: a population-based study," *Journal of Trauma*, vol. 63, no. 5, pp. 1066–1073, 2007.

[2] D. J. Hak, W. R. Smith, and T. Suzuki, "Management of hemorrhage in life-threatening pelvic fracture," *Journal of the American Academy of Orthopaedic Surgeons*, vol. 17, no. 7, pp. 447–457, 2009.

[3] M. Tile, "Pelvic ring fractures: should they be fixed?" *Journal of Bone and Joint Surgery B*, vol. 70, no. 1, pp. 1–12, 1988.

[4] M. C. Moss and M. D. Bircher, "Volume changes within the true pelvis during disruption of the pelvic ring—where does the haemorrhage go?" *Injury*, vol. 27, no. 1, pp. SA21–SA23, 1996.

[5] A. R. Burgess, B. J. Eastridge, J. W. R. Young et al., "Pelvic ring disruptions: effective classification system and treatment protocols," *Journal of Trauma*, vol. 30, no. 7, pp. 848–856, 1990.

[6] M. R. Grimm, M. S. Vrahas, and K. A. Thomas, "Pressure-volume characteristics of the intact and disrupted pelvic retroperitoneum," *Journal of Trauma*, vol. 44, no. 3, pp. 454–459, 1998.

[7] B. L. Riemer, S. L. Butterfield, D. L. Diamond et al., "Acute mortality associated with injuries to the pelvic ring: the role of early patient mobilization and external fixation," *Journal of Trauma*, vol. 35, no. 5, pp. 671–677, 1993.

[8] P. R. Miller, P. S. Moore, E. Mansell et al., "External fixation or arteriogram in bleeding pelvic fracture: initial therapy guided by markers of arterial hemorrhage," *Journal of Trauma*, vol. 54, no. 3, pp. 437–443, 2003.

[9] C. Arvieux, F. Thony, C. Broux et al., "Current management of severe pelvic and perineal trauma," *Journal of Visceral Surgery*, vol. 149, pp. e227–e238, 2012.

[10] W. Chen, Z. Hou, Y. Su et al., "Treatment of posterior pelvic ring disruptions using a minimally invasive adjustable plate," *Injury*, vol. 44, no. 7, pp. 975–980, 2013.

[11] M. D. Bircher, "Indications and techniques of external fixation of the injured pelvis," *Injury*, vol. 27, Supplement 1, pp. 3–19, 1996.

[12] M. Scaglione, P. Parchi, G. Digrandi, M. Latessa, and G. Guido, "External fixation in pelvic fractures," *Musculoskeletal Surgery*, vol. 94, no. 2, pp. 63–70, 2010.

[13] W.-Y. Kirn, T. C. Hearn, O. Seleem, E. Mahalingam, D. Stephen, and M. Tile, "Effect of pin location on stability of pelvic external fixation," *Clinical Orthopaedics and Related Research*, no. 361, pp. 237–244, 1999.

[14] M. J. Gardner and S. E. Nork, "Stabilization of unstable pelvic fractures with supraacetabular compression external fixation," *Journal of Orthopaedic Trauma*, vol. 21, no. 4, pp. 269–273, 2007.

[15] D. Demetriades, M. Karaiskakis, K. Toutouzas, K. Alo, G. Velmahos, and L. Chan, "Pelvic fractures: epidemiology and predictors of associated abdominal injuries and outcomes," *Journal of the American College of Surgeons*, vol. 195, no. 1, pp. 1–10, 2002.

[16] W. D. Dupont and W. D. Plummer Jr., "Power and sample size calculations for studies involving linear regression," *Controlled Clinical Trials*, vol. 19, no. 6, pp. 589–601, 1998.

[17] J. J. Wild Jr., G. W. Hanson, and H. S. Tullos, "Unstable fractures of the pelvis treated by external fixation," *Journal of Bone and Joint Surgery A*, vol. 64, no. 7, pp. 1010–1020, 1982.

[18] T. Pohlemann, C. Krettek, R. Hoffmann, U. Culemann, and A. Gansslen, "Biomechanical comparison of different devices for emergency stabilization of the pelvis," *Unfallchirurg*, vol. 97, no. 10, pp. 503–510, 1994.

[19] M. C. Tucker, S. E. Nork, P. T. Simonian, and M. L. Chip Routt Jr., "Simple anterior pelvic external fixation," *Journal of Trauma*, vol. 49, no. 6, pp. 989–994, 2000.

[20] M. T. Archdeacon, S. Arebi, T. T. Le, R. Wirth, R. Kebel, and M. Thakore, "Orthogonal pin construct versus parallel uniplanar pin constructs for pelvic external fixation: a biomechanical assessment of stiffness and strength," *Journal of Orthopaedic Trauma*, vol. 23, no. 2, pp. 100–105, 2009.

[21] V. Vecsei, "Results of biomechanical examinations of various external fixation mountings in the pelvic region," *Aktuelle Traumatologie*, vol. 18, no. 6, pp. 261–264, 1988.

[22] H.-J. Egbers, F. Draijer, D. Havemann, and W. Zenker, "Stabilisation of the pelvic girdle by external fixation. Biomechanical investigations and clinical experience," *Orthopade*, vol. 21, no. 6, pp. 363–372, 1992.

[23] H. Rieger, S. Winckler, D. Wetterkamp, and J. Overbeck, "Clinical and biomechanical aspects of external fixation of the pelvis," *Clinical Biomechanics*, vol. 11, no. 6, pp. 322–327, 1996.

[24] K. J. Ponsen, G. A. Hoek Van Dijke, P. Joosse, and C. J. Snijders, "External fixators for pelvic fractures: comparison of the stiffness of current systems," *Acta Orthopaedica Scandinavica*, vol. 74, no. 2, pp. 165–171, 2003.

[25] M. J. Gardner, S. Mehta, A. Mirza, and W. M. Ricci, "Anterior pelvic reduction and fixation using a subcutaneous internal fixator," *Journal of Orthopaedic Trauma*, vol. 26, no. 5, pp. 314–321, 2012.

[26] R. Vaidya, R. Colen, J. Vigdorchik, F. Tonnos, and A. Sethi, "Treatment of unstable pelvic ring injuries with an internal anterior fixator and posterior fixation: initial clinical series," *Journal of Orthopaedic Trauma*, vol. 26, no. 1, pp. 1–8, 2012.

[27] J. M. Vigdorchik, A. O. Esquivel, X. Jin et al., "Biomechanical stability of a supra-acetabular pedicle screw internal fixation device (INFIX) vs external fixation and plates for vertically unstable pelvic fractures," *Journal of Orthopaedic Surgery and Research*, vol. 7, article 31, 2012.

11

Evaluation of the Cementation Index as a Predictor of Failure in Coonrad-Morrey Total Elbow Arthroplasty

Manish Kiran,[1] Arpit Jariwala,[2] and Carlos A. Wigderowitz[2]

[1] *University Department of Orthopaedics and Trauma Surgery, TORT Centre, Ninewells Hospital, Dundee DD1 9SY, UK*
[2] *NHS Tayside, Dundee DD1 9SY, UK*

Correspondence should be addressed to Manish Kiran; drmanishkiran@gmail.com

Academic Editor: Padhraig O'Loughlin

Background. The aim of this study is to objectively evaluate the quality of cementation by a novel method called the cementation index and assess its utility as a predictor of failure. *Materials and Methods.* Fifty elbows with primary Coonrad-Morrey total elbow replacement were included. The quality of cementing was assessed by novel methods, the vertical and horizontal cementation index, which were statistically evaluated as predictors of failure. The mean period of followup was 8.08 ± 2.95 years (range: from 5.08 to 10.25 years). *Results.* The mean vertical cementation index of the humerus (vCIH) was 1.22 ± 0.28 and that of the ulna (vCIU) was 1.10 ± 0.18. Radiolucent zones were noted in two cases in the humerus with a horizontal cementation index of 0.21 and 0.14, respectively. Both of the cementation indices were not found to be statistically significant predictors of failure ($P > 0.05$). The five-year survival rate was 94%. *Discussion and Conclusion.* The cementation index, being a ratio, reduces the confounding effect of taking radiographs in different positions of the limb with different magnification in followup radiographs. It is an easy and objective method of assessment of cementation, the results of which need to be validated by a larger study.

1. Introduction

Total elbow replacement is used in the reconstruction of elbows afflicted by rheumatoid arthritis, osteoarthritis, and trauma. There has been a significant improvement in outcome with changes in the implant design, from the initial linked and fully constrained prostheses to the present-day unlinked and linked, semiconstrained implants. Linked prostheses, like the Coonrad-Morrey implant, have been reported to have better long-term functional outcomes than unlinked implants, like the Souter-Strathclyde prosthesis [1, 2]. Aseptic loosening is one of the most common causes of failure of the prosthesis in the long term [3, 4]. Inadequate cementing has been established to contribute to this complication [5, 6]. The aim of this study is to objectively evaluate cementation by a novel method called the cementation index and assess its utility as a predictor of failure.

2. Materials and Methods

Fifty elbows (forty-seven patients), wherein primary total elbow replacement was performed, were included in the study. The Coonrad-Morrey type III prosthesis was used in all cases. The mean age of the patients was sixty-seven years (range from thirty-two to eighty-eight years). The male: female ratio was 20 : 30 elbows. The procedure was performed on the dominant limb in thirty-five elbows and on the right-hand side in thirty-one elbows. The data was retrospectively obtained from clinical case record and radiographs. The diagnoses and indications of surgery are shown in Table 1. The postoperative radiographs were evaluated for the vertical cementation index, calculated by dividing the length of the cement mantle by the length of the humeral and ulnar components separately, and the horizontal cementation index, which was calculated by dividing the length of the radiolucent zone greater than 1 mm, if present, seen at the cement-bone interface, by the total length of the cement-bone interface. The vertical cementation index is shown in Figure 1. The followup data included condition of the surgical wound, infection, neurological deficit, range of movement, stability of the prosthesis in axial compression and varus/valgus stress, severity of pain, shift of the implant tip, and failure of the prosthesis. Multiple logistic regression analysis of age, gender,

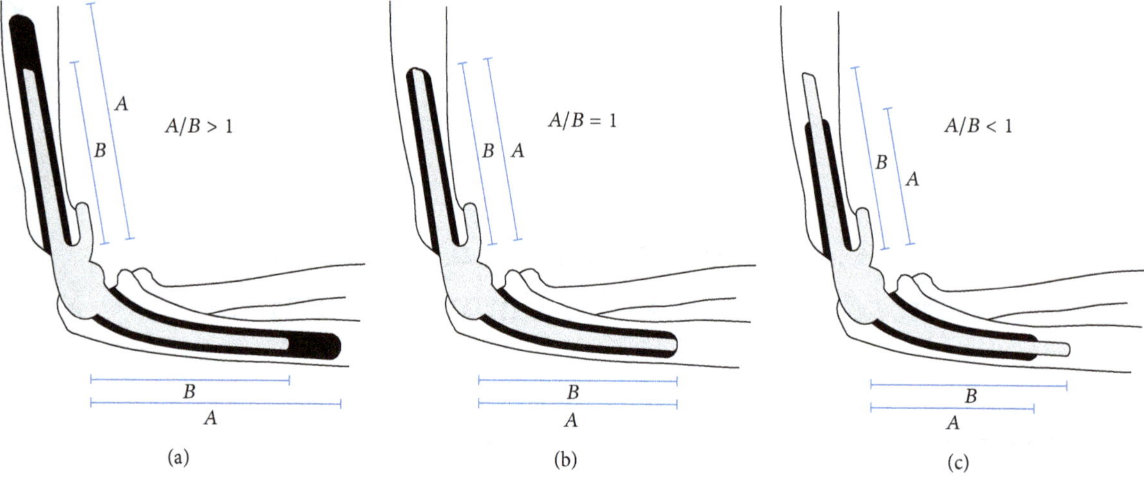

FIGURE 1: Vertical cementation index.

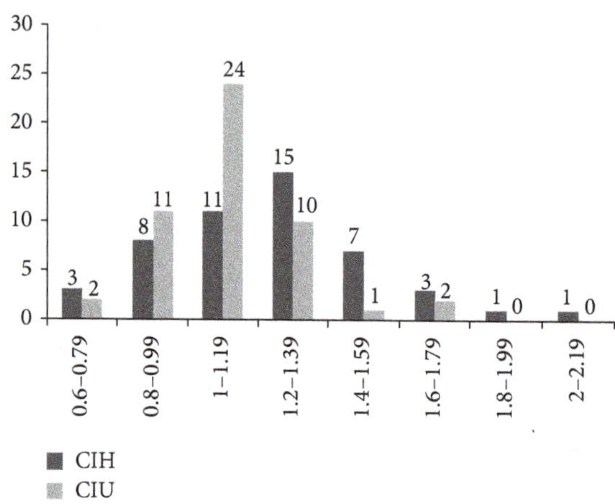

FIGURE 2: Distribution of vertical cementation index.

diagnosis, side operated upon, limb dominance, and cementation index as predictors of failure was done. The functional and radiological outcome was classified according to Morrey's classification [5]. The mean period of followup was 5.08±2.95 years (range from 2.08 to 10.25 years). The mean operative time was 119.08 ± 18.46 minutes (range from 70 to 186 minutes).

3. Results

Failure of the implant was seen in four cases. The reasons for failure are shown in Table 2. Multiple logistic regression analysis showed that age, gender, side operated upon, dominance of limb, and diagnosis were not significant predictors of failure ($P > 0.05$). The mean vertical cementation index of the humerus (vCIH) was 1.22 ± 0.28 (range from 0.7 to 2.1) and that of the ulna (vCIU) was 1.10 ± 0.18 (range from 0.77 to 1.72). The distribution of the two indices is shown in Figure 2. Radiolucent zones were noted in two cases in the humerus with a horizontal cementation index of 0.21 and 0.14, respectively. Both the vertical and horizontal cementation indices were not found to be statistically significant predictors of failure ($P > 0.05$). The implant that failed due to aseptic loosening has a vertical cementation index of 1.8 and a horizontal cementation index of 0.21. The five-year survival rate was 94%. The final results were good in thirty-six elbows, fair in eight elbows, and poor in five elbows.

TABLE 1: Diagnoses and indications for surgery.

Diagnosis*	Indication for surgery*
Rheumatoid arthritis—29 (58)	Pain—36 (72)
Osteoarthritis—5 (10)	Instability—5 (10)
Haemophilia—2 (4)	Comminution—8 (16)
Acute myeloid leukemia—2 (4)	Tumor—1 (2)
Plasmacytoma of distal humerus—1 (2)	
Trauma—11 (22)	

*The values are the number of elbows with the percentage in parenthesis.

4. Discussion

The Coonrad-Morrey prosthesis is an inherently stable linked stemmed implant, due to its toggle-hinge mechanism of

TABLE 2: Reason for failure.

Reason for failure	Number of elbows	Survival in years
Aseptic loosening	1	7.4
Deep infection	2	0.583 0.666
Periprosthetic fracture of the humerus	1	0.916

articulation. Its design has had significant changes in form, articulation, and coating since its introduction in the 1970s. The first design had a high rate of aseptic loosening which was attributed by the designers of the implant and in subsequent series by other authors to inadequate cementation [5, 6]. They put forth the opinion that the constraint in the articulating mechanism and the posterosuperiorly directed vector forces acting on the elbow contributed to loosening [5, 7]. The relatively larger size of the ulnar component in comparison with the ulnar medullary cavity has been postulated to result in inadequate cementation in the ulna [8]. The incidence of aseptic loosening has reduced significantly since the introduction of the anterior flange in the humeral component which can accommodate a bone graft, with some series reporting 100% five-year survivorship of the implant [2]. There have also been changes in the type of titanium coating of the implant and the introduction of the pin-in-pin articulation. Corradi et al. [6] reported a 15-year survivorship of 92.4%. There have been reports of ulnar component loosening in literature due to improper placement of the ulnar component and its impingement on the anterior humeral flange [9]. Morrey et al. [5] believed that inadequate cementation was the cause of aseptic loosening in seven of the eleven cases, which were revised for loosening of the implants. Likewise, Corradi et al. [6] reported one case of inadequate cementation of the ulna, which resulted in loosening and revision, seventeen months after the index procedure. Similarly, Schneeberger et al. [9] also noted inadequate cementation in two humeral components and one ulnar component, resulting in loosening of one humeral and one ulnar component. They opined that the antegrade method of cementing resulted in an inadequate cement mantle and recommended a retrograde method of cementation. Aldridge III et al. [3] noted that the cementation was inadequate in one case and marginal in another. However, this did not result in loosening of the implants. Similarly, Prasad and Dent [2] did not observe any aseptic loosening and reported a 100% survivorship at five years. In our series, we noted a comparable five-year survivorship of the implant. The functional and radiological outcome which was classified according to Morrey's classification [5] was good in a majority of cases in our series. This classification took into account the presence of pain, range of movement, radiological changes like lysis and change in the position of the implant tip, and removal or revision of implants. A painless elbow with a functionally useful range of movement of 100° [7] was achieved in most cases.

Morrey et al. [5] classified the adequacy of cementation as adequate, marginal, and inadequate based on whether the cement mantle crossed the tip of the prosthesis and the width of the radiolucent zone at bone-cement interface. According to this classification, a case with 10% coverage of the implant and one with 90% coverage would both be classified as inadequate cementation, since both of the mantles would not have crossed the tip of the prosthesis. However, one would expect that the clinical outcome of 10% cement coverage would be different from 90% coverage. The cementation index is a novel and objective method of assessment of the coverage of the implant with cement, which circumvents this limitation by providing a numerical value to the degree of cementation of the implant. Since it is a ratio, the effect of taking radiographs in different positions of the limb with different magnification in followup radiographs is reduced, thus ensuring comparability. It is very easy to perform, especially with the new computer based imaging systems. The horizontal component of the index has been validated for assessment of the quality of cementing in the femur [10]. It was not found to be a statistically significant predictor of failure in the present study. This result may not be representative, considering the relatively small number of elbows included in the study. Unlike hip and knee replacements, where a larger number of cases are operated upon, most series of total elbow replacement have between forty to seventy cases. A larger study involving multiple centres would provide adequate number of cases to validate the utility of the cementation index as a predictor of failure.

5. Conclusion

Cementing techniques contribute to the stability and the long-term outcome of the total elbow prostheses. The cementation index is an easy, reproducible, and objective method of assessment of the adequacy of cementation in stemmed prostheses, the results of which need to be validated by a larger study.

Disclosure

Caldicott Guardian approval was obtained, University of Dundee.

Conflict of Interests

None of the authors has any potential or actual personal, financial, political, or competing interest.

References

[1] K. Güttler, I. Landor, P. Vavřík, S. Popelka, A. Sosna, and J. Krásenský, "Total elbow replacement in patients with rheumatoid arthritis," *Acta Chirurgiae Orthopaedicae et Traumatologiae Cechoslovaca*, vol. 73, no. 5, pp. 423–430, 2011.

[2] N. Prasad and C. Dent, "Outcome of total elbow replacement for rheumatoid arthritis: single surgeon's series with Souter-Strathclyde and Coonrad-Morrey prosthesis," *Journal of Shoulder and Elbow Surgery*, vol. 19, no. 3, pp. 376–383, 2010.

[3] J. M. Aldridge III, N. R. Lightdale, W. J. Mallon, and R. W. Coonrad, "Total elbow arthroplasty with the Coonrad/Coonrad-Morrey prosthesis: a 10 to 31-year survival analysis," *Journal of Bone and Joint Surgery B*, vol. 88, no. 4, pp. 509–514, 2006.

[4] D. R. J. Gill and B. F. Morrey, "The Coonrad-Morrey total elbow arthroplasty in patients who have rheumatoid arthritis: a ten to fifteen-year followup study," *Journal of Bone and Joint Surgery A*, vol. 80, no. 9, pp. 1327–1335, 1998.

[5] B. F. Morrey, R. S. Bryan, J. H. Dobyns, and R. L. Linscheid, "Total elbow arthroplasty: a five-year experience at the Mayo Clinic," *Journal of Bone and Joint Surgery A*, vol. 63, no. 7, pp. 1050–1063, 1981.

[6] M. Corradi, M. Frattini, B. Panno, S. Tocco, and F. Pogliacomi, "Linked semi-constrained total elbow prosthesis in chronic arthritis: results of 18 cases," *Musculoskeletal Surgery*, vol. 94, pp. S11–S23, 2010.

[7] B. F. Morrey, L. J. Askew, K. N. An, and E. Y. Chao, "A biomechanical study of normal functional elbow motion," *Journal of Bone and Joint Surgery A*, vol. 63, no. 6, pp. 872–877, 1981.

[8] C. P. Little, A. J. Graham, G. Karatzas, D. A. Woods, and A. J. Carr, "Outcomes of total elbow arthroplasty for rheumatoid arthritis: comparative study of three implants," *Journal of Bone and Joint Surgery A*, vol. 87, no. 11, pp. 2439–2448, 2005.

[9] A. G. Schneeberger, D. C. Meyer, and E. H. Yian, "Coonrad-Morrey total elbow replacement for primary and revision surgery: a 2 to 7.5-year followup study," *Journal of Shoulder and Elbow Surgery*, vol. 16, no. 3, pp. S47–S54, 2007.

[10] M. Umar, V. Patil, and S. Lewthwaite, "Validation of a new grading system for femoral cementation in total hip arthroplasty," *Journal of Bone and Joint Surgery*, vol. 94, no. 37, article 138, 2012.

12

Outcome in Patients with High Body Mass Index following Primary Total Hip Arthroplasty

Zuned Hakim, Claire Rutherford, Elizabeth Mckiernan, and Tony Helm

Royal Preston Hospital, Sharoe Green Lane North, Fulwood, Preston PR2 9HT, UK

Correspondence should be addressed to Zuned Hakim; zuned.hakim@gmail.com

Academic Editor: Werner Kolb

Obesity is becoming a critical problem in the developed world and is associated with an increased incidence of osteoarthritis of the hip. The Oxford Hip Score was used to determine if Body Mass Index (BMI) is an independent factor in determining patient outcome following primary total hip arthroplasty (THA). Using data from 353 operations we found that patients with BMI ≥ 30 had an absolute score that was lower preoperatively and postoperatively compared to those with a BMI < 30. There was no difference in pre- and postoperative point score change within each group; Kendall's rank correlation was 0.00047 (95% CI, −0.073 to 0.074 ($p = 0.99$)) and demonstrated no trend. There was no statistically significant difference in change between those with BMI ≥ 30 and < 30 ($p = 0.65$). We suggest that those with a higher BMI be considered for THA as they can expect the same degree of improvement as those with a lower BMI. Given the on-going increase in obesity these findings could be significant for the future of THA.

1. Introduction

Obesity is becoming a critical problem for healthcare providers in developed nations. In England the proportion of obese adults (BMI ≥ 30) increased between 1993 and 2010 from 13.2% in 1993 to 26.2% in 2010 in men and from 16.4% in 1993 to 26.1% in 2010 in women [1]. Based on existing trends the prevalence of obesity is predicted to increase to 32.1% in men and 31.0% in women by the end of 2012 [2]. Body Mass Index (BMI) is commonly used to estimate body fat using an individual's weight and height [3]. The World Health Organisation defines obesity as a BMI ≥ 30 [4].

The current trend to perform arthroplasty in younger patients who may be overweight poses the question of whether any benefit is to be gained in operating on patients with a BMI ≥ 30.

Cooper et al. and Oliveria et al. identified the association between increasing BMI and increasing incidence of osteoarthritis of the hip [5, 6]. This cohort of patients is, therefore, more likely to require treatment to manage their osteoarthritis, which includes surgical intervention.

The Oxford Hip Score (OHS12) is twelve-question functional outcome score [7]. It is utilised not only for research but also to determine pre- and post-op scores to ascertain improvement in individual patients with zero being the worst outcome and 48 being the best. It has been ratified in previous independent studies and can be considered to be relevant in defining patient satisfaction in elective procedures [8–10]. It is designed to be joint specific minimising the effect of comorbidity [7].

The aim of this study was to observe any difference in Oxford Hip Score between patients undergoing THA with BMI ≥ 30 and < 30 and determine the change in Oxford Hip Score provided by surgery within each group.

2. Method

Between 2012 and 2014, 220 consecutive patients who had undergone THA with a BMI ≥ 30 were identified from Bluespier orthopaedic management software. Over the same time period, 220 consecutive THAs performed in patients with BMI < 30 were identified using the same system. All 440 THAs were performed in the same centre by four consultant surgeons. All were performed via the posterior approach. All implants used were manufactured by Zimmer. Postoperative management was in line with standard departmental protocol. All patients received VTE prophylaxis. Data was missing for 87 of the selected patients. As a result, 176 THAs

Table 1: Preoperative Oxford Hip Scores.

Group	Range	Standard deviation	Median
All	0–39	6.8	14
BMI < 30	0–39	6.8	15
BMI ≥ 30	0–33	6.7	12

(176 patients) were analysed in the group with a BMI ≥ 30 and 177 THAs (177 patients) were analysed in the group with a BMI < 30.

Patient demographics including age, BMI, and ASA grade were collected [11]. Pre- and postoperative Oxford Hip Scores were collected prospectively and data was analysed retrospectively. Preoperative hips scores were recorded in the preoperative assessment clinic up to six weeks prior to surgery. Postoperative hip scores were taken at one year. A change in hip score from pre- and postoperative scores was calculated. All patients underwent elective primary THA. Patients were excluded if they had bilateral hip replacements. All patients that had previously undergone lower limb joint arthroplasty were excluded from the study. All cases were for primary hip osteoarthritis.

The ASA grade was assigned before surgery and relates to the systemic condition of a patient. It is graded from one to five, with one indicating a fit patient, two indicating mild systemic disease, three indicating severe systemic disease, four indicating imminent risk of death due to illness, and five indicating a moribund patient with death as the expected outcome.

Descriptive and statistical analysis was performed using StatsDirect (StatsDirect Ltd., 2013). Mann-Whitney U tests were performed to determine if there was a difference between the two BMI groups with regard to age difference, before and after Oxford Hip Scores and ASA grade. Kendall's rank correlation was calculated for BMI and ASA grade. Statistical significance was set at $p < 0.05$.

3. Result

The median age in the BMI < 30 was 68 (range 56–60) and BMI ≥ 30 was 66 (range 52–74). There was no statistical difference between the two groups ($p = 0.35$).

There were 90 males and 86 females in the <30 BMI group. There were 85 males and 92 females in the ≥30 BMI age group. There was no statistically significant difference in ages between the two BMI groups ($p = 0.55$).

3.1. Preoperative Oxford Scores. The median scores were 14, 15, and 12 for all BMI < 30 and BMI ≥ 30 groups, respectively (Table 1). There was a statistically significant difference between the two BMI groups and preoperative Oxford Hip Score ($p = 0.0002$). A negative correlation exists between BMI and preoperative Oxford Hip Score; Kendall's rank correlation is −0.15 (CI 95%: −0.22 to −0.80 ($p \leq 0.0001$)). This was statistically significant, indicating that an increase in BMI is associated with a worse preoperative Oxford Hip Score (Figure 1).

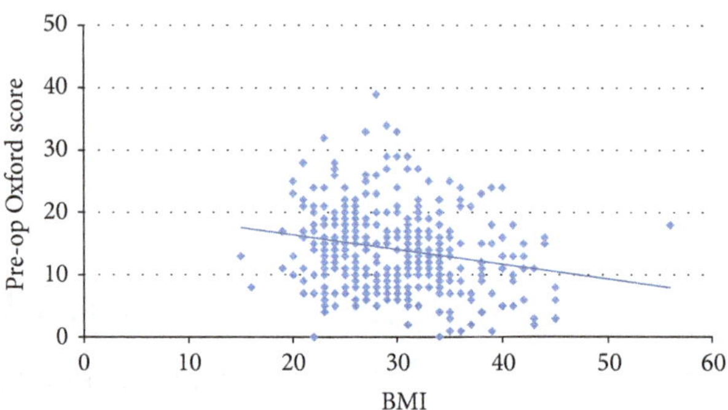

Figure 1: BMI versus pre-op Oxford score.

Table 2: Postoperative Oxford Hip Scores.

Group	Range	Standard deviation	Median
All	8–48	7.1	43
BMI < 30	11–48	4.74	44.5
BMI ≥ 30	8–48	7.29	42

Table 3: Change in Oxford Hip Scores.

Group	Range	Standard deviation	Median
All	−8 to 47	8.1	28
BMI < 30	−8 to 42	6.43	28
BMI ≥ 30	−7 to 47	8.35	28

Table 4: ASA grade.

Group	Range	Standard deviation	Median
All	1 to 4	0.47	2
BMI < 30	1 to 4	0.40	2
BMI ≥ 30	1 to 4	0.49	2

3.2. Postoperative Oxford Scores. The median scores were 43, 44.5, and 42 for all BMI < 30 and BMI ≥ 30 groups, respectively (Table 2). There was a statistically significant difference between the two BMI groups and postoperative Oxford Hip Score ($p = 0.0001$). There was statistically significant negative correlation between BMI and postoperative Oxford Hip Score; Kendall's rank correlation is −0.13 (95% CI, −0.19 to −0.06 ($p = 0.0008$)). This indicates that an increase in BMI is associated with a worse absolute postoperative Oxford Hip Score (Figure 2).

3.3. Change in Oxford Hip Scores. The median change for each group was the same at 28 points (Table 3). There was no statistical difference between the two BMI groups ($p = 0.65$). There was no correlation between BMI and change in Oxford Hip Score; Kendall's rank correlation is 0.00047 (95% CI, −0.073 to 0.074 ($p = 0.9902$)). This demonstrates that there is no relationship between BMI and change in Oxford Hip Score (Figure 3).

3.4. ASA Grade. The median ASA scores were 2 for all groups, respectively (Table 4). There was no statistically significant

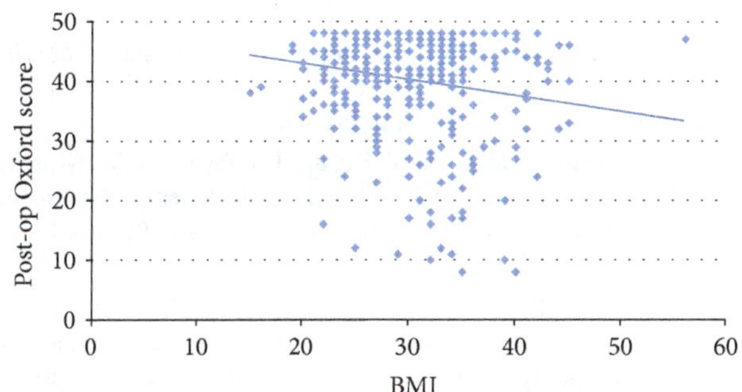

Figure 2: BMI versus post-op Oxford score.

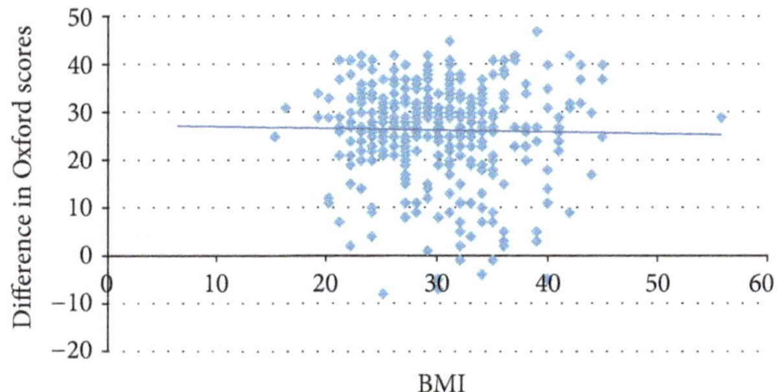

Figure 3: BMI versus difference in Oxford scores.

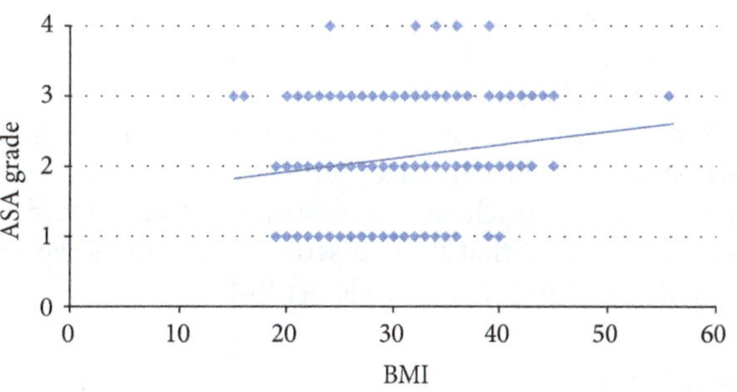

Figure 4: BMI versus ASA grade.

difference between the ASA grade and the two BMI groups ($p = 0.1$). There was a statistically significant correlation between increasing BMI and increasing ASA grade (higher ASA grade indicates worse systemic condition); Kendall's rank correlation is 0.13 (95% CI: 0.065 to 0.19 ($p = 0.007$)) (Figure 4).

Seven cases (1.98%) had a worse OHS12 postoperatively than preoperatively. Of these, 6 were in the BMI ≥ 30 group and only one was in the BMI < 30 group. In this subgroup of patients there was no statistically significant correlation between BMI and change in Oxford Hip Score.

4. Discussion

This paper demonstrates that patients in a higher BMI category have a significantly lower absolute Oxford Hip Score both before and after surgery. Patients with a BMI ≥ 30 experience the same change in Oxford Hip Score as patients with a BMI < 30 (median 28-point difference).

Judge et al. have analysed patient satisfaction with Oxford Hip Score and concluded a 97.6% satisfaction rate with a change of 14 points compared to 81.8% with a change below this threshold. At 6 months they found an absolute score of >35 associated with the highest satisfaction. They also noted that patients with a worse pre-op score still gained the highest satisfaction with a lower post-op score as long as the difference in change was 14 points or more [12]. Our paper did not look specifically at patient satisfaction; however, the improvement in score would suggest, based on current literature, greater satisfaction in our cohort with both groups scoring >35 at 12 months and >14 points increase post-op.

Existing evidence suggests that BMI should not be a discriminatory factor in patient selection for THA. Michalka et al. found that patients with a BMI ≥ 30 gain similar benefit from THA as patients with a BMI < 30 [13]. Andrew et al. assessed the influence of BMI on change in Oxford Hip Score pre- and postoperatively. They concluded that there was no difference between those patients in different BMI categories, suggesting that obese and morbidly obese patients have the same clinical benefit as nonobese patients. They do acknowledge increasing comorbidity such as ischaemic heart disease, diabetes, apnoeic sleep disorders, and hypertension in the obese category, all of which could increase the risk of anaesthesia. However, they conclude the perceived belief that patients with higher BMIs do not clinically benefit following surgery is a misconception. Higher BMIs should not deter the surgeon from performing a THR [14].

This study has several limitations. First, potential bias may exist as some surgeons were more willing to perform THA surgery on those with a higher BMI compared to their colleagues; however, with a relatively equal number of patients in each group we do not suspect bias at the primary care referral level. Second, the type of prosthesis used for each patient was not recorded; therefore, any potential difference in outcome which could be prosthesis-dependent is not known. However, all implants were Orthopaedic Data Evaluation Panel (ODEP) rated and approved for implant and have demonstrated performance within guidelines. Third, complication rates were not assessed in this study. Other papers have reported conflicting outcomes on this. Lübbeke et al. compared the incidence of complications in obese and nonobese patients undergoing primary THA. They found that obesity substantially increased the infection rate in women but not in men and that the incidence of dislocation was higher in obese women than in nonobese women [15]. Andrew et al. identified no difference in complication rate (dislocation, revision rates, increased haemorrhage, deep infection, deep-venous thrombosis, and pulmonary embolism) or radiological change at five years between obese and nonobese patients [14]. We would suggest that an RCT or a prospective cohort study comparing these two groups would go someway in reducing confounding bias and the limitations this study has.

Our study indicates that THA in patients with BMI > 30 does not lead to a reduction in improvement in Oxford Hip Score compared to those with BMI < 30. Patients with a BMI ≥ 30 showed the same increase in Oxford score as those with a BMI < 30 but had lower absolute Oxford Hip Scores both before and after surgery.

We, therefore, recommend that patients with a higher BMI be considered candidates for THA, as they can expect the same degree of change in improvement on Oxford Hip Score. The caveat is that absolute score should not be expected to equal that of patients with a lower BMI.

Conflict of Interests

The authors declare that there is no conflict of interests regarding the publication of this paper.

References

[1] *The NHS Information Centre, Lifestyles Statistics*, Paul Eastwood, Lifestyle Statistics Section Head, 2012, http://www.ic.nhs.uk.

[2] P. Zaninotto, J. Head, E. Stamatakis, H. Wardle, and J. Mindell, "Trends in obesity among adults in England from 1993 to 2004 by age and social class and projections of prevalence to 2012," *Journal of Epidemiology and Community Health*, vol. 63, no. 2, pp. 140–146, 2009.

[3] V. S. Hubbard, "Defining overweight and obesity: what are the issues?" *The American Journal of Clinical Nutrition*, vol. 72, no. 5, pp. 1067–1068, 2000.

[4] N. K. Arden, A. Kiran, A. Judge et al., "What is a good patient reported outcome after total hip replacement?" *Osteoarthritis and Cartilage*, vol. 19, no. 2, pp. 155–162, 2011.

[5] C. Cooper, H. Inskip, P. Croft et al., "Individual risk factors for hip osteoarthritis: obesity, hip injury and physical activity," *American Journal of Epidemiology*, vol. 147, no. 6, pp. 516–522, 1998.

[6] S. A. Oliveria, D. T. Felson, P. A. Cirillo, J. I. Reed, and A. M. Walker, "Body weight, body mass index, and incident symptomatic osteoarthritis of the hand, hip, and knee," *Epidemiology*, vol. 10, no. 2, pp. 161–166, 1999.

[7] D. W. Murray, R. Fitzpatrick, K. Rogers et al., "The use of the Oxford hip and knee scores," *The Journal of Bone and Joint Surgery—British Volume*, vol. 89, no. 8, pp. 1010–1014, 2007.

[8] J. Dawson, R. Fitzpatrick, A. Carr, and D. Murray, "Questionnaire on the perceptions of patients about total hip replacement," *The Journal of Bone & Joint Surgery Series B*, vol. 78, no. 2, pp. 185–190, 1996.

[9] Y. Kalairajah, K. Azurza, C. Hulme, S. Molloy, and K. J. Drabu, "Health outcome measures in the evaluation of total hip arthroplasties—a comparison between the harris hip score and the Oxford hip score," *Journal of Arthroplasty*, vol. 20, no. 8, pp. 1037–1041, 2005.

[10] M. Ostendorf, H. F. van Stel, E. Buskens et al., "Patient-reported outcome in total hip replacement. A comparison of five instruments of health status," *The Journal of Bone & Joint Surgery Series B*, vol. 86, no. 6, pp. 801–808, 2004.

[11] R. D. Dripps, "New classification of physical status," *Anaesthesiology*, vol. 24, article 111, 1963.

[12] A. Judge, N. K. Arden, A. Kiran et al., "Interpretation of patient-reported outcomes for hip and knee replacement surgery: identification of thresholds associated with satisfaction with surgery," *The Journal of Bone & Joint Surgery—British Volume*, vol. 94, no. 3, pp. 412–418, 2012.

[13] P. K. R. Michalka, R. J. K. Khan, M. C. Scaddan, S. Haebich, N. Chirodian, and J. A. Wimhurst, "The influence of obesity on early outcomes in primary hip arthroplasty," *Journal of Arthroplasty*, vol. 27, no. 3, pp. 391–396, 2012.

[14] J. G. Andrew, J. Palan, H. V. Kurup, P. Gibson, D. W. Murray, and D. J. Beard, "Obesity in total hip replacement," *The Journal of Bone and Joint Surgery—British Volume*, vol. 90, no. 4, pp. 424–429, 2008.

[15] A. Lübbeke, R. Stern, G. Garavaglia, L. Zurcher, and P. Hoffmeyer, "Differences in outcomes of obese women and men undergoing primary total hip arthroplasty," *Arthritis & rheumatism*, vol. 57, no. 2, pp. 327–334, 2007.

13

Analysis of the Results of Use of Bone Graft and Reconstruction Cages in a Group of Patients with Severe Acetabular Bone Defects

Ainhoa Toro-Ibarguen, Ismael Auñón-Martín, Emilio Delgado-Díaz, Jose Alberto Moreno-Beamud, Miguel Ángel Martínez-Leocadio, Andrés Díaz-Martín, and Luciano Candel-García

Orthopaedic and Traumatology Surgery, Hospital 12 de Octubre, 28041 Madrid, Spain

Correspondence should be addressed to Ainhoa Toro-Ibarguen; aonia.orot@gmail.com

Academic Editor: Palaniappan Lakshmanan

Introduction. Rings and cages are indicated for use in revision total hip with severe bone loss. *Material and Methods.* A retrospective study was performed on 37 acetabular revision cases with an average age at revision of 67.8 years. According to Paprosky classification, 54% grade II and 46% grade III. We used two types of cages, Protrusio and Contour cage. We used 23 standard liners and 14 dual mobility cups. *Results.* The average follow-up was 5.4 years. The mean Merlé-d'Aubigné score improved from 5.48 to 10.5 points ($P < 0.05$). There were 10 nerve palsies, 6 rings that lost fixation, 10 dislocations, and 4 infections. The need for reoperation for any reason rose to 32% (12/37). Success, defined as a stable reconstruction, was 73%. We found that, using a dual mobility cup cemented into the cage, the dislocation rate and revision rate came down ($P < 0.05$). *Conclusions.* The treatment of severe acetabular defects using bone graft and reconstruction cages is a viable option. The use of a dual mobility cup cemented into the cage could avoid dislocations and the insertion of the ischial flap inside the ischial portion of the acetabulum for further ring stability and protection of the sciatic nerve.

1. Introduction

The demand for primary total hip arthroplasty (THA) is expected to increase over the next several decades, due to the aging population and the obesity crisis [1]. The need for THA is expected to grow 174% to 572,000 primary THAs per year by 2030 in the United States [1]. Consequently, the demand for revision total hip arthroplasty will also increase exponentially. It is estimated that total hip arthroplasty revisions will double every 10 years [2].

The most common indications for acetabular revision include hip instability, aseptic loosening, periprosthetic osteolysis, and infection [2, 3], with the acetabular component involved in >50% of revisions [3]. Acetabular bone loss can be found in any of the revisions of THA and is one of the factors to be taken into account when determining treatment. There are multiple options for the treatment of these defects, each of which have their strengths and weaknesses, as all have common goals such as bone stock rebuild and provide mechanical stability with a maximum host bone contact [4]. Rings and cages are indicated for use in revision THA with severe bone loss, as those described in Paprosky classification, as types II and III [5]. The antiprotrusio cages are designed to manage extended pelvic defects by bridging large bone gaps and protecting the grafts filled to increase the bone stock [6].

We analyze the perioperative and intermediate-term complications and outcome of a consecutive series of 37 reconstruction rings and extensive bone-grafting techniques.

2. Material and Methods

A retrospective single-center study was performed between January 2003 and December 2011. This study included 37 patients who underwent acetabular revision using reconstruction rings, during the inclusion period. There were 25 females and 12 males, with an average age at revision of 67.8 years (range, 29–90 years). 17 were left hips and 20 were right.

In 24 cases (65%), primary hip arthroplasty was indicated because of hip osteoarthritis (Figure 1).

The average time from index arthroplasty to the acetabular revision was 13.4 years (range, 1–27 years). The time from the last procedure to acetabular revision was 7.4 years (range, 0.2–27 years). The number of previous surgeries on the hip in question averaged 1.9 and was 1 (16), 2 (12), 3 (5), 4 (3), and 5 (1). We revised 25 hips for aseptic loosening, one for infection, 3 for acetabular fracture, and eight for recurrent dislocation associated with acetabular loosening.

This procedure was indicated preoperatively based on an evaluation of clinical and radiological records, with potential intraoperative adjustment. A posterolateral approach was used in 32 cases (87%), in one case with femoral trochanteric osteotomy, to obtain better visualization of a Paprosky type IIIb. In 5 cases (13%) the surgeons preferred a Hardinge transgluteal approach. The hip joint was exposed and the acetabular component was removed and the femoral component was tested. Once the acetabulum had been cleaned, the severity of the acetabular defect was graded using the Paprosky classification system [5] (Figure 2).

In four cases angiography was needed to check the anatomical relation between the implant or cement and the pelvic vessels to ascertain their proximity, being the collaboration of vascular surgeons necessary during the intervention. Bone defects were filled with bone graft, using in all cases morselized bones that were small chunks of 0.5 cm, instead of slurry of bone which would make impaction impossible. Morselized allograft bone was firmly impacted with smooth acetabular impaction domes. In two cases structural allografts were used, which were composed of one or more femoral heads. Intraoperatively, the graft was reamed and sized to closely press-fit the residual host bone. Of the 37 cages used in this study, 15 were performed with a Protrusio cage [DePuy Orthopaedics, Inc, Warsaw, IN] and 22 with Contour types [Smith and Nephew Richards, Memphis, TN]. A cage was shaped to provide optimal congruity to the grafted acetabulum. The superior and inferior flanges were bended in order to comply with the individual anatomy of the acetabular region and to maximize the stability of the cage. Iliac fixation was obtained using 2 to 5 cancellous screws, which were placed first in the acetabular dome. The ischiatic flange was fixed using 1 to 3 cancellous screws in 27 reconstruction cages. In 1 cage the inferior flange was slotted into the ischium and in nine cases it was bent to engage the tear drop medially. We used on average 6.6 screws (range, 3–9 screws) to secure the reconstruction cages. After secure fixation of the reconstruction cage, we cemented an all polyethylene acetabular component into the cage in 23 hips. In 14 hips the device used was a dual mobility cup, Polar Cup [Smith and Nephew Richards, Memphis, TN]. The femoral component also was revised in 9 of the 37 cases.

The Postel Merlé D'Aubigné (PMA) score [7] was used to assess patient function. We also noted any medical and surgical complications. According to Goodman et al. [8], we

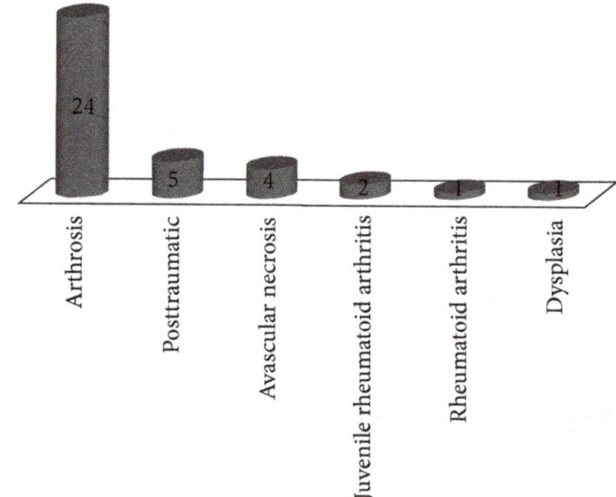

Figure 1: Indications that led to primary hip arthroplasty.

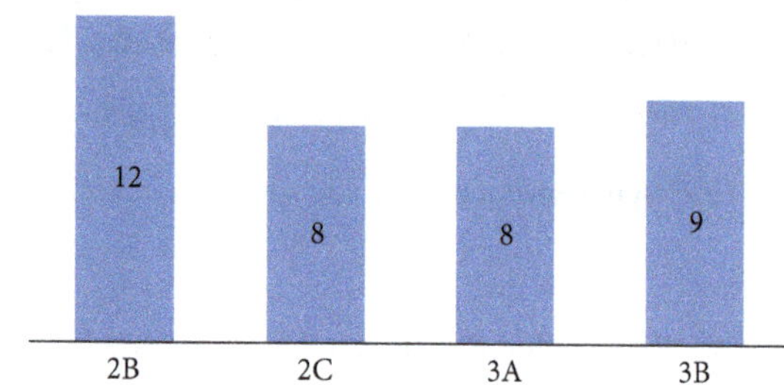

Figure 2: Distribution of the patients depending on the acetabular bone loss using the Paprosky classification.

defined success of the reconstruction as a stable, nondislocating, nonmigrating hip with incorporation of the acetabular bone graft without fracture or resorption that has had no further surgery on the acetabular side. Because several cases required revision of the acetabular cup only, without removal of the reconstruction ring, we also determined a second measure of success in which the acetabular cup was revised, leaving the ring and incorporated bone graft intact.

The radiological assessment was performed on an A/P view of the pelvis and A/P and lateral views of the hip. Failure of an acetabular cage was defined as a change of more than 5° in the inclination of the reinforcement ring, migration of more than 5 mm in either the vertical or horizontal direction, or breakage of the material [9]. The reference point for measuring vertical migration was the inferior aspect of the teardrop, and the Kohler line was the reference for measuring horizontal migration [9]. The bone/graft interface was evaluated using the three-zone classification proposed by DeLee and Charnley [10] to locate radiolucent lines. Radiolucent lines were defined as either simple (less than 1 mm thick, stable, less than 50% of area) or complete (less than 1 mm thick, stable, covering the entire surface area) or complex (2 mm or more in thickness, with or without progression, independent of thickness, location, and extent). The outcome of grafting was evaluated seeing incorporation, resorption, or fracture of the bone graft. Graft incorporation was indicated by continuation of trabecular lines from the graft into host bone without resorption or fracture [11, 12].

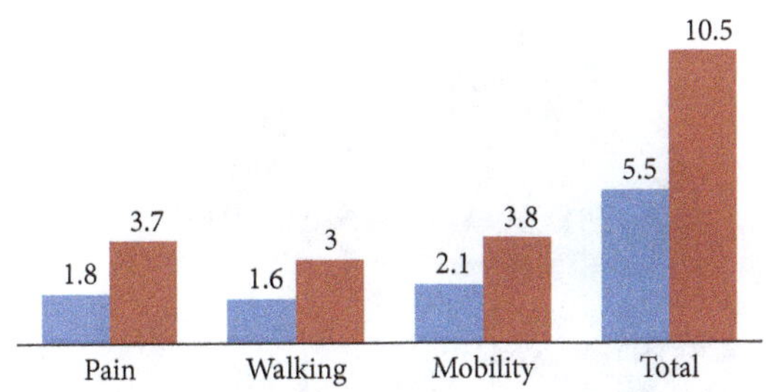

FIGURE 3: Change in the Postel Merlé d'Aubigné from preoperative to follow-up. The PMA pain score went from 1.8 to 3.7, the walking score went from 1.6 to 3.0 and the mobility score went from 2.1 to 3.8, on average.

A critical P value less than 0.05 was used for all statistical comparisons. All analyses were performed using STATA/SE v10.

3. Results

Follow-up averaged 5.4 years; the longest follow-up was 12.5 years. Only one patient died of causes unrelated to the process at a mean follow-up of 24 months.

Preoperative PMA functional scores [7] averaged 5.48 ± 2.41. We observed an improvement ($P < 0.01$) in the postoperative score with an average PMA of 10.55 ± 3.82 (Figure 3). Every component of the PMA changed significantly ($P < 0.001$). There was no significant effect of gender, number of previous surgeries, use of a dual mobility cup, or severity of preoperative bone loss on the functional results. Patients less than 65 years old had better functional scores than patients above 65 years of age ($P < 0.005$).

Thirty-four (92%) structural allografts and morselized cancellous grafts healed uneventfully without fracture or resorption, so that, radiographically, there was a continuous trabecular pattern with host bone. Only 3 patients (8%), those cases with septic acetabular loosening, had progressive radiolucent lines (8%) [10].

We reviewed the 37 patients for any perioperative or intermediate complications. Fourteen of the 37 cases (38%) had no perioperative complications.

There was a 77-year-old woman who was revised at 44 months because of a septic loosening that was associated to recurrent dislocations. The radiograph showed that one of the superior flanges had fractured through the screw holes. A two-stage exchange was deemed necessary with implant of a total femur replacement and a dual mobility cup cemented into a reconstruction cage. At 2 months postoperatively two early dislocations occurred; therefore a new revision to a constrained liner was necessary, with no further complications.

Six rings lost fixation (16%), 3 septic and 3 aseptic loosening: 3 of them were revised and 1 is awaiting revision.

(i) Two revised hips were associated with infection. One of them was the patient explained above. A two-stage exchange was also necessary for the other patient, with implant of a dual mobility cup cemented into a new Contour cage and a total femur replacement. The other septic loosening patient refused to have surgery; he is actually with antibiotherapy.

(ii) There were three aseptic loosenings, of which only one was revised at 84 months. In this case a Protrusio cage lost fixation and impinged the sciatic nerve, so a revision to another cage and neurolysis of the sciatic nerve were necessary. One is awaiting revision. The last one had an early dislocation that was reduced recurrence-free and an aseptic loosening at 36 months postoperatively, but he refused to have surgery.

Two rings possibly were lost with loss of ischial screw fixation in one of them. The other one was a cage with rupture and migration of an ischial screw which impinged the sciatic nerve 2 months postoperatively, requiring the prompt removal of the screw, leaving the cage intact. Both of them had good results in the overall PMA at 104- and 24-month follow-up, respectively. One acetabular cup has become loosened 24 months later and has been revised, leaving the ring intact, with no further complications.

We found no association between the number of previous surgeries and both radiographic failure and loosening undergoing revision. The extent of preoperative bone loss as determined by the Paprosky classifications (type III) [5] was associated with an increased rate of loosening or failure undergoing revision ($P < 0.05$). The acetabular component abduction angles were similar for loosened and unloosened cages (48,7° +/− 5,4° and 48,5° +/− 5,7°, resp.). We found no association between age at revision, number of screws used, size of the reconstruction cage, and use of a dual mobility cup with both radiographic failure and loosening undergoing revision.

There were 4 deep infections (10.8%), three septic acetabular loosenings, explained above, and one further deep infection, successfully treated with irrigation, debridement, and retention of the implants, with no further complications.

Ten hips had dislocations, only one having a dual mobility cup. There were 7 cases of early dislocation (before 3 months postoperatively): 3 of them were reduced without additional surgery and remained recurrence-free. And there were 3 cases of late dislocations (>3 months). The overall postoperative dislocation rate at the end of FU was 27% of which 7 (18.9%) needed further revision. One case was associated with septic loosening as explained above. Another two cases were revised to dual mobility cups, without further complications. In two patients aged 89 and 90, respectively, a resection arthroplasty was left. One of them died of causes unrelated to the process 3 months after the surgery. Another one was revised to a standard cemented liner and dislocated two times again; therefore, another revision was needed to a dual mobility cup, without recurrence. The last patient was a dislocation of a dual mobility cup cemented into a cage 3 months postoperatively. After several attempts to reduction, we found the prosthesis disassembled, so a revision to a constrained liner was necessary in this case. We found an inverse association between the use of dual mobility cups and both dislocation rate ($P < 0.05$) and dislocation undergoing revision ($P < 0.05$).

There were 9 sciatic nerve palsies and 1 femoral nerve palsy. Three cases of sciatic impingement were observed and needed revision: two cases explained above and another case were associated with fracture of the ischium 12 months later with posterior fibrosis of the sciatic nerve that needs neurolysis. The remaining 6 cases, except one, were associated with application of the reconstruction ring on the lateral surface of the ischium and subsequent screw fixation. Full recovery occurred in all cases, except two cases with partial recovery and 1 case with no recovery of the sciatic palsy.

One case had a femoral deep venous thrombosis that provoked an acute arterial ischemia in the popliteal artery. A thrombectomy had to be made.

We observed two material ruptures (screw or cage): the above-mentioned Contour superior flange fracture with septic loosening and the other above mentioned ischial screw fracture that impinged the sciatic nerve needing further revision. The latter one did not cause migration of the cage; therefore it was not necessary to remove it.

In summary, two constrained liners were used because of recurrent dislocations.

The need for reoperation for any reason was 32%, twelve hips (Figure 4).

Given the above criteria for success dictated by Goodman et al. [8] 19 of the 37 hips (51.4%) were successful, and 18 of the 37 hips (48.6%) were deemed to be unsuccessful. However, 8 of these 18 "unsuccessful" rings were left in situ: two patients who refused revision to a new reconstruction cage for loosening cages, 2 patients with one episode of early dislocation that were reduced recurrence-free, 2 revisions for sciatic impingement, where the cages were left intact, one deep infection which was successfully treated with antibiotherapy, and one acetabular cup loosening. In all these "failed" cases, the bone graft and reconstruction ring have been left in situ and thus may be considered successful in the fact that they restored bone stock for future revision, if necessary [8]. Therefore, we could consider that the success rate of this reconstruction is 27 of 37 hips (73%). There were no differences in the outcome or rate of complications when comparing the Protrusio rings and the Contour rings.

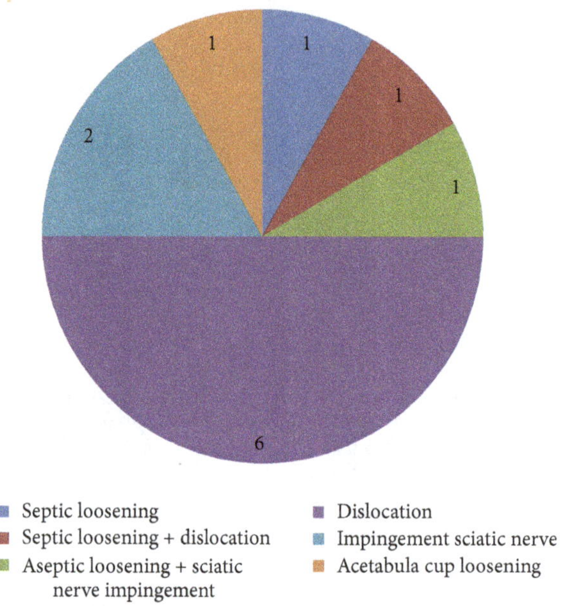

FIGURE 4: Need for reoperation for any reason.

4. Discussion

The presence of severe bone loss is an indication for an acetabular reconstruction with the use of a metal reinforcement ring and bone graft [13–15]. A reinforcement cage is designed to manage extended pelvic defects by bridging large bone gaps and protecting the grafts filled to increase the bone stock in case of future revision [6]. The major advantage of rings and cages is the ability to cement a liner in any position independent of the cage position and the elution of local antibiotics from the cement [2]. The lack of bony ingrowth and biological fixation exposed them to cyclical loading resulting in failure of hardware, typically screw breakage or migration of the ischial flange [8, 13, 16], with this being their major disadvantage. Despite this, midterm results with the use of a cage have been satisfactory, with a survival rate that ranges between 75% with 15-year follow-up [8] and 92,4% for 68 antiprotrusio cages after an average follow-up time of 13 years [17].

We noted a modest improvement in the clinical outcome using the PMA score [7]. Our data regarding pain relief and functional improvement support the observation made by others that improvement in function was limited [8, 12]. Goodman et al. [8] reported a modest functional improvement in their series probably not reflective of reconstruction success given the limitations present preoperatively because of multiple previous surgeries and widespread arthritis of the joints of the lower extremities or debilitating systemic disease or bilateral reconstructions. Therefore, they defined [8] success of reconstruction as a stable, nondislocating, nonmigrating hip that has had no further surgery on the acetabular side. Our data, with a success rate of 73% (27 of 37 hips), are similar to Goodman et al.'s [8], which reported a success rate of 76%.

The results and complications of our study are comparable with other reports describing the use and outcome of reconstruction rings. The perioperative and intermediate rate of complications in our study was 62%, similar to Goodman et al. [8] with 56% (34/61) and higher than Philippe et al. [18] with 38%. The high complication rate associated with these cases reflects the very large acetabular bone deficiencies that must be replaced; the extensive scarring from previous surgery; and the elevated age at revision and high prevalence of local or systemic disorders [8].

Reconstruction with an antiprotrusio cage has a reported failure rate including radiographic loosening that ranges between 0 and 24% [17–25]. The reported rates of revision ranged from 0 to 16% [8, 17–25]. The incidence of failure or radiographic loosening in our study was 16% at an average of 5.4 years postoperatively, with the need for revision for this cause being 8.1% (2.7% without infection). These rates are comparable to other studies like Bostrom et al. [20] with a revision rate of 6% (3% without infection) and an incidence of radiographic loosening of 16% or Goodman et al. [8] which revealed a revision rate of 6.6% and a radiographic loosening or failure of 11.5%. Sembrano and Cheng [26] reported that no single preoperative factor (age, gender) or intraoperative factor (number of screws used, size of the reconstruction cage, and number of previous surgeries or restoration of an optimal center of rotation) predicted cage failure. In fact, in our analysis of different factors, we were not able to identify a single preoperative or intraoperative factor that correlated with failure. We found only one association between preoperative classification of bone loss and radiographic failure and loosening undergoing revision ($P = 0.03$). As Perka and Ludwig [12] reported, we found an increased rate of revision because of cage failure in Paprosky type III defects.

The all-cause rate of acetabular revision described in the literature concerning antiprotrusio cage reconstructions varies from 5% to 24% [20–22, 24]. The need for reoperation for any reason was 32% (twelve hips) in our study, three for failure (one aseptic and two infected, one of them associated with dislocation), six for recurrent dislocation, two for sciatic impingement, and one for cup loosening. Our extremely high rates of revision are probably due to the high number of dislocations (7/37) or sciatic nerve palsies (3/37) that needed revision. It is well known that patients undergoing this form of surgery are at the risk of instability because of many causes, like repeated hip operations, function of abductors [16], position of the components, or cooperation of patient and others. The rate of implant instability during revision of total hip replacement is highly variable in the literature, with recent publications showing a dislocation rate varying from 7.4 to 17.2% [17, 18, 20, 21, 27]. We reported a 39% dislocation rate (9/23) during the analysis of 23 reconstruction cages using a standard cemented liner, a rate that is unacceptably high and should not be accepted in modern orthopaedic practice. There are many probable causes that may have caused this huge dislocation rate in our series. We observed that, by using a dual mobility cup cemented into the cage, our rates improved from 39% to 7.1% (1/14). Schneider et al. [19] observed a 10% (10/96) dislocation rate at a mean follow-up of 41 months in 96 revisions using a reconstruction device associated with a dual mobility cup cemented into the 13 cages, very similar to our series. We observed that the dislocation rate and dislocation undergoing revision decreased using a cemented dual mobility cup into the cage ($P = 0.03$).

We observed a high rate of sciatic nerve palsies (24%) undergoing revision (8.1%); one of them associated with an aseptic loosening of the cage that impinged the sciatic nerve. This could be explained by the following: the acetabular component to be removed often is associated with marked protrusio, fractured and migrated internal fixation, and cement and fibrous adhesions after the previous surgeries can be found. These factors often demand extensive exposure and retraction, which can be associated with stretching of the branches of the sciatic nerve [4, 8, 25]. Fixing the flange to the lateral surface of the ischium with screws, as we did, demands more exposure and retraction near the sciatic nerve; furthermore, the flange could act as an irritant, subsequently leading to sciatica [8]. Slotting the inferior flange into the ischium is a technically demanding procedure but provides several advantages: a more stable fixation of the cage can be obtained in a more horizontal position. Moreover, the risk of sciatic nerve injury can be significantly decreased [4, 8, 25], because the ischiatic flap is inserted inside the ischium.

Finally, we only observed two material ruptures (5.4%). The major concern with standard acetabular cages is the lack of a porous coating for bone ingrowth. Consequently, the potential for biologic, long-term fixation through osseointegration is not predictable, and a high incidence of hardware failure due to screw breakage or ischial flange migration has been reported at midterm follow-up [6]. Our series had a low rate of material rupture, which could explain the high rate of graft uptake in our series. The cages spanning the bone defect allow primary stability and protect the graft from resorption due to mechanical overload, enabling osseous integration [4].

Our study had significant limitations. First, it was a retrospective study without a control group. Second, two reconstruction devices were used in the patients and may have confused the results. Third, midterm follow-up limited our ability to generate definitive conclusions with a power analysis, especially in relation to cup loosening. Fourth, there were only 37, so larger studies with longer follow-up periods are needed.

Although a longer follow-up is required before reaching definitive conclusions, our preliminary results indicate that the treatment of severe acetabular defects by this technique is a viable option and we emphasized the need to use a dual mobility cup cemented into the cage to improve the device stability. Inserting the ischial flange into the ischium could be a possibility to decrease nerve palsy injury and to improve mechanical stability [25].

Conflict of Interests

The authors declare that they have no conflict of interests concerning this paper.

Acknowledgment

Thanks are due to Mr. Martin J. Smyth, B.A., for his help in revising the English language.

References

[1] S. J. Nho, S. M. Kymes, J. J. Callaghan, and D. T. Felson, "The burden of hip osteoarthritis in the United States: epidemiologic and economic considerations," *The Journal of the American Academy of Orthopaedic Surgeons*, vol. 21, supplement 1, pp. S1–S6, 2013.

[2] N. P. Sheth, C. L. Nelson, B. D. Springer, T. K. Fehring, and W. G. Paprosky, "Acetabular bone loss in revision total hip arthroplasty: evaluation and management," *Journal of the*

American Academy of Orthopaedic Surgeons, vol. 21, no. 3, pp. 128–139, 2013.

[3] G. K. Deirmengian, B. Zmistowski, J. T. O'Neil, and W. J. Hozack, "Management of acetabular bone loss in revision total hip arthroplasty," *Journal of Bone and Joint Surgery A*, vol. 93, no. 19, pp. 1842–1852, 2011.

[4] D. Regis, A. Sandri, I. Bonetti, O. Bortolami, and P. Bartolozzi, "Acminimum of 10-year follow-up of the Burch-Schneider cage andcbulk allografts for the revision of pelvic discontinuity," *The Journal of Arthroplasty*, vol. 27, no. 6, pp. 1057.e1–1063.e1, 2012.

[5] W. G. Paprosky, P. G. Perona, and J. M. Lawrence, "Acetabular defect classification and surgical reconstruction in revision arthroplasty: a 6-year follow-up evaluation," *Journal of Arthroplasty*, vol. 9, no. 1, pp. 33–44, 1994.

[6] D. Regis, A. Sandri, and I. Bonetti, "Acetabular reconstruction with the Burch-Schneider antiprotrusio cage and bulk allografts: minimum 10-year follow-up results," *BioMed Research International*, vol. 2014, Article ID 194076, 9 pages, 2014.

[7] R. Merle D'Aubigné, "Numerical classification of the function of the hip," *Revue de Chirurgie Orthopédique et Réparatrice de l'appareil Moteur*, vol. 56, pp. 481–486, 1970.

[8] S. Goodman, H. Saastamoinen, N. Shasha, and A. Gross, "Complications of ilioischial reconstruction rings in revision total hip arthroplasty," *Journal of Arthroplasty*, vol. 19, no. 4, pp. 436–446, 2004.

[9] F. Bonnomet, P. Clavert, P. Gicquel, Y. Lefèbvre, and J.-F. Kempf, "Reconstruction by graft and metallic reinforcement device in severe aseptic acetabular loosening: 10 years survivorship analysis," *Revue de Chirurgie Orthopedique et Reparatrice de l'Appareil Moteur*, vol. 87, no. 2, pp. 135–146, 2001.

[10] J. G. DeLee and J. Charnley, "Radiological demarcation of cemented sockets in total hip replacement," *Clinical Orthopaedics and Related Research*, vol. 121, pp. 20–32, 1976.

[11] T. Azuma, H. Yasuda, K. Okagaki, and K. Sakai, "Compressed allograft chips for acetabular reconstruction in revision hip arthroplasty," *Journal of Bone and Joint Surgery Series B*, vol. 76, no. 5, pp. 126–137, 1994.

[12] C. Perka and R. Ludwig, "Reconstruction of segmental defects during revision procedures of the acetabulum with the Burch-Schneider anti-protrusio cage," *Journal of Arthroplasty*, vol. 16, no. 5, pp. 568–574, 2001.

[13] E. Winter, M. Piert, R. Volkmann et al., "Allogeneic cancellous bone graft and a burch-schneider ring for acetabular reconstruction in revision hip arthroplasty," *Journal of Bone and Joint Surgery—Series A*, vol. 83, no. 6, pp. 862–867, 2001.

[14] T. J. Gill, J. B. Sledge, and M. E. Müller, "The Burch-Schneider anti-protrusio cage in revision total hip arthroplasty: indications, principles and long-term results," *Journal of Bone and Joint Surgery*, vol. 80, no. 6, pp. 946–953, 1998.

[15] A. Bergmann, E. Heisel, and E. Fritsch, "Erfahrungen mit metallischen Abstützringen in Kombination mit zementierten Polyäthylenpfannen bei Hüftendoprothesenwechseln und mögliche Alternativen," *Orthop Praxis*, vol. 27, pp. 206–211, 1991.

[16] Y. Kosashvili, D. Backstein, O. Safir, D. Lakstein, and A. E. Gross, "Acetabular revision using an anti-protrusion (ilio-ischial) cage and trabecular metal acetabular component for severe acetabular bone loss associated with pelvic discontinuity," *Journal of Bone and Joint Surgery*, vol. 91, no. 7, pp. 870–876, 2009.

[17] A. Coscujuela-Mañá, F. Angles, C. Tramunt, and X. Casanova, "Burch-Schneider antiprotrusio cage for acetabular revision: a 5- to 13-year follow-up study," *Hip International*, vol. 20, no. S7, pp. S112–S118, 2010.

[18] R. Philippe, O. Gosselin, J. Sedaghatian et al., "Acetabular reconstruction using morselized allograft and a reinforcement ring for revision arthroplasty with Paprosky type II and III bone loss: survival analysis of 95 hips after 5 to 13 years," *Orthopaedics and Traumatology: Surgery and Research*, vol. 98, no. 2, pp. 129–137, 2012.

[19] L. Schneider, R. Philippot, B. Boyer, and F. Farizon, "Revision total hip arthroplasty using a reconstruction cage device and a cemented dual mobility cup," *Orthopaedics and Traumatology: Surgery and Research*, vol. 97, no. 8, pp. 807–813, 2011.

[20] M. P. Bostrom, A. P. Lehman, R. L. Buly, S. Lyman, and B. J. Nestor, "Acetabular revision with the contour antiprotrusio cage: 2- to 5-year followup," *Clinical Orthopaedics and Related Research*, no. 453, pp. 188–194, 2006.

[21] H. Pieringer, V. Auersperg, and N. Böhler, "Reconstruction of severe acetabular bone-deficiency: the Burch-Schneider antiprotrusio cage in primary and revision total hip arthroplasty," *The Journal of Arthroplasty*, vol. 21, no. 4, pp. 489–496, 2006.

[22] D. J. Berry and M. E. Muller, "Revision arthroplasty using an anti-protrusio cage for massive acetabular bone deficiency," *Journal of Bone and Joint Surgery Series B*, vol. 74, no. 5, pp. 711–715, 1992.

[23] M. Kerboull, M. Hamadouche, and L. Kerboull, "The Kerboull acetabular reinforcement device in major acetabular reconstructions," *Clinical Orthopaedics and Related Research*, no. 378, pp. 155–168, 2000.

[24] K. Kawanabe, H. Akiyama, E. Onishi, and T. Nakamura, "Revision total hip replacement using the Kerboull acetabular reinforcement device with morsellised or bulk graft," *Journal of Bone and Joint Surgery—Series B*, vol. 89, no. 1, pp. 26–31, 2007.

[25] J. Lamo-Espinosa, J. Duart Clemente, P. Díaz-Rada, J. Pons-Villanueva, and J. R. Valentí-Nín, "The Burch-Schneider antiprotrusio cage: medium follow-up results," *Musculoskeletal Surgery*, vol. 97, no. 1, pp. 31–37, 2013.

[26] J. N. Sembrano and E. Y. Cheng, "Acetabular cage survival and analysis of factors related to failure," *Clinical Orthopaedics and Related Research*, vol. 466, no. 7, pp. 1657–1665, 2008.

[27] A. L. Whaley, D. J. Berry, and W. Scott Harmsen, "Extra-large uncemented hemispherical acetabular components for revision total hip arthroplasty," *Journal of Bone and Joint Surgery—Series A*, vol. 83, no. 9, pp. 1352–1357, 2001.

Elution Characteristics of Vancomycin, Gentamicin, and Vancomycin/Gentamicin Combination from Calcium Phosphate Cement

Masataka Uchino,[1] Ken Sugo,[2] Kouji Naruse,[1] Kentaro Uchida,[3] Noriko Hirakawa,[1] Masahiro Toyama,[1] Genyou Miyajima,[1] and Ken Urabe[1]

[1] *Department of Orthopaedic Surgery, Kitasato University Medical Center, 6-100 Arai, Kitamoto, Saitama 364-8501, Japan*
[2] *HOYA Technosurgical Corporation, 1-1-110 Tsutsujigaoka, Akishima, Tokyo 196-0012, Japan*
[3] *Department of Orthopaedic Surgery, Kitasato University School of Medicine, 1-15-1 Kitasato, Minami-ku, Sagamihara, Kanagawa 252-0375, Japan*

Correspondence should be addressed to Ken Urabe; kenurabe@med.kitasato-u.ac.jp

Academic Editor: Werner Kolb

The antibiotic elution profiles from calcium phosphate cement (CPC) used for treating infection sites after total joint arthroplasty vary depending on the type and number of impregnated antibiotics. The purpose of this study was to develop a method for efficiently eluting vancomycin hydrochloride (VCM) and gentamicin sulfate (GM) from CPC. Examination of the antibiotic elution profiles of CPC impregnated with either VCM (CPC/V) or GM (CPC/G) or both (CPC/VG) revealed that the early elution of VCM from CPC/VG was impaired compared to CPC/V. However, the elution of GM from CPC/VG was similar or higher compared to CPC/G. Scanning electron microscopy showed that the pore structure of CPC markedly differed depending on the type and number of antibiotics present. The pore size of CPC/VG was smaller compared to CPC/V but was larger compared to CPC/G. Thus, the inhibition of the early elution of VCM, which is a larger molecule than GM, was attributed to the decreased pore size of CPC/VG. These findings suggest that when dual treatment with VCM and GM is required for infection following total joint arthroplasty, each antibiotic should be individually impregnated into CPC to maximize the elution efficiency of VCM.

1. Introduction

Periprosthetic joint infection after total joint arthroplasty is a serious complication that requires prompt treatment. The two-stage exchange procedure is as an effective treatment option for such infections. The first stage of the procedure involves removal of the prosthetic components and bone cement, debridement of necrotic and granulation tissues, and insertion of an antibiotic-impregnated cement spacer. After treatment with intravenous antibiotics, revision total joint arthroplasty is performed in the second stage. The use of antibiotic-impregnated cement spacers is considered to be the optimal method for the localized delivery of antibiotics. However, it has been shown that a treatment failure rate for patients with methicillin-resistant *S. aureus* (MRSA) or methicillin-resistant *S. epidermidis* (MRSE) infection is higher than the reported rate including patients infected with both nonresistant and resistant organisms [1]. The prevalence of infection caused by MRSA and MRSE has increased in orthopedic patients [2]. Better localized delivery system of antibiotics should be considered for the treatment of MRSA and MRSE.

Recent studies have demonstrated that antibiotics-impregnated calcium phosphate cement (CPC) releases large amounts of antibiotics over long periods [3–5]. We previously compared the elution profiles of vancomycin hydrochloride (VCM) from CPC and PMMA in vitro and found that 8.1-fold more VCM was eluted from CPC than from PMMA in the first 24 h [6]. Therefore our institution uses both antibiotics-impregnated PMMA and CPC in the first stage

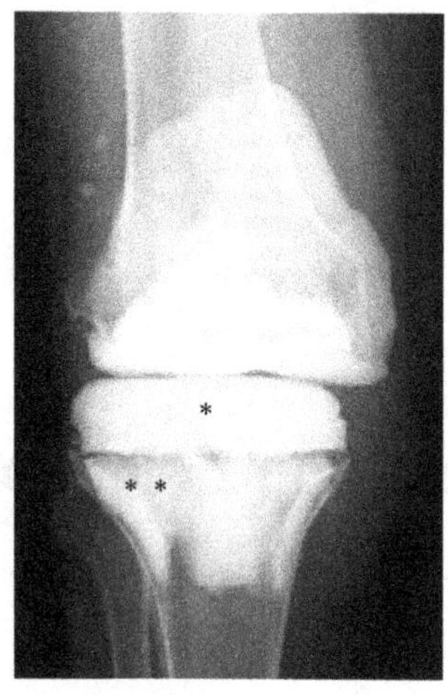

FIGURE 1: Combination use of antibiotics-impregnated PMMA and CPC in the first stage of the two-stage exchange procedure in our institution. *: PMMA. **: CPC.

of the two-stage exchange procedure for the treatment of periprosthetic joint infection as shown in Figure 1.

In the case that the causative microorganism is not detected although physical, hematological, and radiological findings show periprosthetic joint infection, administration of some types of antibiotics should be considered to kill both nonresistant and resistant organisms. In the present study, we confirmed that two types of antibiotics showed the different elution patterns from CPC when each antibiotic was impregnated into CPC separately. We examined whether CPC impregnated with two types of antibiotics with two different elution patterns showed the same elution profiles of each antibiotic to CPC impregnated with each antibiotic alone. Based on these findings, we established a methodology to simultaneously release two types of antibiotics from CPC with similar elution patterns to antibiotics impregnated in CPC alone.

2. Materials and Methods

2.1. Materials. CPC (Biopex-R Advance) was obtained from HOYA Technosurgical Corp. (Tokyo, Japan). Injectable VCM and gentamicin sulfate (GM) were purchased from Shionogi (Osaka, Japan) and Nichi-Iko Pharmaceutical (Toyama, Japan), respectively. All other chemicals were obtained from Wako Pure Chemical Industries (Osaka, Japan).

2.2. Preparation of Test Specimens for Double Antibiotic Therapy. VCM and GM were impregnated into CPC to prepare test specimens in triplicate. Briefly, CPC powder (12 g), VCM (0.3 g), 40 mg/mL GM (2.0 mL), and solvent (0.8 mL) were uniformly mixed to make a paste, which was then applied to a truncated cone-shape silicone mold. The paste was hardened by incubation for 3 h in a chamber at 37°C and 95% relative humidity. Once hardened, the molds were removed to obtain the test specimens, which were designated as CPC/VG. In addition, reference specimens of CPC impregnated with either VCM or GM, designated as CPC/V and CPC/G, were

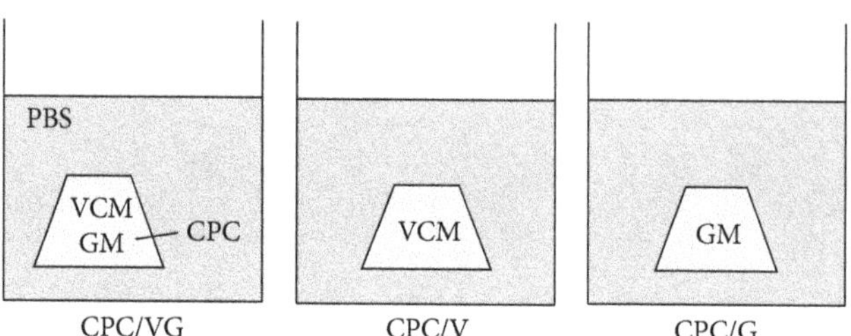

FIGURE 2: Schematic illustration of the protocol used to measure the elution of VCM and GM from the three types of antibiotic-impregnated CPC specimens.

prepared in the same manner as for CPC/VG, but without the addition of GM or VCM, respectively. For CPC/V, CPC powder (12 g), VCM (0.3 g), and solvent (2.8 mL) were mixed into a paste and treated as above. To prepare CPC/G, CPC powder (12 g), GM (2.0 mL), and solvent (0.8 mL) were used.

2.3. Antibiotic Elution. The test and reference specimens of impregnated CPC (1 g) were immersed in 10 mL sterile phosphate-buffered saline (PBS(-)) (Figure 2) and were then incubated at 37°C for 16 weeks. PBS(-) was replaced daily. Eluates were collected on days 1, 3, 7, and 14 and weeks 4, 8, 12, and 16. VCM and GM were detected by high-performance liquid chromatography (HPLC) on the day of collection.

2.4. Determination of VCM Concentration. A series of standard solutions of differing known concentrations of VCM in PBS(-) were prepared and injected into a CAPCELL-PAK C18 UG120 column (5 μm, φ4.6 mm × 25 cm; Shiseido, Tokyo, Japan) of an Elite LaChrom HPLC system (Hitachi High-Technologies, Tokyo, Japan) equipped with a L-2455 Diode Array Detector (Hitachi High-Technologies). The HPLC conditions were as follows: column temperature 30°C; mobile phase A, triethylamine buffer (pH 3.2)/acetonitrile/tetrahydrofuran = 92/7/1 (v/v); isocratic elution, phase A (20 min); flow rate, 1 mL/min; wavelength, 280 nm; and injection volume, 20 μL. The peak area of VCM in each standard solution was measured and plotted against the VCM concentration to generate a calibration curve. The concentration of VCM in each eluate sample was then determined by HPLC under the same conditions using the standard calibration curve.

2.5. Determination of GM Concentration. A series of standard solutions of differing known concentrations of GM in PBS(-) separately are injected into a CAPCELL-PAK C18 UG120 column (5 μm, φ4.6 mm × 25 cm) of an Elite LaChrom HPLC system (Hitachi High-Technologies) equipped with a L-2480 Fluorescence Detector (Hitachi High-Technologies). The three peak areas, which corresponded to the C1, C1a, and C2 components of GM, in each standard GM solution were measured and plotted against the GM concentration to generate a calibration curve. The concentration of GM in each eluate sample was then determined by HPLC using the standard calibration curve. As GM has no specific UV absorption, postcolumn derivatization with o-phthalaldehyde was used to form fluorescent products for the determination of GM concentration, according to a method described by Anhalt [7].

2.6. Pore Structure and Porosimetry Analyses. The relationship between the pore structure and antibiotic elution profiles of the test and reference specimens was analyzed and compared. To prepare CPC/VG, CPC powder (3 g), VCM (0.075 g), GM (0.5 mL), and solvent (0.2 mL) were mixed uniformly to prepare a paste, which was then placed in a cylindrical acrylic mold and hardened by incubation for 3 h at 37°C and 95% relative humidity. The molds were removed to obtain the specimens. CPC/V and CPC/G test specimens were prepared in the same manner as that used for CPC/VG. CPC/V was prepared using CPC powder (3 g), VCM (0.075 g), and solvent (0.7 mL), and CPC/G was prepared using CPC powder (3 g), GM (0.5 mL), and solvent (0.2 mL). The obtained specimens were immersed in 20 mL PBS(-) and incubated at 37°C for 24 h. The PBS(-) was then replaced with 20 mL acetone for dehydration of the specimens. After 10 min, the specimens were removed from the acetone and then dried at room temperature. Thin sections (1-2 mm thickness) of each specimen were prepared using a microtome for scanning electron microscopy (SEM) analysis (S-4300, Hitachi High-Technologies) and the analysis of pore size using a mercury porosimetry (AutoPore IV9520, Micromeritics, Norcross, GA, USA).

3. Results and Discussion

3.1. VCM Elution from CPC. The elution of VCM from CPC was monitored by measuring the concentration of the released antibiotic over a 16-week period (Figure 3). The elution continued for several weeks, although the concentration gradually decreased after reaching a peak at 24 h. The elution of VCM during the first 7 days was reduced by approximately two-thirds from CPC impregnated with both VCM and GM (CPC/VG) compared to CPC/V. As the elution of VCM from CPC/VG was clearly inhibited, the target MIC and associated antibacterial effect would not be achieved with this material at sites of periprosthetic joint infection. All tests were run in triplicate and averaged. A triplicate test is enough, because, in such experiment system, there are few errors so that error bars in the figure hide in the closed circles.

3.2. GM Elution from CPC. The time course for the elution of GM from CPC/G and CPC/VG was also examined (Figure 4). In contrast to the elution profile of VCM, that of GM was nearly identical from both single- and double-impregnated CPC throughout the measurement period. As shown in Figures 3 and 4, approximately 4-fold higher amounts of VCM were eluted from CPC compared to GM. All tests were run in triplicate and averaged. A triplicate test is enough, because, in such experiment system, there are few errors so that error bars in the figure hide in the closed circles.

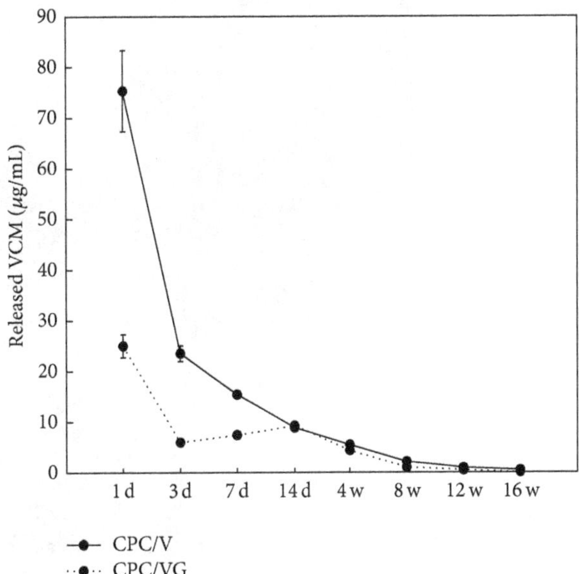

FIGURE 3: Elution of VCM from CPC/V and CPC/VG. Measurements were performed on the indicated days/weeks. Data are presented as the mean ± standard deviation of triplicate experiments.

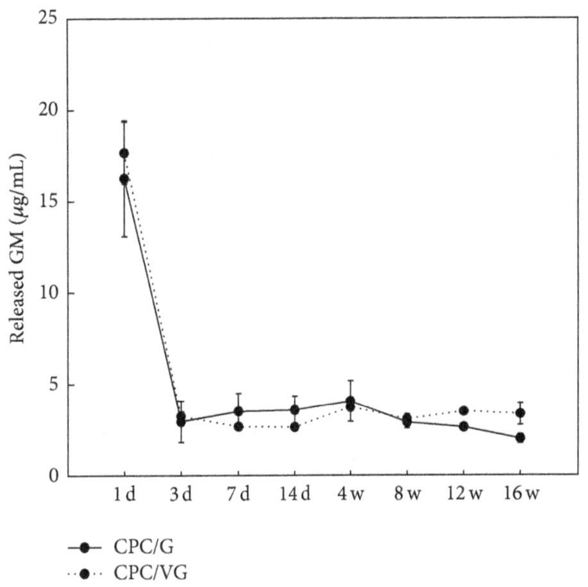

FIGURE 4: Elution of GM from CPC/G and CPC/VG. Measurements were performed on the indicated days/weeks. Data are presented as the mean ± standard deviation of triplicate experiments.

3.3. SEM Observation. Innumerable pores are present on the surface and within CPC and act as passages for antibiotic elution [8]. To investigate why the elution patterns of VCM and GM from CPC differed depending on the type and number of impregnated antibiotics, we therefore analyzed the pore structure of the various antibiotic-impregnated CPC specimens by SEM. The SEM images differed markedly between the CPC/V, CPC/G, and CPC/VG specimens (Figure 5). The surface and interior of CPC/V were comprised of

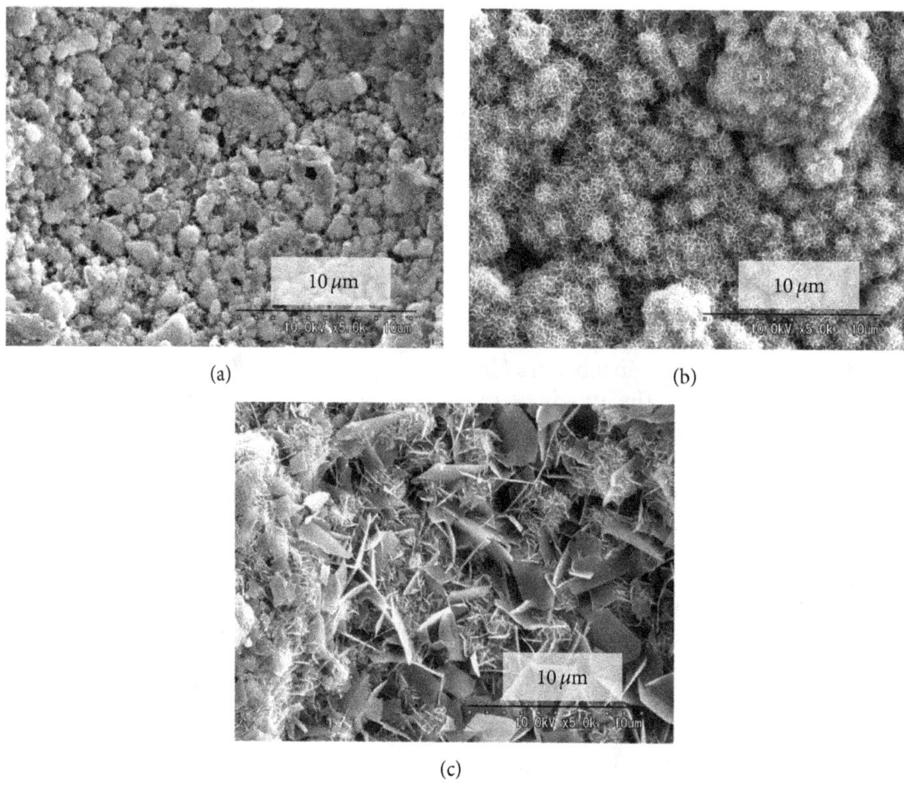

(a) (b) (c)

FIGURE 5: SEM images of the surfaces of CPC/V (a), CPC/VG (b), and CPC/G (c).

cobblestone-like microstructures, whereas CPC/G contained numerous needle-like projections. Interestingly, CPC/VG appeared to have a structure that combined the CPC/V and CPC/G characteristics, in which the cobblestone-like microstructures were covered in smaller needle-like projections.

3.4. Porosimetry Analysis. Mercury porosimetry was used to measure the pore size distribution of the antibiotic-impregnated CPC specimens (Figure 6). Consistent with the SEM analysis, the pore size was found to change depending on the type and number of impregnated antibiotics. Specifically, impregnation with VCM increased the pore size of CPC, whereas GM decreased the pore size of CPC. In CPC/VG, the average pore was intermediate in size between the larger pores observed in CPC/V and the smaller pores found in CPC/G. The results of the porosimetry analysis suggest that the reduced elution of VCM from CPC impregnated with VCM and GM under double antibiotic therapy conditions was due to the decrease in CPC pore size. Conversely, based on the increase in CPC/G pore size after impregnation with VCM, the elution of GM would be expected to be enhanced from CPC/VG; however, as demonstrated from the GM elution profile presented in Figure 4, the amount of GM in the eluate was not markedly affected. The differential effects on the elution of VCM and GM in response to the change in pore size may be explained by the sizes of these antibiotics. Compared with VCM, which has a MW of approximately 1450, the MW of GM is only 480. Thus, the increase in pore size resulting from the introduction of VCM into CPC/G would not be expected to markedly affect the elution of the relatively small GM, whereas the decrease in pore size resulting from the introduction of GM into CPC/V appears to have markedly decreased the elution of the larger VCM. This result is the problem of pore size

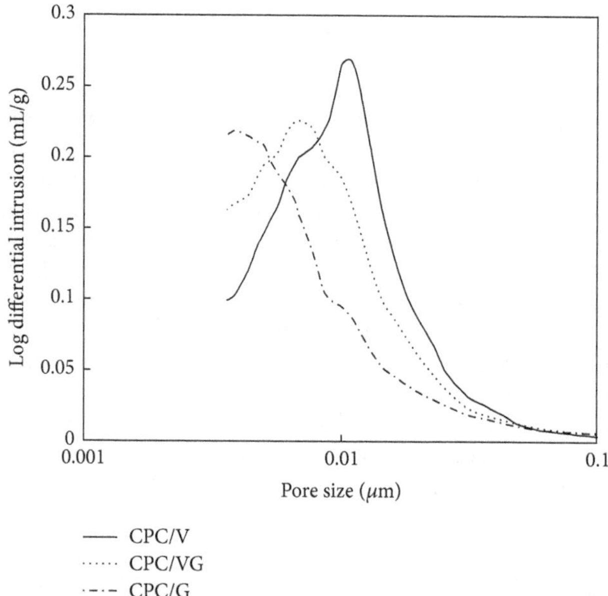

FIGURE 6: Results of mercury porosimetry analysis for CPC/V, CPC/G, and CPC/VG.

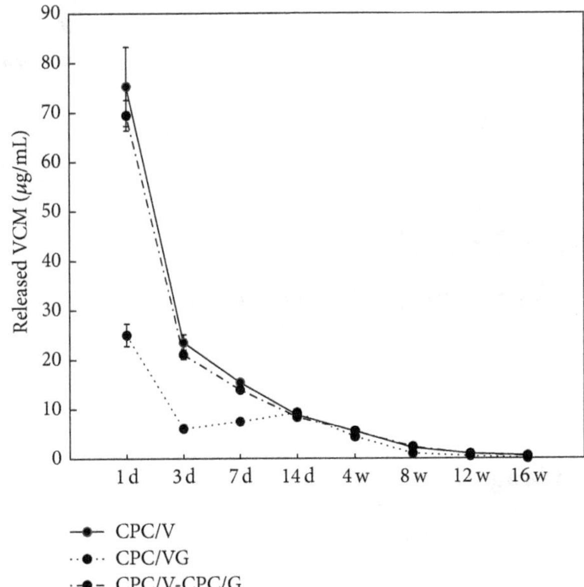

FIGURE 7: Elution profiles of VCM from CPC/V, CPC/VG, and CPC/V-CPC/G. Measurements were performed on the indicated days/weeks. Data are presented as the mean ± standard deviation of triplicate experiments.

and not an antagonistic interaction between VCM and GM, according to another preliminary experiment. It indicated that the residual titer of VCM (0.3 g), after mixing with 2.0 mL of GM (40 mg/mL), showed 99.7% (37°C, 24 h). The reduction of VCM, as described in this paper, could not be observed only by combining both antibiotics.

3.5. Improved Antibiotic Elution System. As the above results demonstrated that the elution of VCM from CPC was markedly reduced when both GM and VCM were impregnated into CPC, we attempted to increase the elution of VCM by using single antibiotic-impregnated CPC specimens, CPC/V and CPC/G, immersed together in PBS(-), designated as CPC/V-CPC/G. The elution profile of VCM from CPC/V located in close proximity to CPC/G was monitored over a 16-week period (Figure 7). As can be seen from the VCM elution curve, the elution profiles of VCM from CPC/V and CPC/V-CPC/G were nearly identical, whereas that from CPC/VG was comparatively reduced by approximately two-thirds. Therefore, the inhibition of VCM elution from CPC was clearly alleviated using this approach. All tests were run in triplicate and averaged. A triplicate test is enough, because, in such experiment system, there are few errors so that error bars in the figure hide in the closed circles.

4. Conclusions

The present findings demonstrate that the impregnation of CPC with both VCM and GM inhibits the early elution of VCM when compared to CPC impregnated with VCM only. Notably, the pore size of CPC impregnated with VCM and GM was smaller than that found in CPC/V, suggesting that this decrease in pore size impaired the elution of the relatively large VCM molecule. When dual antibiotic treatment with VCM and GM is used for infection after total joint arthroplasty, CPC impregnated with VCM and GM individually should be used.

Conflict of Interests

The authors declare that there is no conflict of interests regarding the publication of this paper.

References

[1] F. Leung, C. J. Richards, D. S. Garbuz, B. A. Masri, and C. P. Duncan, "Two-stage total hip arthroplasty: how often does it control methicillin-resistant infection?" *Clinical Orthopaedics and Related Research*, vol. 469, no. 4, pp. 1009–1015, 2011.

[2] W. E. Shams and R. P. Rapp, "Methicillin-resistant staphylococcal infections: an important consideration for orthopedic surgeons," *Orthopedics*, vol. 27, no. 6, pp. 565–568, 2004.

[3] O. Kisanuki, H. Yajima, T. Umeda, and Y. Takakura, "Experimental study of calcium phosphate cement impregnated with dideoxy-kanamycin B," *Journal of Orthopaedic Science*, vol. 12, no. 3, pp. 281–288, 2007.

[4] T. Sasaki, Y. Ishibashi, H. Katano, A. Nagumo, and S. Toh, "In vitro elution of vancomycin from calcium phosphate cement," *The Journal of Arthroplasty*, vol. 20, no. 8, pp. 1055–1059, 2005.

[5] M. Suzuki, T. Tsukeoka, Y. Tsuneizumi et al., "Mechanical strength and in vitro antibiotic release profile of antibiotics-loaded calcium phosphate bone paste," *Clinical Orthopaedic Surgery*, vol. 39, no. 3, pp. 309–314, 2004 (Japanese).

[6] K. Urabe, K. Naruse, H. Hattori et al., "In vitro comparison of elution characteristics of vancomycin from calcium phosphate cement and polymethylmethacrylate," *Journal of Orthopaedic Science*, vol. 14, no. 6, pp. 784–793, 2009.

[7] J. P. Anhalt, "Assay of gentamicin in serum by high pressure liquid chromatography," *Antimicrobial Agents and Chemotherapy*, vol. 11, no. 4, pp. 651–655, 1977.

[8] S. Sugiyama, M. Itokazu, T. Akaike, Y. Nonomura, and K. Shimizu, "Drug delivery system for antibiotics using calcium phosphate cement," *Orthopedic Surgery*, vol. 55, no. 3, pp. 357–362, 2004 (Japanese).

15

Analysis of Contoured Anatomic Plate Fixation versus Intramedullary Rod Fixation for Acute Midshaft Clavicle Fractures

Juliann Kwak-Lee,[1] Elke R. Ahlmann,[1] Lingjun Wang,[2] and John M. Itamura[3]

[1] *Los Angeles County + University of Southern California Medical Center, 1200 N. State Street, GNH 3900, Los Angeles, CA 90033, USA*
[2] *Department of Orthopedics, Los Angeles County + University of Southern California Medical Center, 1200 N. State Street, GNH 3900, Los Angeles, CA 90033, USA*
[3] *Keck School of Medicine, Kerlan-Jobe at White Memorial Medical Center, 1700 Cesar E. Chavez Avenue, Suite 1400, Los Angeles, CA 90033, USA*

Correspondence should be addressed to Elke R. Ahlmann; ahlmann2002@yahoo.com

Academic Editor: Ely Steinberg

The recent trend has been toward surgical fixation of displaced clavicle fractures. Several fixation techniques have been reported yet it is unclear which is preferable. We retrospectively reviewed one hundred one consecutive patients with acute midshaft clavicle fractures treated operatively at a level-1 trauma center. Thirty-four patients underwent intramedullary pin fixation and 67 had anatomic plate fixation. The outcomes we assessed were operative time, complications, infection, implant failure, fracture union, range of motion, and reoperation rate. There were 92 males and 9 females with an average age of 30 years (range: 14–68 years). All patients were followed to healing with an average followup of 20 months (range: 15–32 months). While fracture union by six months ($P = 0.8729$) and range of motion at three months ($P = 0.6139$) were similar, the overall healing time for pin fixation was shorter ($P = 0.0380$). The pin group had more infections ($P = 0.0335$) and implant failures ($P = 0.0245$) than the plate group. Intramedullary pin fixation may have improved early results, but there was no long term difference in overall rate of union and achievement of full shoulder motion. The higher rate of implant failure with pin fixation may indicate that not all fracture patterns are amenable to fixation using this device.

1. Introduction

Clavicle fractures are common injuries accounting for 5–10% of all fractures [1–3]. The majority of fractures (70–80%) are located within the middle third of the shaft [1, 2, 4]. Traditionally, acute midclavicular fractures have been treated nonoperatively with either sling or figure-of-eight bandage, with a reported less than 1% rate of fracture nonunion [5–8]. Until recently, operative indications typically included open fractures, tenting of the skin, neurovascular injuries, and concomitant shoulder girdle injuries [9, 10]. However, more recent studies have reported nonunion rates of 4–29% [11–16] and malunion rates of 14–36% [9, 14, 17–19] with displaced clavicle fractures. One study demonstrated that shoulder biomechanics were significantly altered by malunion of the clavicle [19]. Patients complained of weakness, rapid fatiguability, loss of endurance, numbness, and paraesthesias with overhead activities and deficits in functional cosmesis. Studies that have used patient-based outcome measures have described unsatisfactory outcome rates of 25–30%, with complications including neurologic symptoms and functional deficits [2, 9, 12, 15, 19]. Improved patient outcomes, earlier return to function, decreased nonunion and malunion rates, and better cosmesis have all been reported with operative fixation of acute clavicle fractures [13, 16, 17, 20]. Based on these recent studies, the trend has moved towards surgical stabilization of selected clavicle fractures, with operative indications including significant shortening or distraction

(>1.5 centimeters), displacement greater than 100%, and the presence of a zed fragment [10, 17, 21].

Several fixation methods have been reported including plate fixation [9, 17, 21], intramedullary pin fixation [22–25], and placement of intramedullary threaded k-wires [20, 26] and elastic intramedullary nails [6, 27]. Plate fixation has emerged as a popular technique. Placement of the plate has been a subject of debate with common locations including superior, anterior, or inferior surfaces of the clavicle. Several biomechanical studies evaluating plate placement concluded that anteroinferior plates may fail at a lower load than superiorly placed plates [28, 29]. Typically low contact dynamic compression (LCDC) plates or reconstruction plates have been used [14, 21]; however, precontoured plates designed to parallel the S-shaped curve of the clavicle have recently become popular alternatives [9, 17, 30]. Disadvantages of plate fixation include extensive soft tissue dissection which may result in damage to the superior clavicular nerves resulting in paresthesias, as well as implant prominence due to the superficial location of the plate [31, 32].

A less invasive alternative gaining popularity is intramedullary pin fixation. This technique utilizes a limited incision for fracture reduction and a separate small incision for pin placement through the lateral clavicle. Only a limited number of studies with small numbers of patients have evaluated the clinical outcome of this method of fixation [22–25, 33].

The purpose of this study is to evaluate whether one method of fixation (either pin or plate fixation) is preferable over the other in terms of complication rates, intraoperative variables, return to full shoulder motion, and time to fracture union for the treatment of acute midshaft clavicle fractures.

2. Patients and Methods

A retrospective review of the upper extremity trauma database was conducted to identify all operatively treated clavicle fractures at our institution from 2006 to 2010. All patients who presented with clavicle fractures with either displacement ≥100%, shortening of ≥1.5 centimeters, and/or the presence of a vertical zed fragment are counseled and offered surgical fixation. A total of 125 patients with clavicle fractures who underwent open reduction internal fixation of the clavicle were identified. All patients with concomitant shoulder girdle injuries, that is, floating shoulders (7 patients), clavicle fractures of the distal third or proximal third (7 patients), and less than one year of followup were excluded (10 patients). This left a total of 101 patients with isolated operatively treated midshaft clavicle fractures available for review.

Retrospective chart review was performed for operative time, estimated blood loss, intraoperative and postoperative complications, shoulder range of motion, and length of time to fracture healing.

Digital plain radiographs of the clavicle taken at initial injury and at each followup visit were reviewed by a single investigator (ERA) for initial injury fracture pattern, Orthopaedic Trauma Association (OTA) Classification [34], implant-related complications, and evidence of fracture healing. The initial injury radiographs were reviewed for the presence or absence of a zed fragment. The amount of initial fracture shortening and displacement were measured using a digital ruler. The clavicle fracture was deemed radiographically healed when there was evidence of bridging callous and obliteration of the initial fracture lines.

TABLE 1: Injury mechanism distribution.

Mechanism of injury	Number of patients
Sports	30
Fall from bicycle	27
Ground level fall	17
Motorcycle	15
No data	5
Fall from height	2
Hit by car	2
Motor vehicle accident	2
Assault	1
Total	**101**

There were 92 males and 9 females with an average age of 29.7 years (range: 14 to 68 years). The majority of injuries were due to low energy trauma (Table 1). There were 47 right (47%) and 54 left (53%) sided injuries, of which 50 (50%) affected the dominant side extremity. The average time from injury to surgery was 12.8 days (range: 1 to 43 days). Sixty-seven patients (66%) underwent plate fixation and 34 (34%) underwent intramedullary pin placement. The average length of followup was 20 months (range: 15 to 32 months). Patient demographics are summarized in Table 2.

All surgical procedures were performed by or under the supervision of two upper extremity trauma surgeons. One surgeon exclusively performed plate fixation while the second surgeon performed both plate and pin fixation surgeries. The surgical indications for fracture fixation included open fracture, presence of a zed fragment, >100% vertical displacement, shortening of >1.5 cm, and skin tenting.

All 67 clavicle plate fixation procedures were performed in a similar fashion through an incision centered over the superior aspect of the clavicle, taking care to dissect and preserve the cutaneous supraclavicular nerves whenever possible. Acumed anatomic contoured clavicle plates (Acumed USA, Hillsboro, OR) were used on all 67 patients and all were positioned over the superior surface of the clavicle (Figures 1(a)-1(b)). All fractures were fixed with three 3.5 mm screws (6 cortices of fixation) on either side of the fracture site. Occasionally, in order to aid in reduction of small fracture fragments or zed fragments, 2.0 mm Modular Hand System screws (Synthes, Inc., West Chester, PA) were additionally used.

Thirty-four patients underwent intramedullary pin fixation by a single surgeon using a standardized technique of a limited incision for fracture reduction and a separate small incision for pin placement through the lateral clavicle. Twenty-nine patients had fixation using the Rockwood Clavicle Pin (Depuy Orthopaedics, Warsaw, IN) and five patients had placement of the Acumed Clavicle Rod (Acumed USA, Hillsboro, OR). Both pin fixation methods were performed

TABLE 2: Patient demographics and fracture patterns.

Demographics	Pin (range)	Plate (range)	P value
No. of patients	34	67	0.1135
Age (years)	27.6 (14–59)	31.7 (16–68)	0.1453
Gender: male	29	63	0.1843
Gender: female	5	4	0.2194
Dominant extremity fracture	17	33	0.7287
Time from injury to surgery (days)	11.8 (3–26)	13.4 (1–42)	0.6349
Length of followup (months)	19 (15–26)	22 (18–32)	0.2578
Fracture pattern			
OTA 15-B1	12	15	
OTA 15-B2	16	34	0.3492
OTA 15-B3	6	18	
Average displacement (mm)	18.4 (9–30)	20.6 (7–47)	0.1649
Average shortening (mm)	21.6 (7–37)	20.2 (7–37)	0.3631

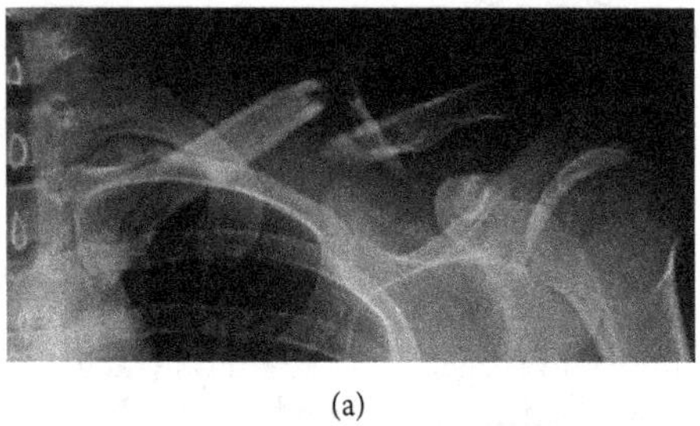

(a)

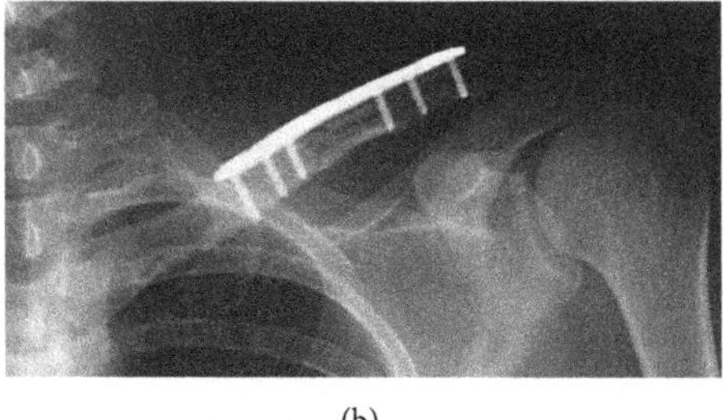

(b)

FIGURE 1: (a) AP radiograph of the shoulder demonstrates the intercalary fragment in the midshaft clavicle fracture representing the zed fragment and >100% fracture displacement. (b) Postoperative radiograph of the same patient after fracture fixation using the Acumed contoured clavicle plate.

according to the manufacturers' recommended technique and both pins function in a similar manner (Figures 2(a)–2(c)).

Postoperatively patients were placed in a shoulder sling for 10 days and subsequently allowed to perform passive and active range of motion exercises from 0 to 90 degrees of shoulder elevation under the direction of a physical therapist. Six weeks postoperatively, all patients were then allowed to perform active and passive range of motion, including overhead activities. Patients were told to refrain from participating in sports for a total of 6 months from the time of operative fixation. Those patients who underwent intramedullary pin fixation were told that they would have to undergo a second procedure from removal of the pin at a minimum of three months postoperatively or when there was evidence of healing of the fracture. Clavicle plates were not routinely removed after fracture union.

Statistical analysis was performed using GraphPad Prism software (GraphPad Software, Inc., San Diego, CA). Chi-square test and Student's t-test were used to determine differences in demographic data, intraoperative measures, rate of fracture healing, and range of motion. Fisher's exact test was used to determine differences in the distribution of fracture patterns and the rate of complications between the two groups. A P value of less than 0.05 was considered significant.

3. Results

Operative times were measured from incision to skin closure. In the pin group, the average operative time was 99.5 min (range 43–169 min) while in the plate group, the average operative time was significantly longer with an average of 131.8 min (range 30–246 min) ($P = 0.0007$). Estimated blood loss between the two procedures showed no difference ($P = 0.4709$).

The complications for pin and plate fixation are described in detail in Table 3. In the intramedullary pin group, there was a significantly increased rate of implant failure ($P = 0.0245$). All 3 failures consisted of the rod backing out through the skin and required either removal or reinsertion of the pin if the fracture was not fully healed. The fracture pattern of these three patients showed comminution and the presence of zed fragments. The one failure after plate fixation was breakage of the plate 3 weeks postoperatively as a result of a fall during a seizure episode. This patient underwent a second procedure for removal of the plate and repeat fixation using a new Acumed clavicle plate. The pin group also demonstrated a significantly higher rate of implant-associated infection than those treated with plate fixation ($P = 0.0335$). As plate fixation techniques included a larger incision and more dissection, 11 of 67 patients (16.4%) developed numbness

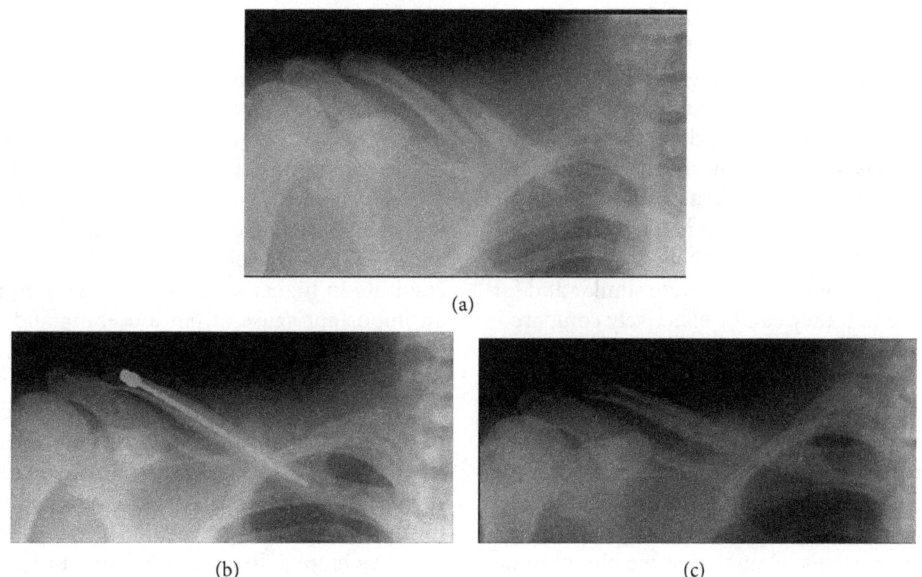

(a)

(b) (c)

FIGURE 2: (a) AP radiograph of the clavicle showing a midshaft clavicle fracture with displacement and 2.3 cm shortening. (b) Postoperative radiograph of the same patient after fracture fixation using the Rockwood clavicle. (c) Followup radiograph taken 3 months postoperatively after fracture union and removal of the Rockwood clavicle pin.

TABLE 3: Clinical results and complications of pin versus plate fixation.

Complications	Pin (no. of patients)	%	Plate (no. of patients)	%	*P* value
Infection	4	11.8	1	1.5	0.0335
Implant failure	3	8.8	1	1.5	0.0245
Nonunion after 6 months	3	8.8	4	6	0.8729
Failed implant removal	3	8.8	0	0	0.5472
Adhesive capsulitis	1	2.9	0	0	0.8720
Symptomatic implant	0	0	2	2.9	0.6949
DVT	0	0	1	1.5	0.8483
Incisional symptoms	0	0	11	16.4	0.0275

DVT: deep venous thrombosis.

or hypersensitivity over their incision sites which was not seen after pin fixation ($P = 0.0275$). Two patients (2.9%) developed implant prominence or symptomatic implants, yet neither desired to have subsequent surgery for plate removal.

Unique to the pin group, 76% of patients (26 of 34 patients) underwent a second surgery for pin removal as recommended. Three of these patients (8.8%) had failed implant removal with breakage of the pin and subsequent implant retention. All three patients had a 2.5-millimeter rod.

Full range of motion at 3-month followup was similarly achieved in both groups with 18 of 34 patients (52.9%) in the pin group and 39 of 67 patients (58.2%) in the plate group ($P = 0.6139$). One patient in the pin group (2.9%) developed postoperative adhesive capsulitis, which resulted in a delay in regaining full shoulder motion. This patient did eventually attain full motion by six months postoperatively. All patients in this series regained full shoulder motion by 6 months.

There was a significantly longer time to fracture union in those patients who underwent plate fixation with an average of 14.6 weeks (range 6–33.5 weeks) compared to pin fixation at 9.5 weeks (range 6–24 weeks) ($P = 0.0380$). Fracture nonunion at 6 months (26 weeks) was 6.0% (4 of 67) in the plate group and 8.8% (3 of 34) in the pin group ($P = 0.8729$). In both groups, all fractures that did not heal within six months were in patients who were heavy smokers; these patients did eventually heal their fractures by their latest followup.

4. Discussion

Management of patients with displaced midshaft clavicle fractures has evolved over the last 10 years with a move away from nonoperative treatment to the use of various fixation devices including the intramedullary pin and plate fixation. Yet the ideal method of treatment still remains unclear. We therefore compared intraoperative variables, complications, function, and fracture healing in patients treated with intramedullary pin devices and anatomic contoured plates determine if one method is preferable to the other.

We acknowledge several limitations of this study. First, owing to the nonrandomized retrospective design we did not control for potentially confounding variables such as patient demographics and fracture pattern. We did, however, determine that there were no significant differences (P values >0.05) between patients who underwent pin fixation and those who had plate fixation with regards to age, gender distribution, hand dominance, sidedness of the fracture, time to surgery, fracture pattern, and length of followup. This indicates that the two groups of patients were similar and for this reason we believe that they can be effectively compared. Second, there is inherent selection bias in the choice of surgical implant when performing a retrospective analysis. In this series, one surgeon only performed plate fixation; the other initially performed mainly pin fixation and then moved toward primarily performing plate fixation. One would be led to believe that this bias would skew the plate group toward more comminuted fractures and the pin group toward more simple fracture patterns. Nonetheless we observed no difference in the distribution of fracture patterns between the two groups ($P > 0.05$) such that selection bias based on fracture pattern is less likely.

The standard technique of plate fixation has advanced with the design of the precontoured plate which better fits the curve of the clavicle and was developed to reduce some of the common complications associated with this fixation technique including implant prominence. Despite the use of contoured plates, two patients in our series (3%) did report symptoms of discomfort associated with implant prominence, yet neither wished to undergo a further surgical procedure for plate removal. This is lower than the rate of plate prominence previously reported which has ranged from 7 to 32% with precontoured plates [17, 35]. A study evaluating the clinical applicability of the Acumed locking clavicle plate reported that this plate is adequately shaped for the fixation of fractures in the medial three-fifths of the clavicular shaft [30]. However, not all patients with a fracture located in the lateral two-fifths of the clavicular shaft had anatomic fit of the plate. This may explain why a certain proportion of patients may still have implant prominence despite the use of an "anatomic" plate.

Another complication in our series primarily seen with plate fixation was a symptomatic incision, including both hypersensitivity and numbness. Although during our surgical approach we routinely dissect, neurolyse, and protect the supra- and infraclavicular nerves, 16.4% of patients in the plate group still reported skin numbness or hypersensitivity around their surgical incision. It is possible that intraoperative traction and/or stretching of the nerves over the plate may still occur in a certain proportion of patients and lead to this complication.

The S-shaped clavicle poses a problem for intramedullary pin insertion with sufficient engagement length into the curved medullary canal and may potentially explain why a higher rate of implant failure was seen in our series after pin fixation. A biomechanical study evaluating pin fixation in simple midshaft clavicle fractures reported that stability of fracture fixation is closely related to the length of intramedullary pin engagement [36]. The intramedullary pin functions as an internal splint that maintains alignment of the fracture without rigid fixation [20, 22, 37] and thus is not designed for axially and rotationally unstable fracture patterns. Since the pin functions as a load sharing device having no rigid fixation, a longer leverage of bending moment is needed to improve stability of the fracture fixation [20]. However, using a large and rigid intramedullary pin has the problem of a short engaged length in both the curved medullary canal of the clavicle and the medial fracture fragment, resulting in higher stress at the bone-pin interface, which is an important cause of pin loosening and failure of fixation [22]. Thus in the presence of significant comminution or a zed fragment at the fracture site, there is even less engaged length of the pin in the medullary canal further limiting the amount of fixation. Several biomechanical analyses of the Rockwood clavicle pin confirmed this as the pin was reported to be inadequate for fixation when rotational stiffness was required [38, 39]. All three patients in our series who developed loosening of the Rockwood clavicle pin had segmental comminution making them rotationally and axially unstable and thus less appropriate for pin fixation. It is for this reason that we now only perform intramedullary pin fixation for simple fractures with adequate cortical apposition.

Our patients who had loss of fixation additionally developed infection as the pin backed out of the lateral end of the clavicle to a point that the device became superficial resulting in skin breakdown and erosion of the lateral fixation nut through the skin. This then led to bacterial seeding of the implant with the development of purulent drainage and an abscess at the pin entry site. One additional patient who did not have implant failure also developed an abscess over the superficial lateral fixation nut. Mudd et al. [24] reported similar problems with lateral prominence of the implant resulting in skin necrosis and infection in four of 18 patients (22%) while Strauss et al. [25] reported 3 of 16 (19%) patients developed posterior skin breakdown due to implant prominence. We did note less prominence and a decrease in related complications once we started using a high-speed burr to smooth the sharp lateral end of the rod and make it flush with the nut. We recommend taking into consideration the patient's habitus and soft tissue coverage over the posterolateral acromion when considering intramedullary pin fixation as this device may be prominent and problematic for thin patients.

Pin fixation for clavicle fractures is less invasive. Extensive soft tissue dissection is spared and the periosteum remains intact. This may allow abundant callus formation and better healing of the fracture, which is perhaps reflected in our faster healing rate with plate fixation, although ultimately there was no difference in the overall rate of union when compared to plate fixation. There were three patients in the pin group (8.8%) and four patients (6%) in the plate group with delayed union who had not healed their fractures by 6 months. All patients were smokers and ultimately healed their fractures by 18 months after surgery. These rates are comparable to those reported in the literature with delayed union and nonunion rates of 0–6% [23–25] and 0–17% [13, 23–25], respectively, for intramedullary pin fixation and 0–4% [17, 21, 37] and 2–4% [17, 35, 40], respectively, for plate fixation.

Both intramedullary pins and contoured clavicle plates are reasonable choices for fixation of midshaft clavicle fractures. The less invasive technique of intramedullary pin fixation may have improved early results with shorter operative times and faster overall fracture healing, but in the long term there was no significant difference in overall rate of union and achievement of full shoulder motion between the two groups. The higher rate of implant failure associated with pin fixation may indicate that this device is not suitable for all fracture patterns. We recommend plate fixation for fractures with significant comminution or a zed fragment. Pin fixation should be reserved for simple fractures with good cortical apposition as this technique is both more technically challenging and requires adequate bone purchase thus making it less suitable for rotationally and axially unstable fracture patterns.

Disclosure

Each author certifies that his or her institution has approved the human protocol for this investigation and that all investigations were conducted in conformity with ethical principles of research and that informed consent for participation in the study was obtained. See Guidelines for Authors for a complete description of levels of evidence (Level of Evidence: Therapeutic Level III).

Conflict of Interests

Dr. Kwak-Lee, Dr. Ahlmann, and Lingjun Wang certify that they have no commercial associations (e.g., consultancies, stock ownership, equity interest, patent/licensing arrangements, etc.) that might pose a conflict of interest in connection with the submitted article. Dr. Itamura is a speaker for Acumed.

References

[1] M. D. McKee, "Clavicle fractures," in *Rockwood and Green's Fractures in Adults*, pp. 1106–1143, Lippincott Williams & Wilkins, Hagerstown, Md, USA, 7th edition, 2010.

[2] A. Nordqvist, C. J. Petersson, and I. Redlund-Johnell, "Midclavicle fractures in adults: end result after conservative treatment," *Journal of Orthopaedic Trauma*, vol. 12, no. 8, pp. 572–576, 1998.

[3] F. Postacchini, S. Gumina, P. de Santis, and F. Albo, "Epidemiology of clavicle fractures," *Journal of Shoulder and Elbow Surgery*, vol. 11, no. 5, pp. 452–456, 2002.

[4] A. Nordqvist and C. Petersson, "The incidence of fractures of the clavicle," *Clinical Orthopaedics and Related Research*, vol. 300, pp. 127–132, 1994.

[5] K. Andersen, P. O. Jensen, and J. Lauritzen, "Treatment of clavicular fractures: figure-of-eight bandage versus a simple sling," *Acta Orthopaedica Scandinavica*, vol. 58, no. 1, pp. 71–74, 1987.

[6] C. S. Neer, "Nonunion of the clavicle," *Journal of the American Medical Association*, vol. 172, pp. 1006–1011, 1960.

[7] C. M. Robinson and D. A. Cairns, "Primary nonoperative treatment of displaced lateral fractures of the clavicle," *Journal of Bone and Joint Surgery A*, vol. 86, pp. 1359–1365, 2004.

[8] C. R. Rowe, "An atlas of anatomy and treatment of midclavicular fractures," *Clinical Orthopaedics and Related Research*, vol. 58, pp. 29–42, 1968.

[9] M. D. McKee, L. M. Wild, and E. H. Schemitsch, "Midshaft malunions of the clavicle," *Journal of Bone and Joint Surgery A*, vol. 85, no. 5, pp. 790–797, 2003.

[10] M. Zlowodzki, B. A. Zelle, P. A. Cole, K. Jeray, and M. D. McKee, "Treatment of acute midshaft clavicle fractures: systematic review of 2144 fractures. On behalf of the Evidence-Based Orthopaedic Trauma Working Group," *Journal of Orthopaedic Trauma*, vol. 19, no. 7, pp. 504–508, 2005.

[11] M. R. Brinker, T. B. Edwards, D. P. O'Connor, and C. M. Robinson, "Estimating the risk of nonunion following nonoperative treatment of a clavicular fracture," *Journal of Bone and Joint Surgery A*, vol. 87, no. 3, pp. 676–677, 2005.

[12] J. M. Hill, M. H. McGuire, and L. A. Crosby, "Closed treatment of displaced middle-third fractures of the clavicle gives poor results," *Journal of Bone and Joint Surgery B*, vol. 79, no. 4, pp. 537–541, 1997.

[13] D. B. Judd, M. P. Pallis, E. Smith, and C. R. Bottoni, "Acute operative stabilization versus nonoperative management of clavicle fractures," *American Journal of Orthopedics*, vol. 38, no. 7, pp. 341–345, 2009.

[14] V. Kulshrestha, T. Roy, and L. Audige, "Operative versus nonoperative management of displaced midshaft clavicle fractures: a prospective cohort study," *Journal of Orthopaedic Trauma*, vol. 25, no. 1, pp. 31–38, 2011.

[15] J. Nowak, M. Holgersson, and S. Larsson, "Sequelae from clavicular fractures are common: a prospective study of 222 patients," *Acta Orthopaedica*, vol. 76, no. 4, pp. 496–502, 2005.

[16] V. Smekal, A. Irenberger, P. Struve, M. Wambacher, D. Krappinger, and F. S. Kralinger, "Elastic stable intramedullary nailing versus nonoperative treatment of displaced midshaft clavicular fractures: a randomized, controlled, clinical trial," *Journal of Orthopaedic Trauma*, vol. 23, no. 2, pp. 106–112, 2009.

[17] Canadian Orthopaedic Trauma Society, "Nonoperative treatment compared with plate fixation of displaced midshaft clavicular fractures," *Journal of Bone and Joint Surgery*, vol. 89, pp. 1–10, 2007.

[18] K. Y. Chan, J. B. Jupiter, R. D. Leffert, and R. Marti, "Clavicle malunion," *Journal of Shoulder and Elbow Surgery*, vol. 8, no. 4, pp. 287–290, 1999.

[19] M. D. McKee, E. M. Pedersen, C. Jones et al., "Deficits following nonoperative treatment of displaced midshaft clavicular fractures," *Journal of Bone and Joint Surgery A*, vol. 88, no. 1, pp. 35–40, 2006.

[20] E. J. Zenni, J. K. Krieg, and M. J. Rosen, "Open reduction and internal fixation of clavicular fractures," *Journal of Bone and Joint Surgery A*, vol. 63, no. 1, pp. 147–151, 1981.

[21] M. D. McKee, J. G. Seiler, and J. B. Jupiter, "The application of the limited contact dynamic compression plate in the upper extremity: an analysis of 114 consecutive cases," *Injury*, vol. 26, no. 10, pp. 661–666, 1995.

[22] D. Boehme, R. J. Curtis Jr., J. T. DeHaan, S. P. Kay, D. C. Young, and C. A. Rockwood Jr., "Non-union of fractures of the mid-shaft of the clavicle. Treatment with a modified Hagie intramedullary pin and autogenous bone-grafting," *Journal of Bone and Joint Surgery A*, vol. 73, no. 8, pp. 1219–1225, 1991.

[23] C. Chu, S. Wang, and L. Lin, "Fixation of mid-third clavicular fractures with knowles pins: 78 patients followed for 2–7 years," *Acta Orthopaedica Scandinavica*, vol. 73, no. 2, pp. 134–139, 2002.

[24] C. D. Mudd, K. J. Quigley, and L. B. Gross, "Excessive complications of open intramedullary nailing of midshaft clavicle fractures with the Rockwood Clavicle Pin," *Clinical Orthopaedics and Related Research*, vol. 469, no. 12, pp. 3364–3370, 2011.

[25] E. J. Strauss, K. A. Egol, M. A. France, K. J. Koval, and J. D. Zuckerman, "Complications of intramedullary Hagie pin fixation for acute midshaft clavicle fractures," *Journal of Shoulder and Elbow Surgery*, vol. 16, no. 3, pp. 280–284, 2007.

[26] F. A. Grassi, M. S. Tajana, and F. D'Angelo, "Management of midclavicular fractures: comparison between nonoperative treatment and open intramedullary fixation in 80 patients," *Journal of Trauma*, vol. 50, no. 6, pp. 1096–1100, 2001.

[27] M. Mueller, C. Rangger, N. Striepens, and C. Burger, "Minimally invasive intramedullary nailing of midshaft clavicular fractures using titanium elastic nails," *The Journal of Trauma*, vol. 64, no. 6, pp. 1528–1534, 2008.

[28] M. R. Iannotti, L. A. Crosby, P. Stafford, G. Grayson, and R. Goulet, "Effects of plate location and selection on the stability of midshaft clavicle osteotomies: a biomechanical study," *Journal of Shoulder and Elbow Surgery*, vol. 11, no. 5, pp. 457–462, 2002.

[29] C. Robertson, P. Celestre, A. Mahar, and A. Schwartz, "Reconstruction plates for stabilization of mid-shaft clavicle fractures: Ddifferences between nonlocked and locked plates in two different positions," *Journal of Shoulder and Elbow Surgery*, vol. 18, no. 2, pp. 204–209, 2009.

[30] J. I. Huang, P. Toogood, M. R. Chen, J. H. Wilber, and D. R. Cooperman, "Clavicular anatomy and the applicability of precontoured plates," *Journal of Bone and Joint Surgery A*, vol. 89, no. 10, pp. 2260–2265, 2007.

[31] C. Collinge, S. Devinney, D. Herscovici, T. DePasquale, and R. Sanders, "Anterior-inferior plate fixation of middle-third fractures and nonunions of the clavicle," *Journal of Orthopaedic Trauma*, vol. 20, no. 10, pp. 680–686, 2006.

[32] J. Poigenfurst, G. Rappold, and W. Fischer, "Plating of fresh clavicular fractures: results of 122 operations," *Injury*, vol. 23, no. 4, pp. 237–241, 1992.

[33] C. P. Kleweno, A. Jawa, J. H. Wells et al., "Midshaft clavicular fractures: comparison of intramedullary pin and plate fixation," *Journal of Shoulder and Elbow Surgery*, vol. 20, no. 7, pp. 1114–1117, 2011.

[34] J. L. Marsh, T. F. Slongo, J. Agel et al., "Fracture and dislocation classification compendium—2007: Orthopaedic Trauma Association Classification, Database and Outcomes Committee," *Journal of Orthopaedic Trauma*, vol. 21, supplement 10, pp. S1–S133, 2007.

[35] C. VanBeek, K. J. Boselli, E. R. Cadet, C. S. Ahmad, and W. N. Levine, "Precontoured plating of clavicle fractures: decreased hardware-related complications?" *Clinical Orthopaedics and Related Research*, vol. 469, no. 12, pp. 3337–3343, 2011.

[36] T. Harnroongroj and Y. Jeerathanyasakun, "Intramedullary pin fixation in clavicular fractures: a study comparing the use of small and large pins," *Journal of Orthopaedic Surgery*, vol. 8, no. 2, pp. 7–11, 2000.

[37] M. Demirhan, K. Bilsel, A. C. Atalar, E. Bozdag, E. Sunbuloglu, and A. Kale, "Biomechanical comparison of fixation techniques in midshaft clavicular fractures," *Journal of Orthopaedic Trauma*, vol. 25, no. 5, pp. 272–278, 2011.

[38] D. S. Drosdowech, S. E. E. Manwell, L. M. Ferreira, D. P. Goel, K. J. Faber, and J. A. Johnson, "Biomechanical analysis of fixation of middle third fractures of the clavicle," *Journal of Orthopaedic Trauma*, vol. 25, no. 1, pp. 39–43, 2011.

[39] T. Renfree, B. Conrad, and T. Wright, "Biomechanical comparison of contemporary clavicle fixation devices," *Journal of Hand Surgery*, vol. 35, no. 4, pp. 639–644, 2010.

[40] O. Böstman, M. Manninen, and H. Pihlajamäki, "Complications of plate fixation in fresh displaced midclavicular fractures," *The Journal of Trauma*, vol. 43, no. 5, pp. 778–783, 1997.

16

Clinical and Radiographic Outcomes with a Hydroxyapatite and Porous Coated Cup Design

John Wang, James DiPietro, Mathias Bostrom, Bryan Nestor, Douglas Padgett, and Geoffrey Westrich

Hospital for Special Surgery, 535 East 70th Street, New York, NY 10021, USA

Correspondence should be addressed to Geoffrey Westrich; westrichg@hss.edu

Academic Editor: Neal L. Millar

Press-fit, hydroxyapatite-coated acetabular cup designs may offer a lower incidence of loosening and migration than older designs. Our study evaluated the initial clinical and radiographic success of a cementless acetabular shell in a large cohort of primary total hip arthroplasty (THA) patients. We queried our institution's prospectively collected registry for a series of 771 primary THAs (695 patients) implanted with this cup by 4 high-volume arthroplasty surgeons. Of the 613 hips with minimum 2-year followup, average HHS (Harris Hip Score) was 93.6, WOMAC (Western Ontario and McMaster Universities Osteoarthritis Index) was 87.6, and VAS (Visual Analog Scale) pain score was 1.2. While there was a 2% reoperation rate (12 hips), none of the cups were revised for aseptic loosening. No radiolucencies were found and there was no evidence of acetabular loosening. At early followup, this newer cementless acetabular cup implant design exhibits high survivorship and clinical success.

1. Introduction

When cementless acetabular cups were initially introduced in primary total hip arthroplasty (THA), studies showed mixed clinical outcomes, with problems such as failure of the locking system of the liner and the thinness of the polyethylene. Newer generations of press-fit acetabular components have been used with increasing frequency and high success rates [1–3]. Its advantages over previous generation cementless cup designs include the elimination of screw/cup fretting and corrosion, decreased neurovascular injury risk, and elimination of screw holes. Mid- and long-term studies have shown it to have favorably low rates of osteolysis and loosening [4–15].

However, in an effort to improve on the performance of press-fit cups, attention has turned towards the use of hydroxyapatite coating (HA) in conjunction with the porous coating found on most commercially available acetabular cups. Previous designs of HA-coated acetabular shells have shown mixed results at mid-term followup [3]. Studies have demonstrated that HA-coated, porous acetabular components significantly enhanced bone ongrowth in the presence of wear particles, preventing migration and reducing osteolysis [16]. HA-coated porous and sintered beaded components provided a more effective seal against the ingress of wear debris when compared with cemented cups [1]. However, other studies have shown that HA-coating has no effect on the revision rate of cementless cups [17]. Some of the unfavorable results could be attributed to manufacturing techniques such as the quality of powder, roughness of implants, method of spray coating, and the thickness of coating.

In this study, we report on a large, retrospective consecutive series of the Stryker Trident acetabular shell (Stryker Orthopedics, Mahwah, NJ). The Trident shell is a press-fit, porous, HA-coated acetabular design. We hypothesized that this newer cementless shell design would lead to excellent bone ongrowth and patient outcomes at early followup.

2. Materials and Methods

We queried our prospectively collected registry for a consecutive series of 771 primary total hip arthroplasties in 695 patients implanted with a Stryker Trident acetabular shell

TABLE 1: Published data on outcomes of similar cementless primary THAs.

Manuscript	Implant used	Number of hips	Mean age	Mean Followup (years)	Revision (acetabular aseptic loosening)	Revision (all cause)	Dislocation	Osteolysis
Anseth et al. (2010) [18]	Harris-Galante I/II	113	54	17.2	2 (1.8%)	4 (3.5%)	NR	2 (1.8%)
Baker et al. (2010) [19]	ABG I	69	53	15	8 (11.6%)	8 (11.6%)	0	10 (14.5%)
Belmont et al. (2008) [12]	Trispike (DePuy)	223	71.8	20	9 (4%)	26 (11.7%)	1 (0.45%)	17 (7.6%)
Della Valle et al. (2009) [13]	Harris-Galante I	204	52	20.6	5 (4%)	10 (8.1%)	5/124	NR
Chen et al. (2006) [20]	Duraloc	145	56.2	6.7	0 (0%)	2 (1.4%)	9/148 (6.1%)	3 (2%)
Streit et al. (2012) [21]	Fitmore	89	49	12	0 (0%)	5/81, 2 liner exchange	1/81	0 (0%)
Berli et al. (2007) [22]	Morscher	112		14.7	2.5%	4.7%		
Della Valle et al. (2004) [23]	Trilogy	308	64	4–7	1 (0.3%)	8 (2.4%)	NR	12 (5%)
Sugano et al. (2012) [24]	Biolox forte	93	56	12.4	1 (1.1%)	2 (2.2%) (cup only)	1 (1.1%)	0 (0%)
de Witte et al. (2011) [25]	CementLess Spotorno	102	55.9	11.8	9 (8.8%)	10 (cup)	NR	NR
Stefl et al. (2012) [26]	Harris-Galante I	120	NR	23.3	1 (0.8%)	22 (18.3%)	NR	8 (6.7%)
Gottliebsen et al. (2012) [27]	Mallory-Head	77 HA coated 73 non-HA coated	57 (HA) 63 (non-HA)	11	HA coated: 0 (0%) Non-HA coated: 7 (9.6%)	HA coated: 0% Non-HA: 9.6%	NR	NR

during the period of January 2006 to December 2007. The Stryker Trident acetabular shell is manufactured of titanium with an improved locking mechanism and a hydroxyapatite outer coating to improve bony ongrowth and incorporation. The standard technique utilized for cup implantation was line to line reaming since the cup outer diameter is approximately 1.7 mm larger than the base diameter with the HA-coating.

The surgeries were performed by the four senior authors (Mathias Bostrom, Bryan Nestor, Douglas Padgett, and Geoffrey Westrich), who are all high-volume arthroplasty surgeons. All patients underwent a combination of spinal and epidural anesthesia for postoperative pain management. Patients were placed in a lateral decubitus position with the operative side facing up, and all surgeries were done using a standard posterolateral approach with soft tissue repair. Exclusion criteria barred patients that had undergone revision hip surgery and that had less than 2-year followup from our study.

Diagnosis, age, gender, implant data, postoperative complications, and revisions were collected for all patients with a minimum followup of two years. Clinical outcome measures included HHS, WOMAC, and VAS pain scores preoperatively, at 6 weeks after surgery, and annually thereafter. Radiographic analysis was performed to assess cup position and radiolucencies. Radiographic analysis was conducted by an orthopedic surgery fellow in adult reconstruction (John Wang). Osteointegration of the acetabular component was evaluated by assessing bony ongrowth on two orthogonal X-ray views, namely, the AP pelvis and Lowenstein's cross-table lateral views. Clinical and radiographic findings were compared to published data on outcomes of similar cementless primary THAs (Table 1).

3. Results

In this patient cohort, the main indications for primary hip replacement were osteoarthritis, avascular necrosis, and post-traumatic arthritis; however, a detailed list of preoperative diagnoses is available in Table 2. During the study period, 30 patients out of the 771-patient cohort died, leaving 741 hips for analysis. Of this group, 613 hips had completed two-year minimum follow-up visits (83% followup), and the average followup was 3 years (range 2–5.1 years; median 2.95 years). Of the 613 patients in the final study group, 349 patients had right hip replacements and 264 had left hip replacements. In addition, there were 319 women and 294 men in the remaining study cohort. A polyethylene liner was used in 64% of the acetabular shells and a ceramic liner was used in the remaining 36% of shells.

TABLE 2: Detailed list of preoperative diagnoses.

Diagnosis	Number of patients
Osteoarthritis	671
Avascular necrosis	28
Posttraumatic arthritis	21
Childhood hip problem	15
Dysplasia	12
Rheumatoid arthritis	9
Osteonecrosis	6
Hip fracture	5
Multiple epiphyseal dysplasia	2
Septic arthritis	1
Paget's disease	1

At the latest followup the clinical outcomes were excellent, with an average HHS score of 93.6 (31–100), an average WOMAC score of 87.6 (13–100), and an average VAS pain score of only 1.2 (0–10). No differences in outcomes scores on the HHS/WOMAC/or VAS were noted between the patients that received polyethylene or ceramic liners ($P < 0.05$).

The overall reoperation rate was 2% or (12/613) with 12 hips requiring reoperation. The reasons for revision were as follows: 7 instability (1.14%), 3 periprosthetic fractures (0.49%), 1 infection (0.16%), and 1 heterotopic ossification (0.16%). The seven cases of instability were all treated with revision to a constrained acetabular liner from the same manufacturer. The three cases of periprosthetic fracture all involved the femur and none of the fractures involved the acetabular component. The femur fractures were treated with open reduction and internal fixation. The one revision for infection was treated with a two-stage protocol. The first stage involved explantation of the prosthesis with an extensive debridement and insertion of an antibiotic impregnated cement spacer followed by six weeks of intravenous antibiotics. The second stage involved a reimplantation of a new prosthesis. The one revision for heterotopic ossification involved repeat arthrotomy of the hip joint with excision of the heterotopic bone to improve range of motion followed by postoperative radiation treatment. No revisions were performed for aseptic loosening of the acetabular component during our study. Mean abduction and anteversion angles at latest followup were 45.7 degrees (std. dev. ±6.6) and 24.5 degrees (std. dev. ±7.9), respectively. Radiographic analysis of AP pelvis X-rays revealed no radiolucencies at the bone-implant interface and no evidence of loosening or cup migration.

4. Discussion

Since the introduction of cemented total hip arthroplasties, attention has been focused on improving the mechanical failure rates of acetabular components. While early followup of cemented acetabular components was favorable, longer followups showed increased failure and loosening rates [4–6]. Earlier uncemented designs focused on initial mechanical fixation and stability of the acetabular components to the pelvis. However, high failure rates were evident with followup due to lack of osteointegration [7–9]. Newer acetabular shell designs featuring press-fit for initial mechanical stability and porous-coating for osteointegration have shown improved failure rates at mid- and long-term followups [10–12]. More recently, hydroxyapatite coating has been added to the porous coating in an attempt to improve on the biological fixation. Calcium hydroxyapatite is a naturally occurring substance found in bone and enamel and has been used clinically for over 30 years. It is well accepted that HA exhibits osteoconductive properties which improves early bone ongrowth and mechanical fixation of implants [15]. Hydroxyapatite's purported benefits include better and faster bone ongrowth, the formation of a barrier against wear debris, and allowing for less intimate fit between the cup and the acetabulum for ongrowth. While acetabular designs involving smooth surfaces and HA-coating have shown high early failure rates [13–15], numerous short-term studies have indicated that HA is capable of reducing early migration of the components as compared to the uncoated implants [28, 29]. A few longer-term studies have shown high clinical survival rates with no radiographic signs of failure in revision settings at mid-term followup [30–32]. However, longer-term follow-up studies are sparse, and concerns remain about HA-coated acetabular implants.

This study demonstrates excellent clinical and radiographic results with a contemporary press-fit acetabular component with an HA-coating. Our results compare favorably with the results of other studies from manufacturers with similar uncemented contemporary acetabular shells such as the Trilogy and Duraloc (see Table 1). Our 1.8% revision rate was unrelated to the fixation of the cup and at latest followup, all the Trident acetabular shells had excellent osteointegration to the acetabulum with no radiographic evidence of radiolucencies or cup migration.

5. Conclusions

In this study, a large cohort was able to be retrospectively reviewed. The results at short-term followup showed no radiographic or clinical evidence of failure or loosening. All revisions were performed for reasons other than failure or loosening. Although the length of followup is short, the early results are very encouraging. No early failure mechanisms or causes for concern were identified. Although our short-term results were promising, we clearly advocate further long-term follow-up studies of this patient cohort.

Conflict of Interests

Geoffrey Westrich is a Consultant for Stryker Orthopedics.

References

[1] D. P. Gwynne-Jones, N. Garneti, C. Wainwright, J. A. Matheson, and R. King, "The Morscher press fit acetabular component: a nine- to 13-year review," *Journal of Bone & Joint Surgery B*, vol. 91, no. 7, pp. 859–864, 2009.

[2] R. T. Spak and S. A. Stuchin, "Cementless porous-coated sockets without holes implanted with pure press-fit technique: average 6-year follow-up," *Journal of Arthroplasty*, vol. 20, no. 1, pp. 4–10, 2005.

[3] G. P. Grobler, I. D. Learmonth, B. P. Bernstein, and B. J. Dower, "Ten-years results of a press-fit, porous-coated acetabular component," *Journal of Bone & Joint Surgery B*, vol. 87, no. 6, pp. 786–789, 2005.

[4] A. Paulsen, A. B. Pedersen, S. P. Johnsen, A. Riis, U. Lucht, and S. Overgaard, "Effect of hydroxyapatite coating on risk of revision after primary total hip arthroplasty in younger patients: findings from the Danish Hip Arthroplasty Registry," *Acta Orthopaedica*, vol. 78, no. 5, pp. 622–628, 2007.

[5] M. J. Coathup, J. Blackburn, A. E. Goodship, J. L. Cunningham, T. Smith, and G. W. Blunn, "Role of hydroxyapatite coating in resisting wear particle migration and osteolysis around acetabular components," *Biomaterials*, vol. 26, no. 19, pp. 4161–4169, 2005.

[6] K. R. Schulte, J. J. Callaghan, S. S. Kelley, and R. C. Johnston, "The outcome of Charnley total hip arthroplasty with cement after a minimum twenty-year follow-up. The results of one surgeon," *Journal of Bone & Joint Surgery A*, vol. 75, no. 7, pp. 961–975, 1993.

[7] S. M. Madey, J. J. Callaghan, J. P. Olejniczak, D. D. Goetz, and R. C. Johnston, "Charnley total hip arthroplasty with use of improved techniques of cementing. The results after a minimum of fifteen years of follow-up," *Journal of Bone & Joint Surgery A*, vol. 79, no. 1, pp. 53–64, 1997.

[8] W. F. Mulroy, D. M. Estok, and W. H. Harris, "Total hip arthroplasty with use of so-called second-generation cementing techniques. A fifteen-year-average follow-up study," *Journal of Bone & Joint Surgery A*, vol. 77, no. 12, pp. 1845–1852, 1995.

[9] C. A. Engh, W. L. Griffin, and C. L. Marx, "Cementless acetabular components," *Journal of Bone & Joint Surgery B*, vol. 72, no. 1, pp. 53–59, 1990.

[10] W. N. Capello, R. A. Colyer, C. B. Kernek, J. V. Carnahan, and J. J. Hess, "Failure of the Mecron screw-in ring," *Journal of Bone & Joint Surgery B*, vol. 75, no. 5, pp. 835–836, 1993.

[11] J. D. Bruijn, J. L. Seelen, R. M. Feenstra, B. E. Hansen, and F. P. Bernoski, "Failure of the Mecring screw-ring acetabular component in total hip arthroplasty. A three to seven year follow-up study," *Journal of Bone & Joint Surgery A*, vol. 77, no. 5, pp. 760–766, 1995.

[12] P. J. Belmont Jr., C. C. Powers, S. E. Beykirch, R. H. Hopper Jr., C. A. Engh Jr., and C. A. Engh, "Results of the anatomic medullary locking total hip arthroplasty at a minimum of twenty years: a concise follow-up of previous reports," *Journal of Bone & Joint Surgery A*, vol. 90, no. 7, pp. 1524–1530, 2008.

[13] C. J. Della Valle, N. W. Mesko, L. Quigley, A. G. Rosenberg, J. J. Jacobs, and J. O. Galante, "Primary total hip arthroplasty with a porous-coated acetabular component: a concise follow-up, at a minimum of twenty years, of previous reports," *Journal of Bone & Joint Surgery A*, vol. 91, no. 5, pp. 1130–1135, 2009.

[14] M. Al Muderis, U. Bohling, U. Grittner, L. Gerdesmeyer, and J. Scholz, "Cementless total hip arthroplasty using the spongiosa-I fully coated cancellous metal surface: a minimum twenty-year follow-up," *Journal of Bone & Joint Surgery A*, vol. 93, no. 11, pp. 1039–1044, 2011.

[15] W. N. Capello, J. A. D'Antonio, M. T. Manley, and J. R. Feinberg, "Hydroxyapatite in total hip arthroplasty. Clinical results and critical issues," *Clinical Orthopaedics and Related Research*, no. 355, pp. 200–211, 1998.

[16] T. V. Swanson, "Early results of 1000 consecutive, posterior, single-incision minimally invasive surgery total hip arthroplasties," *Journal of Arthroplasty*, vol. 20, no. 7, supplement 3, pp. 26–32, 2005.

[17] L. D. Dorr, Z. Wan, M. Song, and A. Ranawat, "Bilateral total hip arthroplasty comparing hydroxyapatite coating to porous-coated fixation," *Journal of Arthroplasty*, vol. 13, no. 7, pp. 729–736, 1998.

[18] S. D. Anseth, P. A. Pulido, W. S. Adelson, S. Patil, J. C. Sandwell, and C. W. Colwell, "Fifteen-year to twenty-year results of cementless Harris-Galante porous femoral and Harris-Galante porous I and II acetabular components," *Journal of Arthroplasty*, vol. 25, no. 5, pp. 867–691, 2010.

[19] P. N. Baker, I. A. McMurtry, G. Chuter, A. Port, and J. Anderson, "THA with the ABG I prosthesis at 15 years: excellent survival with minimal osteolysis," *Clinical Orthopaedics and Related Research*, vol. 468, no. 7, pp. 1855–1861, 2010.

[20] C. J. Chen, J. S. Xenos, J. P. McAuley, A. Young, and C. A. Engh Sr., "Second-generation porous-coated cementless total hip arthroplasties have high survival," *Clinical Orthopaedics and Related Research*, vol. 451, pp. 121–127, 2006.

[21] M. R. Streit, K. Schröder, M. Körber et al., "High survival in young patients using a second generation uncemented total hip replacement," *International Orthopaedics*, vol. 36, no. 6, pp. 1129–1136, 2012.

[22] B. J. Berli, G. Ping, W. Dick, and E. W. Morscher, "Nonmodular flexible press-fit cup in primary total hip arthroplasty: 15-year followup," *Clinical Orthopaedics and Related Research*, vol. 461, pp. 114–121, 2007.

[23] A. G. Della Valle, A. Zoppi, M. G. E. Peterson, and E. A. Salvati, "Clinical and radiographic results associated with a modern, cementless modular cup design in total hip arthroplasty," *Journal of Bone & Joint Surgery A*, vol. 86, no. 9, pp. 1998–2003, 2004.

[24] N. Sugano, M. Takao, T. Sakai, T. Nishii, H. Miki, and K. Ohzono, "Eleven- to 14-year follow-up results of cementless total hip arthroplasty using a third-generation alumina ceramic-on-ceramic bearing," *Journal of Arthroplasty*, vol. 27, no. 5, pp. 736–741, 2012.

[25] P. B. de Witte, R. Brand, H. G. W. Vermeer, H. J. L. van der Heide, and A. F. W. Barnaart, "Mid-term results of total hip arthroplasty with the CementLess Spotorno (CLS) system," *Journal of Bone & Joint Surgery A*, vol. 93, no. 13, pp. 1249–1255, 2011.

[26] M. D. Stefl, J. J. Callaghan, S. S. Liu, D. R. Pedersen, R. C. Johnston, and D. D. Goetz, "Primary cementless acetabular fixation at a minimum of twenty years of follow-up: a concise update of a previous report," *Journal of Bone & Joint Surgery A*, vol. 94, no. 3, pp. 234–239, 2012.

[27] M. Gottliebsen, O. Rahbek, P. F. Ottosen, K. Søballe, and M. Stilling, "Superior 11-year survival but higher polyethylene wear of hydroxyapatite-coated Mallory-Head cups," *HIP International*, vol. 22, no. 1, pp. 35–40, 2012.

[28] M. T. Manley, W. N. Capello, J. A. D'Antonio, A. A. Edidin, and R. G. T. Geesink, "Fixation of acetabular cups without cement in total hip arthroplasty. A comparison of three different implant surfaces at a minimum duration of follow-up of five years," *Journal of Bone & Joint Surgery A*, vol. 80, no. 8, pp. 1175–1185, 1998.

[29] J. Thanner, J. Kärrholm, P. Herberts, and H. Malchau, "Porous cups with and without hydroxylapatite-tricalcium phosphate

coating: 23 matched pairs evaluated with radiostereometry," *Journal of Arthroplasty*, vol. 14, no. 3, pp. 266–271, 1999.

[30] S. D. Cook, K. A. Thomas, J. E. Dalton, T. K. Volkman, T. S. Whitecloud III, and J. F. Kay, "Hydroxylapatite coating of porous implants improves bone ingrowth and interface attachment strength," *Journal of Biomedical Materials Research*, vol. 26, no. 8, pp. 989–1001, 1992.

[31] A. Dorairajan, R. M. Reddy, and S. Krikler, "Outcome of acetabular revision using an uncemented hydroxyapatite-coated component: two- to five-year results and review," *Journal of Arthroplasty*, vol. 20, no. 2, pp. 209–218, 2005.

[32] W. L. Jaffe, H. B. Morris, J. P. Nessler, M. Naughton, and J. Shen, "Hydroxylapatite-coated acetabular shells with arc deposited titanium surface roughening and dual radius design," *Bulletin of the NYU Hospital for Joint Diseases*, vol. 65, no. 4, pp. 257–262, 2007.

17

The Biological Effects of Combining Metals in a Posterior Spinal Implant: *In Vivo* Model Development Report of the First Two Cases

Christine L. Farnsworth,[1] Peter O. Newton,[1,2] Eric Breisch,[3] Michael T. Rohmiller,[1] Jung Ryul Kim,[4] and Behrooz A. Akbarnia[2,5]

[1] *Division of Orthopedics, Rady Children's Hospital-San Diego, 3020 Children's Way, MC 5054, San Diego, CA 92123, USA*
[2] *Department of Orthopaedic Surgery, University of California San Diego, San Diego, CA 92103, USA*
[3] *Department of Pathology, Rady Children's Hospital San Diego, San Diego, CA 92123, USA*
[4] *Department of Orthopaedic Surgery, Chonbuk National University Hospital, Jeonbuk 561-712, Republic of Korea*
[5] *San Diego Center for Spinal Disorders, La Jolla, CA 92037, USA*

Correspondence should be addressed to Christine L. Farnsworth; cfarnsworth@rchsd.org

Academic Editor: Federico Canavese

Study Design. Combinations of metal implants (stainless steel (SS), titanium (Ti), and cobalt chrome (CC)) were placed in porcine spines. After 12 months, tissue response and implant corrosion were compared between mixed and single metal junctions. *Objective.* Model development and an attempt to determine any detriment of combining different metals in posterior spinal instrumentation. *Methods.* Yucatan mini-pigs underwent instrumentation over five unfused lumbar levels. A SS rod and a Ti rod were secured with Ti and SS pedicle screws, SS and Ti crosslinks, SS and CC sublaminar wires, and Ti sublaminar cable. The resulting 4 SS/SS, 3 Ti/Ti, and 11 connections between dissimilar metals per animal were studied after 12 months using radiographs, gross observation, and histology (foreign body reaction (FBR), metal particle count, and inflammation analyzed). *Results.* Two animals had constructs in place for 12 months with no complications. Histology of tissue over SS/SS connections demonstrated 11.1 ± 7.6 FBR cells, 2.1 ± 1.7 metal particles, and moderate to extensive inflammation. Ti/Ti tissue showed 6.3 ± 3.8 FBR cells, 5.2 ± 6.7 particles, and no to extensive inflammation (83% extensive). Tissue over mixed components had 14.1 ± 12.6 FBR cells and 13.4 ± 27.8 particles. Samples surrounding wires/cables versus other combinations demonstrated FBR (12.4 ± 13.5 versus 12.0 ± 9.6 cells, $P = 0.96$), particles (19.8 ± 32.6 versus 4.3 ± 12.7, $P = 0.24$), and inflammation (50% versus 75% extensive, $P = 0.12$). *Conclusions.* A nonfusion model was developed to study corrosion and analyze biological responses. Although no statistical differences were found in overlying tissue response to single versus mixed metal combinations, galvanic corrosion between differing metals is not ruled out. This pilot study supports further investigation to answer concerns when mixing metals in spinal constructs.

1. Introduction

Metal spinal implants are not routinely removed, so corrosion over potentially several decades is a concern [1, 2]. Any movement between metal surfaces, even on the microscopic level, results in etching of the softer surface and often produces wear debris. As the metallic debris oxidizes or corrodes, the particles harden, causing abrasion and more severe etching, resulting in a cycle of implant destruction. Corrosion complications in spinal surgery are related to both loss of implant integrity and biological responses and include infection, toxicity, deterioration of construct strength, and pain [3]. Spine surgeons have experience with visualizing debris and darkened tissue surrounding implants that have been removed routinely or due to a clinical concern [4–6]. There is certainly the potential of motion existing between metal components of a construct designed to stabilize a spine following surgical intervention, both before a bony fusion is complete and following bony healing. Concern of corrosion increases when mixing two different metals in a biological, electrolytic system where an oxidation reaction, boosted by temperature, creates the ideal environment for galvanic corrosion. With the increased clinical use of titanium (Ti) and potential use of Ti in combination with existing stainless steel (SS) implants, there is increased concern amongst surgeons of galvanic corrosion related to mixing these metal classes. In addition to the concern of fretting corrosion caused by micromotion between components, galvanic corrosion could potentially occur within a spinal implant where SS or chromium (serving as an anode) is in physical contact with Ti (the cathode) within an *in vivo* environment acting as a conducting electrolyte.

Clinical studies of corrosion of explanted spinal implants as well as animal model studies including tissue response at metal junctions have been done [5–12]. A general consensus seems to have been reached that SS implants have a more significant risk of corrosion than Ti; however, in these investigations all components were of a single metal (SS or Ti). Clinical studies and reviews still tend to advise against mixing metal materials and those with different surface finishes [11, 13]. *In vitro* studies of spinal constructs including both SS and Ti components following cyclical mechanical testing at biological temperatures in either serum or saline solutions suggest that corrosion in SS-Ti interfaces is the same [14] or even less [15] than in SS only. Other *in vitro* studies using similar biological environments have been shown to produce similar levels of corrosion in mixed metal components as in an *in vivo* environment [16]. However, *in vitro* studies cannot elucidate any information about tissue response to corrosion. Metal particulate (Ti) placed at the level of a spinal arthrodesis in an *in vivo* model (rabbit) has been shown to increase cellular inflammatory response, osteoclastic response, and osteolysis [9, 10]; however, implants were not available to be evaluated for corresponding corrosion. There are no known studies showing corrosive effects on implants at metallic junctions and overlying *in vivo* tissue response to spinal implants composed of different metals. This study evaluated implants and the surrounding tissue of mixed versus single metal combinations (Ti and SS rods with SS, cobalt chrome (CC) and Ti sublaminar wires, SS and Ti cross links, and SS and Ti screws with SS and Ti connectors) twelve months following posterior spinal instrumentation using a Yucatan minipig model.

2. Materials and Methods

The institutional animal care and use committee approved and provided oversight for this study. Seven Yucatan minipigs approaching the age of skeletal maturity (12–14 months of age, 26–49 kg, and two female and five male) were acquired and housed for at least one week preoperatively to acclimate. Mini-pigs were housed both pre- and postoperatively in controlled climate inside individual pens.

2.1. Surgical Protocol. To assure adequate surgical analgesic plasma levels, twelve to nineteen hours prior to surgery, a patch of skin between the shoulder blades of the animal was clipped, swabbed with alcohol, and a fentanyl transdermal patch (100 micrograms/hour) was affixed. The patch was left in place until three to four days post-op. Any breakthrough pain was treated with buprenorphine, 0.01 mg/kg IM.

Animals were deprived from solid food for twelve to fifteen hours prior to surgery (water remained available *ad lib*) to decrease aspiration risk. The mini-pigs were weighed immediately prior to the surgical procedure and sedated by an intramuscular (IM) injection into the neck muscles behind an ear of a cocktail of 25 mg/kg ketamine, 2 mg/kg xylazine, and 0.05 mg/kg atropine. Once sedated, the animals were placed prone for dorsoventral (DV) and laterally recumbent on the left side for lateral radiographs, and then they were shaved over the lower back and grounding pad site. Preoperative antibiotics consisted of IM cefazolin (1 gram) given 30 minutes prior to surgery for wound prophylaxis. A maintenance infusion of lactated Ringer's solution was given at a rate of 5–10 cc/kg/hr through an over-the-needle catheter placed in an ear vein. Induction began with propofol, 2 mg/kg, administered through the intravenous line. Direct laryngoscopy to intubate the trachea using a 6.0 or 6.5 mm inner diameter, cuffed endotracheal tube was performed. After securing the endotracheal tube, mechanical ventilation was started and anesthesia was maintained with volatilized isoflurane (1.5–3%). Following this, each animal was positioned in the prone (or dorsal) position and the lower back prepped with betadine. A transcutaneous pulse oximeter was applied to the tongue or ear, a rectal probe was inserted to monitor temperature, and a heating blanket was applied to maintain normothermia. Heart rate, oxygen saturation, and temperature were constantly monitored.

Following achievement of an adequate level of anesthesia, a posterior approach was used to visualize the lower thoracic and entire lumbar spine using sterile surgical techniques. Instrumentation sites were prepared over five levels. All SS and Ti implants were commercially available for spine surgery (DePuy Spine, Inc, Raynham, MA), but the CC wires were experimental. The appropriate rod length was measured and one 4.75 mm Ti rod and one 4.75 mm SS rod were cut and placed adjacent to the spinous process (SS on the left and Ti on the right side, Figure 1, where L1 refers to the most proximal surgical vertebral level and L5, the most distal). No attempt was made to bend the rods to match the natural sagittal contour of the spines. Rods were secured in place with the following construct: Ti pedicle screw (4.75 mm × 25 mm long) at Level 1 with Ti offset connector on the left and SS connector on the right, SS cross link at Level 1-2, SS sublaminar wire (18 gauge, or 1.0 mm diameter) at Level 2, a single Ti sublaminar cable (1.0 mm diameter) at Level 3, CC sublaminar wire (MP35N, 1.0 mm diameter) at Level 4, Ti cross link at Level 4-5, and SS pedicle screw (4.75 mm × 25 mm long) at Level 5. All sublaminar wires and cables were placed from distal to proximal around the lamina. This construct resulted in 4 SS/SS connections, 3 Ti/Ti connections, and 11 connections between dissimilar metals per animal. No fusion was done in order to maximize any possible corrosive responses.

Following surgery, administration of anesthesia was terminated and the animal recovered in a padded pen. Radiographs were taken as detailed below. Once the animal

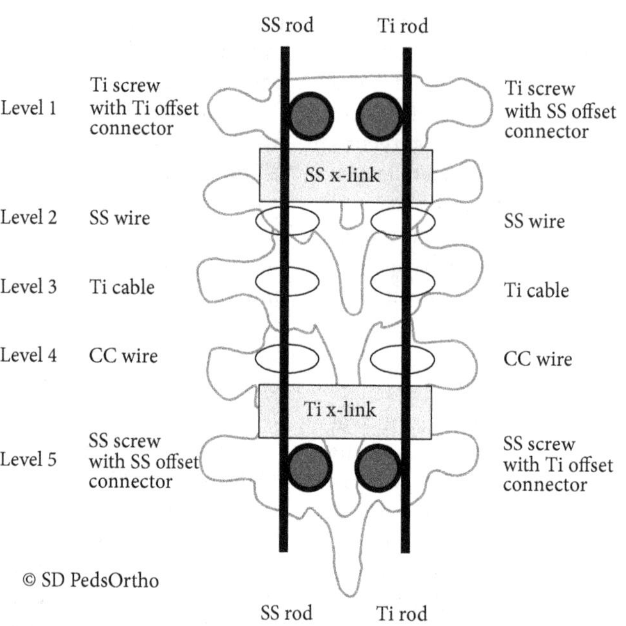

Figure 1: Schematic depiction of implanted construct.

exhibited sufficient tone and was breathing independently, the endotracheal tube was removed. Postoperative antibiotics consisted of sulfamethoxazole and trimethoprim (SMZ), 50 mg/kg PO BID for 5 days post-op. When the implants had been in place for one year, the animal were weighed, sedated as detailed above, and euthanized with Beuthanasia-D delivered intravenously in a dose of 90 mg/kg of phenobarbital. The entire lumbar spine along with the implants was harvested *en bloc*.

2.2. Radiographic Analysis. Plain radiographs (DV and lateral) were taken immediately prior to surgery (following sedation), immediately following surgery while still under surgical anesthesia, at 3, 6, 9, and 12 months post-op (of sedated animals) and following harvest. The location and integrity of the implants, along with any post-op fusion, were evaluated for each of the instrumented segments. Cobb angles of the instrumented regions were measured from lateral radiographs at each time point. Also, the distance between each rod and sublaminar wires/cable (rod-to-wire distance) was measured from the immediate postoperative lateral radiographs and analyzed to determine any trend in risk for neurological deficit. To eliminate the radiographic magnification effect, rod diameter (4.75 mm) served to calibrate all measurements.

2.3. Gross Observation. Photographs were taken of the entire spine with overlying tissue and qualitative observations recorded about the integrity of the tissue, color of the tissue and rod-wire contact areas, presence of loose metallic material, and condition of the wires (intact or broken, eroded, etc.). Overlying tissue, screw connectors, and sublaminar wires were removed from each Ti and SS rod at each level. Both rods from each spine had photographs taken at each level of contact with a metal component and qualitative observations were recorded (coloring, etching of the surface, and loose material).

2.4. Histological Analysis. Tissue samples directly overlying the rods alone and at each metallic contact were dissected away from eleven locations over the SS rod and eleven locations over the Ti rod, taking care to avoid any contact of scalpel blades with any of the metal implants. These samples were immediately placed in 10% neutral buffered formalin in labeled collection tubes. Following fixation, the tissue samples were submitted for routine paraffin embedment. Paraffin blocks were sectioned at 4 microns, and the sections were placed on glass slides. Slides were stained with hematoxylin and eosin (H&E) then examined under light microscopy to qualitatively determine the histopathology of the tissues. Evaluation of the slides included foreign body reaction (FBR, giant cells/macrophages in six 100x microscopic fields), metal particle count (particles $>3.3\,\mu$m in six 100x fields), and inflammation (graded 0 = not present to 2 = extensively present). Histological classifications were compared between tissue over single metal combinations (SS + SS, Ti + Ti) and over each combination of different metals (SS + Ti, SS + CC, Ti + CC) and between tissue over wire combinations and nonwire combinations.

2.5. Corrosion Analysis. Following removal of all tissue, the constructs were thoroughly rinsed in distilled water with care taken to avoid any metal contact with the constructs. They were then affixed to laminated sheets of the construct diagram and sterilized via ethylene oxide. Constructs were photographed then disassembled. Each component was again photographed and viewed, recording any discoloration or etching of the metal.

Just prior to surgery and at 3, 6, 9, and 12 (just before to euthanizing) months post-op, each animal had 3 mL of blood drawn from an ear vein via a butterfly catheter. Blood was placed in metal free collection tubes (royal blue top) and the serum was extracted and stored frozen (−20°C). Metal level analysis of the serum was not performed as there were only two animals at the 12-month survival period and the analysis was deemed to be not very meaningful for such a small sample size.

2.6. Data Collection and Analysis/Statistical Methods. Qualitative data was collected from the radiographic, visual observation, and histological evaluations as described above. The continuous dependent variables (FBR cells and number of metal particles in slides of overlying tissue) were compared between mixed versus single metal and wire versus other combinations using repeated measures analysis of variance (ANOVA). Chi-square comparisons of mixed versus single metal and wire versus other contacts were made for the histological parameter of inflammation. Significance was set at $P < 0.05$. A sample size of $n = 7$ was used due to the pilot nature of this project, so the power for the statistical analyses will be expectedly very low.

Table 1: Surgical parameters.

	P12	P2
	Male	Male
Levels instrumented	T12, T13, L1, L2, L3	L1, L2, L3, L4, L5
Length of surgery	125 min.	140 min.
Weight gain	26%	48%
Length increase	6%	19%
Implants in place	12 months	12 months
Blood loss	10 cc	<20 cc

Table 2: Radiographic parameters, kyphosis measured from lateral radiographs.

	P12	P2
Pre-op kyphosis	25°	19°
Immediate post-op kyphosis	4°	0°
3 months post-op	23°	17°
6 months post-op	33°	13°
9 months post-op	25°	12°
12 months post-op	34°	11°
After harvest	29°	11°

3. Results

3.1. Surgical Procedure. Four (one female and three male) animals had neurological dysfunction immediately postoperatively which did not resolve after two days. The first two surgeries had additional Ti supralaminar (most cephalad level) and SS infralaminar hooks attached bilaterally to the rods in two vertebral levels proximal to those outlined in Figure 1. Upon inspection of the spine following harvest, all four hooks in both animals had fractured and pulled through the laminae. In addition, a sublaminar wire technique was used in these first two animals in which the SS and CC double wires were passed through the sublaminar space then secured around the rods, leaving a double wire around the laminae. Since it was felt that these techniques resulted in neurologic deficit both times, all remaining cases were performed without hooks and using a single sublaminar wiring technique. Following these adjustments to the implant protocol, there were two additional neurologic insults that occurred in the immediate postoperative period. One deficit was clearly due to a pedicle screw placement impinging on the spinal cord, seen immediately on postoperative radiographs. The other neurological deficit was determined to be due to a CC wire that did not conform to the anterior surface of the lamina, extending over 1.5 cm into the canal. These four animals were euthanized and not included in further analyses.

Five months post-op, one female mini-pig developed a Group E Streptococcus (common in "streptococcal lymphadenitis of swine") surgical site infection, for which it was treated with aggressive irrigation and debridement of the wound under sedation (immediately and again one week later) with twice daily cleaning of the wound and a twenty-day course of antibiotics (Naxcel, 200 mg IM daily). The infection did not resolve, so the animal was euthanized almost 7 months following implant placement. This animal was also excluded from all further analyses.

Surgical times for the remaining two male animals were 125 minutes and 140 minutes, with blood loss of <20 cc in the two animals (Table 1). The recovery periods were unremarkable and animals were returned to regular pen and activity levels within two days. Body weight increased by 26 and 48% (from 49 and 40 kg pre-op to 61.5 and 59 kg, resp.) and body length increased by 6 and 19% (from 92.5 and 80 cm pre-op to 98 and 95 cm, resp.) over the 12 months following surgery.

3.2. Radiographic Analysis. Radiographs taken immediately post-op showed appropriately placed implant constructs (Figure 2). All implants remained intact and in place for the full twelve months. No intervertebral fusion developed at any of the surgical levels. In the 3-month post-op X-rays, lucency was seen around all of the screws (right and left and proximal and distal) indicating that there was motion of the screws within the bone. Lucency remained the same or increased in the 6-, 9-, and 12-month post-op films; however, screws did not pull out (Figure 3). Pre-op X-rays of the surgical levels showed some kyphosis "naturally" present (19 and 25°) which was eliminated by placement of the implant construct (post-op kyphosis was 4° kyphosis and 0°, Table 2). Kyphosis returned by the 3-month post-op films, with both animals returning to within 2° of the pre-op sagittal contour. There was some evidence of vertebral body wedging created by posterior tethering of growth by the implant construct in one animal (P2).

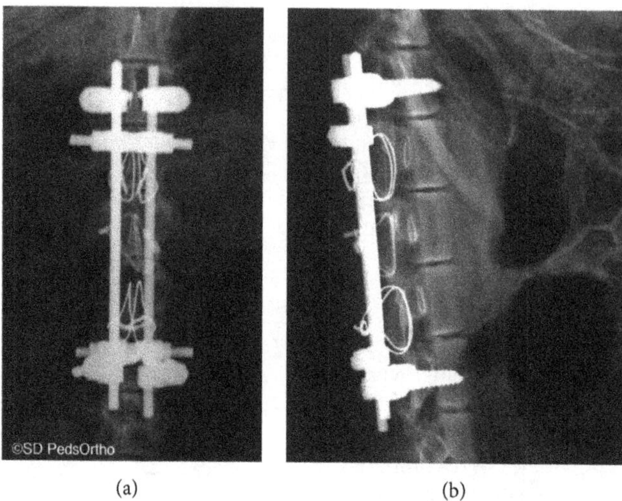

(a) (b)

FIGURE 2: Dorsoventral (a) and lateral (b) radiographs taken immediately following placement of implant construct.

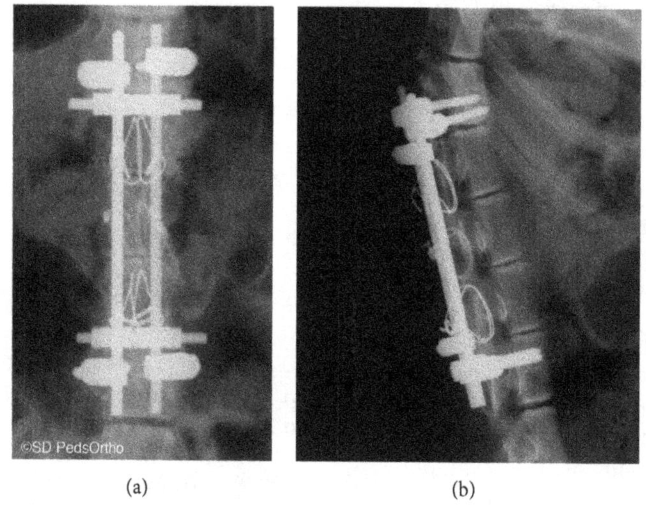

(a) (b)

FIGURE 3: Dorsoventral (a) and lateral (b) radiographs taken 12 months following placement of implant construct (prior to harvest). Lucency around screws is especially seen on the lateral view, both in proximal and distal pair of screws.

Rod-wire distance measurements (average ± stdev, adjusted for magnification) for the animals remaining in the study for the full 12-month period ($n = 2$) were 10.35 ± 0.48 mm for SS wires, 9.00±2.27 for Ti cables, and 11.73±0.06 for CC wires (Figure 4 shows an example). This demonstrated that the Ti cables protruded into the canal by 1 to 2 mm less than the SS and CC wires, conforming more readily to the posterior wall of the spinal canal. In the one single animal that did have a neurological deficit with single wires, rod-wire distances were 12.34 for SS wires, 11.81 for Ti cable, and 17.42 for CC wires. The one CC wire indicated with a solid arrow in Figure 4 was over 19 mm.

3.3. Gross Observation. By gross observation, all implants and wires remained intact and in place. Muscle tissue over the implants for the two spines was generally pink and normal in appearance, with slight tissue discoloration noted over a few of the implants (P12: very little discoloration, P2: yellow coloring over the SS rod + Ti screw and SS rod + SS wire junctions and slight graying over the Ti rod + SS x-link junction). There was some "scarring" (white, glistening tissue) surrounding all metal components. No loose metal particles were detectable in any of the specimens by gross observation.

There was some scratching of the SS and Ti rods in P12, mainly with the Ti cable junction on the SS rod. However, there was no obvious discoloration of any of the implants from P12 or P2.

3.4. Histological Analysis. Figure 5 shows the typical appearance of histological samples including fibrosis, necrosis (pyknotic nuclei and necrotic debris), foreign body reaction (granuloma, giant multinucleated cells), and presence of metal particles. A summary of the histological data for single metal (SS and Ti) and mixed metal combinations is

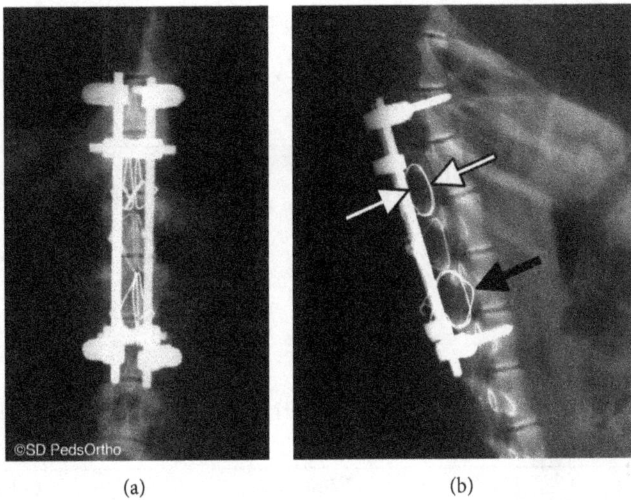

(a) (b)

FIGURE 4: Dorsoventral (a) and lateral (b) radiographs taken immediately post-op. This animal sustained a neurological deficit post-op which did not resolve. An example of a rod-to-wire distance measurement is shown on the lateral radiograph as distance between two outlined arrows, and CC wire deemed to be the cause of the neurological deficit is shown by a solid black arrow.

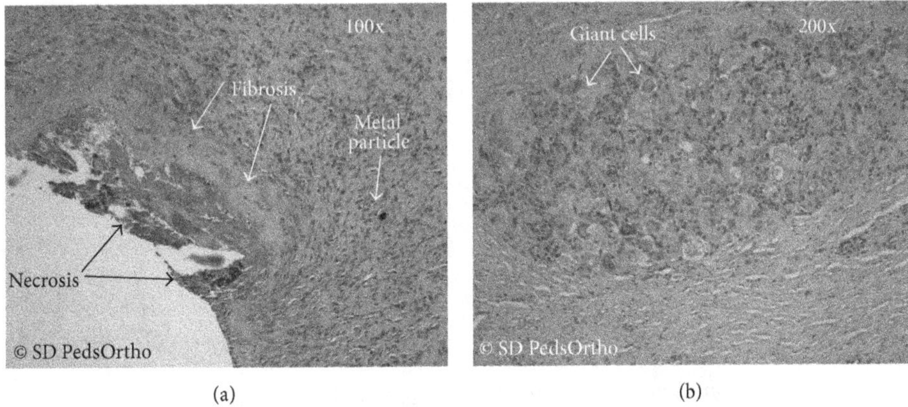

(a) (b)

FIGURE 5: H&E stained slides: (a) from tissue overlying a SS rod with SS crosslink junction showing fibrosis, necrosis, and a metal particle, (b) from tissue overlying a SS rod with CC sublaminar wire, giant cells showing foreign body reaction.

presented in Table 3. Histology of tissue over SS connections ($n = 8$) demonstrated 11.1 ± 7.6 FBR cells, 2.1 ± 1.7 metal particles, and moderate to extensive inflammation. When Ti components were linked ($n = 6$), tissue histology showed 6.3 ± 3.8 FBR cells, 5.2 ± 6.7 metal particles, and no to extensive inflammation (83% extensive). Tissue over mixed metal components ($n = 22$) had 14.1 ± 12.6 FBR cells and 13.4 ± 27.8 metal particles. Although it appears that there are more FBR cells and metal particles in mixed metal combinations than in SS or Ti alone, this is not significantly proven ($P = 0.347$, and 0.381, resp.). Samples surrounding sublaminar wires/cables versus other combinations (Table 4) demonstrated FBR (12.4 ± 13.5 versus 12.0 ± 9.6 cells, $P = 0.96$), metal particles (19.8 ± 32.6 versus 4.3 ± 12.7, $P = 0.24$), and inflammation (50% versus 75% extensive, $P = 0.12$). The number of metal particles in overlying tissue was on average 5 times higher in wire metal combinations, but this was not a significant finding ($P = 0.241$).

3.5. Corrosion Analysis. Figure 6 shows one set of components twelve months after implantation. All yellow, orange, or red discoloration is likely due to tissue remaining on the implants. We did not scrub the implants due to the risk of scratching the surfaces. No erosion of the rods is seen, with only some surface scratching at the SS rod to SS crosslink junction, mainly in one animal (P2). The Ti rod had darker discoloration at the metal junctions than the SS rod but was not scratched.

4. Discussion

Despite the fact that surgical techniques for sublaminar hook and wire/cable placement currently employed in the pediatric population for spinal deformity correction were performed in this mini-pig model by spine surgeons with many years of experience performing sublaminar wires, the first two cases resulted in neurological deficit. A revised technique was

TABLE 3: Histological results of tissue overlying metal junctions comparing single metal and mixed metal combinations (values are average ± standard deviation).

	SS ($n = 8$)	Ti ($n = 6$)	Mixed ($n = 22$)	P value
Foreign body reaction (number of cells in 6 100x fields)	11.1 ± 7.6	6.3 ± 3.8	14.1 ± 12.7	0.347
Metal particles (number of particles in 6 fields)	2.1 ± 1.7	5.2 ± 6.7	13.4 ± 27.8	0.381
Inflammation (average score) (0 = not present, 2 = extensively present)	1.8 ± 0.4	1.7 ± 0.8	1.6 ± 0.6	0.711

TABLE 4: Histological results of tissue overlying metal junctions comparing wire and other types of combinations (values are average ± standard deviation).

	Wire ($n = 12$)	Other ($n = 24$)	P value
Foreign body reaction (number of cells in 6 100x fields)	12.4 ± 13.5	12.0 ± 9.6	0.956
Metal particles (number of particles in 6 fields)	19.8 ± 32.7	4.3 ± 12.7	0.241
Inflammation (average score) (0 = not present, 2 = extensively present)	1.8 ± 0.4	1.7 ± 0.8	0.711

applied, which provided improved neurological outcomes. However, the Yucatan mini-pig was still found to be susceptible to neurological deficit when the sublaminar wires/cables do not conform well to the posterior canal. This was especially the case with use of CC wire, in which the surgeons found it much more difficult to precisely contour and control the shape due to the high yield strength of the metal. This shows how relatively stenotic and neurologically sensitive the Yucatan mini-pig is as a model for sublaminar wire placement. Sublaminar hooks were found not to be a viable technique in this animal model due to the fragile laminar bone and the forces applied as the spine returned to its normal kyphosis. Clearly, studying sublaminar wiring techniques for use in the clinical population using this animal model is not optimal.

Immediately post-op, the regular kyphotic contour of the lumbar spine was removed in all the animals as the spine was instrumented with straight rods. Within the first three months following surgery, most of the normal kyphotic contour returned as the spine returned to its natural position via flexion through the unfused intervertebral discs. This return of kyphosis was accomplished at the expense of screw loosening, as seen on radiographs. Sublaminar hooks, used in the first two animals, pulled out as the spine returned to its kyphotic contour resulting in vertebral fracture, whereas the pedicle screws loosened but did not pull out substantially, allowing a nontraumatic return of the normal kyphotic contour. Pedicle screws were therefore found to be a safer technique than hooks for vertebral fixation in this model that we have proposed to use to study corrosion. No fusion occurred over the 12-month survival period, allowing maximal opportunity for motion of the implant construct with possible related corrosion effects.

Corrosion in orthopedic implants has been correlated with decrease in implant integrity, tissue reaction, infection, and pain [6, 13, 17–20]. More specifically, corrosion due to micromotion in spine implants has been blamed for late onset pain and drainage from the instrumentation site. Wimmer and Gluch report on eight patients with radiographic lucency around pedicle screws, six of which had a discharging sinus and pain between 12 and 34 months post-op. Instrumentation was removed from these six patients, and overlying tissue was found to be necrotic and stained with metallosis. They theorize that micromotion between implant components causes metal debris, metal debris, resulting in a foreign body reaction, formation of a false membrane and subsequent late onset fluid drainage [21]. Likewise, Dubousset et al. attribute late onset infection to micromotion of the instrumentation [22]. However, Richards suspected late drainage following spinal instrumentation is caused by intraoperative seeding that remains subclinical for at least 12 months [23]. Likewise, Clark and Shufflebarger found that drainage appearing at least one year following surgery was a granulomatous reaction caused not by fretting corrosion but by the late activation of bacteria introduced at the time of surgery. They prolonged the culture time from 72 hours (1 of 10 cultures was positive) to 7 days (11 of 12 cultures were positive) [24]. More recently, Ho et al. reported that last onset infections in this population are likely due to many factors, including past medical history, use of blood transfusions, and not using a postoperative drain. Specifically, the number of anchor points or levels of instrumentation, which would correspond to the number of metal connections, was not associated with delayed infections [25]. In addition to corrosion resulting from micromotion, corrosion due to having two metals of different types in

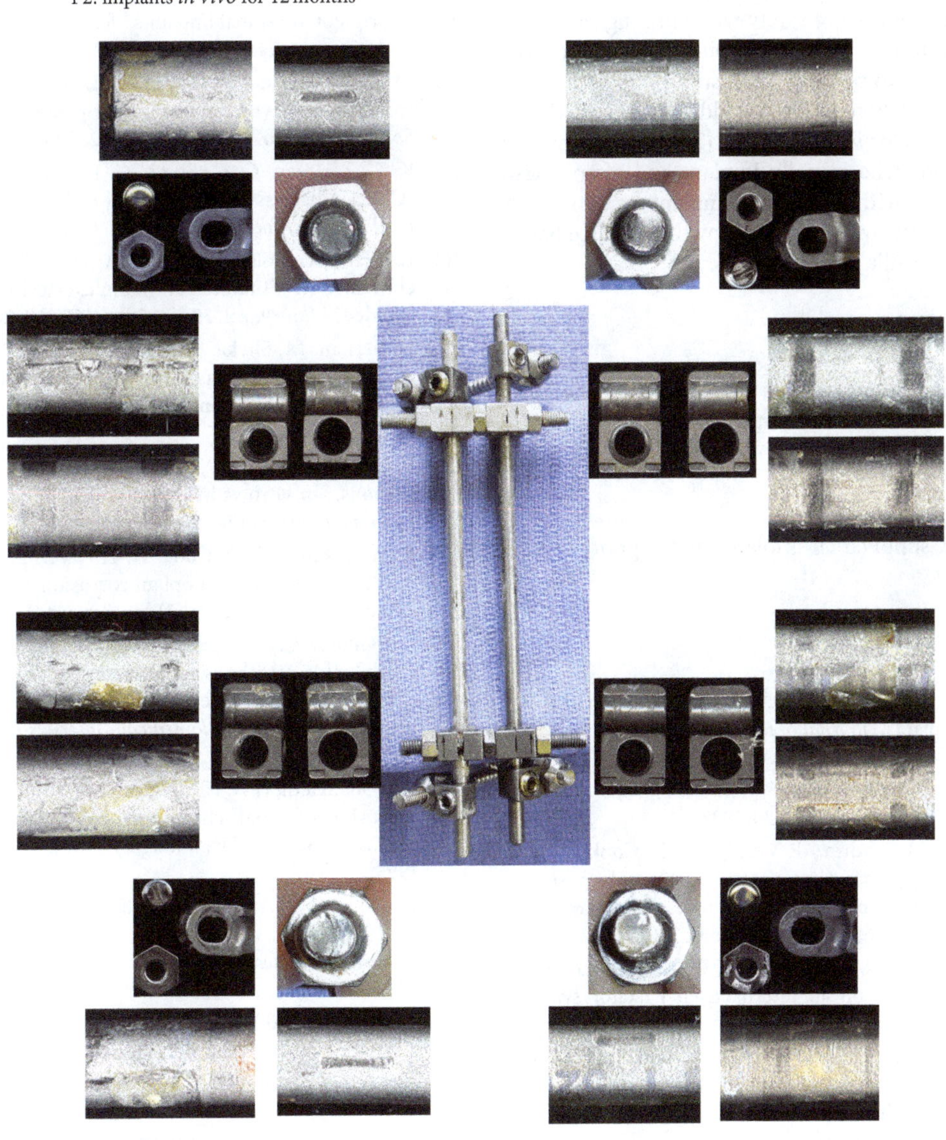

Figure 6: Explanted components from one animal following twelve months *in vivo*. These are arranged in the same orientation as in Figure 1.

contact with each other has been shown to be a clinical problem in hip prostheses [18].

In the current *in vivo* study, there were no obvious or catastrophic tissue consequences resulting from the contact of differing metals in spinal implants in this animal model over a year. Tissue samples over the single metal combinations and mixed metal combinations had similar levels of foreign body reaction, metal particles, fibrosis, and inflammation. Also, no significant differences were found in overlying tissue response to wires versus other types of combinations in this preliminary study; however, there is a suggestion that wires moving over a rod produce more metal particles than fixed metal junctions, regardless of the type of metal wires or rod. Though it remains best to err on the side of caution, this study does not offer support that mixed metal combinations are any more dangerous, or cause a more severe physiological reaction at the tissue level, than combining components of the same metal.

At this time, most surgeons remain hesitant to combine stainless steel with titanium or cobalt chrome metal in orthopedic implants for fear of increased complication rates [11, 13]. This study must be considered preliminary work and the lack of statistical differences noted is likely due to the small sample size and limited statistical power. In addition to the valuable, but limited, data on the effect of corrosion in a biological environment, valuable lessons have been learned regarding the limitation of this animal model to study spinal techniques including the fragile laminar bone that will not tolerate sublaminar hooks exerting substantial forces and the neurological sensitivity of this animal model to sublaminar wiring. Further study with greater numbers is needed to answer the clinical concern of safety when mixing metals in spinal constructs, and we hope these pilot data will inform others who may wish to perform such studies. *In vivo* study such as this is ultimately required, in addition to ASTM and ISO testing standards for *in vitro* testing [26], and is clinically relevant to surgeons who initially implant and often revise patients particularly with nonfusion implant systems such as distraction based growing rods or growth guidance based procedures such as Shilla or Luque trolley.

Conflict of Interests

The authors declare that there is no conflict of interests regarding the publication of this paper.

Acknowledgment

DePuy Spine, Inc. supplied all implants and support for the research study.

References

[1] J. J. Jacobs, J. L. Gilbert, and R. M. Urban, "Corrosion of metal orthopaedic implants," *Journal of Bone and Joint Surgery A*, vol. 80, no. 2, pp. 268–282, 1998.

[2] J. Black, "Does corrosion matter?" *Journal of Bone and Joint Surgery B*, vol. 70, no. 4, pp. 517–520, 1988.

[3] W. J. Gaine, S. M. Andrew, P. Chadwick, E. Cooke, and J. B. Williamson, "Late operative site pain with isola posterior instrumentation requiring implant removal: infection or metal reaction?" *Spine*, vol. 26, no. 5, pp. 583–587, 2001.

[4] U. Vieweg, D. van Roost, H. K. Wolf, C. A. Schyma, and J. Schramm, "Corrosion on an internal spinal fixator system," *Spine*, vol. 24, no. 10, pp. 946–951, 1999.

[5] L. Aulisa, A. di Benedetto, A. Vinciguerra, and P. Tranquilli-Leali, "Corrosion of the Harrington's instrumentation and biological behaviour of the rod-human spine system," *Biomaterials*, vol. 3, no. 4, pp. 246–248, 1982.

[6] S. Cook, M. Asher, S.-M. Lai, and J. Shobe, "Reoperation after primary posterior instrumentation and fusion for idiopathic scoliosis: toward defining late operative site pain of unknown cause," *Spine*, vol. 25, no. 4, pp. 463–468, 2000.

[7] Y. Mochida, T. W. Bauer, H. Nitto, H. E. Kambic, and G. F. Muschler, "Influence of stability and mechanical properties of a spinal fixation device on production of wear debris particles in vivo," *Journal of Biomedical Materials Research*, vol. 53, no. 3, pp. 193–198, 2000.

[8] H. Senaran, P. Atilla, F. Kaymaz, E. Acaroglu, and A. Surat, "Ultrastructural analysis of metallic debris and tissue reaction around spinal implants in patients with late operative site pain," *Spine*, vol. 29, no. 15, pp. 1618–1623, 2004.

[9] B. W. Cunningham, C. M. Orbegoso, A. E. Dmitriev et al., "The effect of spinal instrumentation particulate wear debris: an in vivo rabbit model and applied clinical study of retrieved instrumentation cases," *Spine Journal*, vol. 3, no. 1, pp. 19–32, 2003.

[10] N. J. Hallab, B. W. Cunningham, and J. J. Jacobs, "Spinal implant debris-induced osteolysis," *Spine*, vol. 28, no. 20, pp. S125–S138, 2003.

[11] J. S. Kirkpatrick, R. Venugopalan, P. Beck, and J. Lemons, "Corrosion on spinal implants," *Journal of Spinal Disorders and Techniques*, vol. 18, no. 3, pp. 247–251, 2005.

[12] M. L. Villarraga, P. A. Cripton, S. D. Teti et al., "Wear and corrosion in retrieved thoracolumbar posterior internal fixation," *Spine*, vol. 31, no. 21, pp. 2454–2462, 2006.

[13] K. C. Zartman, G. C. Berlet, C. F. Hyer, and J. R. Woodard, "Combining dissimilar metals in orthopaedic implants: revisited," *Foot & Ankle Specialist*, vol. 4, no. 5, pp. 318–323, 2011.

[14] P. J. Høl, A. Mølster, and N. R. Gjerdet, "Should the galvanic combination of titanium and stainless steel surgical implants be avoided?" *Injury*, vol. 39, no. 2, pp. 161–169, 2008.

[15] H. Serhan, M. Slivka, T. Albert, and S. D. Kwak, "Is galvanic corrosion between titanium alloy and stainless steel spinal implants a clinical concern?" *Spine Journal*, vol. 4, no. 4, pp. 379–387, 2004.

[16] L. C. Lucas, P. Dale, R. Buchanan, Y. Gill, D. Griffin, and J. E. Lemons, "In vitro vs in vivo corrosion analyses of two alloys," *Journal of Investigative Surgery*, vol. 4, no. 1, pp. 13–21, 1991.

[17] K. A. Thomas, S. D. Cook, A. F. Harding, and R. J. Haddad Jr., "Tissue reaction to implant corrosion in 38 internal fixation devices," *Orthopedics*, vol. 11, no. 3, pp. 441–451, 1988.

[18] J. L. Gilbert, C. A. Buckley, and J. J. Jacobs, "In vivo corrosion of modular hip prosthesis components in mixed and similar metal combinations. The effect of crevice, stress, motion, and alloy coupling," *Journal of Biomedical Materials Research*, vol. 27, no. 12, pp. 1533–1544, 1993.

[19] B. F. Shahgaldi, F. W. Heatley, A. Dewar, and B. Corrin, "In vivo corrosion of cobalt-chromium and titanium wear particles," *Journal of Bone and Joint Surgery B*, vol. 77, no. 6, pp. 962–966, 1995.

[20] L. C. Lucas, R. A. Buchanan, and J. E. Lemons, "Investigations on the galvanic corrosion of multialloy total hip prostheses," *Journal of Biomedical Materials Research*, vol. 15, no. 5, pp. 731–747, 1981.

[21] C. Wimmer and H. Gluch, "Aseptic loosening after CD instrumentation in the treatment of scoliosis: a report about eight cases," *Journal of Spinal Disorders*, vol. 11, no. 5, pp. 440–443, 1998.

[22] J. Dubousset, H. Shuffleberger, and D. Wenger, "Late infection with CD instrumentation," *Orthopaedic Transactions*, vol. 18, article 121, 1994.

[23] S. Richards, "Delayed infections following posterior spinal instrumentation for the treatment of idiopathic scoliosis," *Journal of Bone and Joint Surgery A*, vol. 77, no. 4, pp. 524–529, 1995.

[24] C. E. Clark and H. L. Shufflebarger, "Late-developing infection in instrumented idiopathic scoliosis," *Spine*, vol. 24, no. 18, pp. 1909–1912, 1999.

[25] C. Ho, D. J. Sucato, and B. S. Richards, "Risk factors for the development of delayed infections following posterior spinal fusion and instrumentation in adolescent idiopathic scoliosis patients," *Spine*, vol. 32, no. 20, pp. 2272–2277, 2007.

[26] M. Hahn, R. Nassutt, G. Delling, O. Mahrenholtz, E. Schneider, and M. Morlock, "The influence of material and design features on the mechanical properties of transpedicular spinal fixation implants," *Journal of Biomedical Materials Research*, vol. 63, no. 3, pp. 354–362, 2002.

18

Experiences of a Peripheral Unit in Using a Tripolar Constrained Acetabular Component for Recurrent Dislocations following Total Hip Joint Replacements

Mohammed S. Arshad, Shashi Godey, Arun Kumar, and Martyn Lovell

University Hospital of South Manchester, Southmoor Road, Manchester M23 9LT, UK

Correspondence should be addressed to Mohammed S. Arshad; shebi@doctors.org.uk

Academic Editor: Shyu-Jye Wang

Primary total hip arthroplasty is a successful procedure, although complications such as dislocation can occur. In certain patient populations if this is recurrent, it can be difficult to manage effectively. We present a retrospective analysis of our experience of using a capture/captive cup over an 8-year period for frail elderly patients who presented with recurrent hip dislocations. Our findings show no redislocations in our cohort and a survival analysis demonstrates just less than half surviving at 2 years after surgery. Furthermore, Harris Hip Scores were generally calculated to be good. A constrained acetabular component provides durable protection against additional dislocations without substantial deleterious effects on component fixation. Such components should be considered especially in a group of patients with comorbidities or those who are fragile, elderly, and low-demand in nature.

1. Introduction

Primary total hip arthroplasty (THA) is a renowned and successful procedure. Complications such as dislocation can occur and variable rates are reported but there is a cumulative increase which may approach 5% [1–7]. Recurrence is seen in up to two-thirds of cases with the problem persisting after revision surgery in about half [1, 8, 9]. Numerous risk factors have been documented which include increasing age, reduced cerebral capabilities, neuromuscular disorders, abductor deficiency, and mal-positioning of components at time of surgery [10–12]. Surgical solutions to correct, reverse, or manage such factors have on the whole produced mixed and inconclusive results, whether it is altering a mal-positioned component, using cup augments, increasing femoral head size, converting to a bipolar hemiarthroplasty, or reconstructing adjacent tissues [13–20].

Studies have advocated the use of a "capture/captive cup" (CC) (Figure 1) or constrained acetabular component to effectively manage dislocations [21–25]. By capturing the head and locking it within the acetabular component, forces causing dislocation are redistributed to the locking mechanism and liner-shell and shell-bone interfaces [24]. Thus such devices provide immediate stability and are a welcome solution to a debilitating complication, although the procedure has been associated with some setbacks, mainly a reduced range of motion, possible loosening, or dissociation of the component from the pelvis which requires either open reduction or revision [25, 26]. We present our experience of using a constrained cup in managing recurrent dislocations in low-demand patients.

2. Materials and Methods

A retrospective case-note review of all patients who underwent revision of their acetabular component using a tripolar Trident acetabular cup (Stryker-Howmedica-Osteonics, Rutherford, New Jersey) between 2005 and 2013 (identified through a local database) was undertaken by two orthopaedic surgeons. It was recognised that a constrained liner was offered to patients who had undergone recurrent dislocations ($n \geq 2$). A small number of our cohort had undergone further

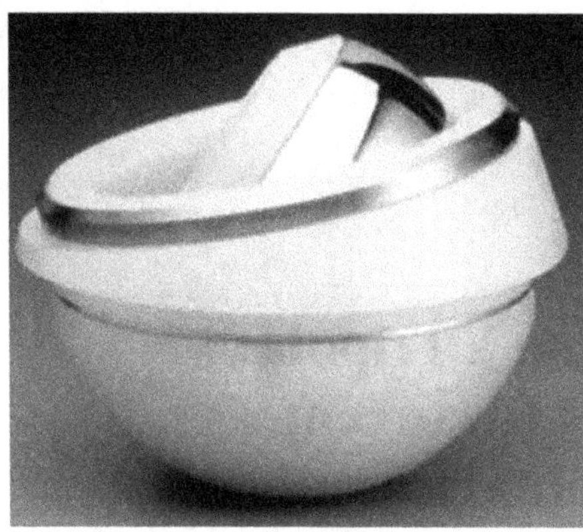

Figure 1: Photograph demonstrating a capture/captive cup (tripolar Trident acetabular cup: Stryker-Howmedica-Osteonics, Rutherford, New Jersey).

procedures following on from their primary THA: THA revision ($n = 3$); posterior lip augmentation device (PLAD) ($n = 3$).

In total 43 patients who received a constrained acetabular component were identified. The mean age of our cohort was 76.5 years (range 53–93 years). Our male to female ratio was 19 : 24. A majority of our patients (93%) had undergone their primary surgery due to osteoarthritis. The remaining patients ($n = 3$) required a THA for a fractured neck of femur, nonunion of a fractured neck of femur, and a previous septic arthritis. Analysis of documentation revealed that 84% of patients had undergone either a trochanteric osteotomy ($n = 14$) or Hardinge (anterolateral) approach ($n = 29$) during primary surgery.

All 43 patients were followed up after their procedure; however, at the time of data analysis, 23 patients had died due to their comorbidities, 5 patients were lost to follow-up, and 2 patients were excluded for further analysis due to dementia and ongoing investigation for a psychiatric illness. Following initial analysis of all patients, the 13 remaining patients were reviewed further, specifically observing their postoperative pain scores and mobility status along with any recent radiographic abnormalities. Additionally, relevant questions were asked in order to calculate a Harris Hip Score [27] which was then graded [28].

For our cohort of remaining patients, pain levels were also documented according to a visual analogue score (VAS). Radiographs were reviewed by an orthopaedic surgeon to assess acetabular component failure in terms of stability by identifying features of loosening. Our cemented cups were analysed using DeLee and Charnley's criteria [29] and Tompkin et al.'s criteria were applied to uncemented cups [30].

3. Results

The mean time from previous surgery (whether primary or revision) to receiving a capture cup was 74 months (range 6 months–252 months). In 9% of cases ($n = 4$), the capture cup was uncemented; the remainder were cemented (Figure 2). Additionally, 6 of our patients had also undergone revision of their femoral component during the same session of surgery. These findings are summarised in Table 1. Many of our patients (>50%) had a monoblock Charnley femoral stem and thus the capture cup avoided a femoral component revision.

Table 1: Summary of data analysis of the 43 patients identified in our study. All patients underwent a capture/captive cup procedure for recurrent dislocations ($n \geq 2$). CC = capture/captive cup, PLAD = posterior lip augmentation device, and THA = total hip arthroplasty.

43 patients	
Alive	13
Dead	23
Lost to follow-up	5
Psychiatric illness	2
Cause of primary surgery	
Osteoarthritis	40
Neck of femur fracture	1
Neck of femur fracture nonunion	1
Secondary to septic arthritis	1
Further surgery after primary total hip arthroplasty (THA)	
THA revision (prior to CC)	3
PLAD (prior to CC)	3
Femoral component revision (at time of CC)	6
Capture/captive cup (CC)	
Uncemented	4
Cemented	39
Surgical approach	
Trochanteric osteotomy	14
Hardinge	29

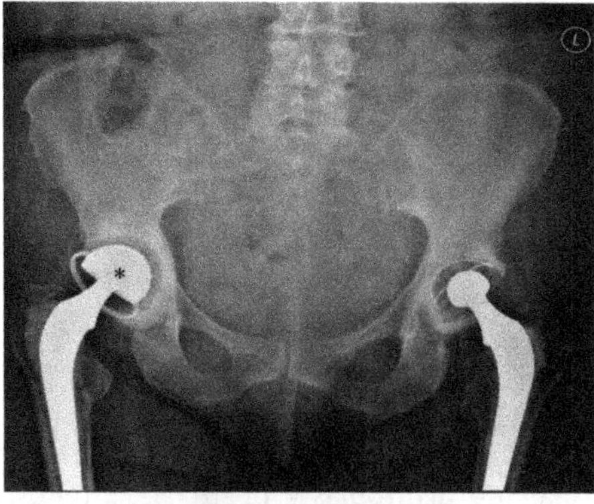

Figure 2: Radiograph demonstrating the use of a cemented capture/captive cup for the right hip*.

Overall, our follow-up mean time was 26 months (range 1 month–68 months). A Kaplan-Meier plot of survival based on follow-up times (Figure 3) demonstrates that, one year after surgery, the survival was 62% and, at 2 years, was 48%. Of those patients who are currently alive, a VAS was recorded during their last follow-up. A mean score of 2.8 (range 0–8) was noted. The median Harris Hip Score [27] was 80.2 points (range 43.2–96.6) resulting in "good" grade on average (Table 2). In terms of mobility only, during their last follow-up, 5 patients were mobilising independently, 4 patients were

TABLE 2: Harris Hip Scores (and grading) of surviving patients (n = 13) after undergoing a capture/captive cup.

	Harris Hip Score	Grade	
Median	80.2	Poor	2
		Fair	3
Range	43.2–96.6	Good	3
		Excellent	5

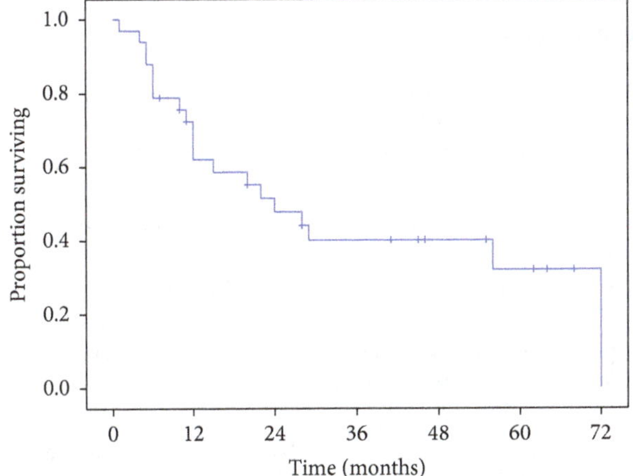

FIGURE 3: Graph demonstrating a Kaplan-Meier plot of survival (based on follow-up times) for patients undergoing a capture/captive cup.

mobilising with support, and 4 patients were unable to do so or were struggling and required more than a stick or crutch.

Radiographic analysis of these patients revealed that all cemented cups were satisfactory in that no loosening was evident as per DeLee and Charnley zones [29]. As per Tompkin et al.'s criteria [30], 75% of our uncemented cups were stable (n = 3) with the other cup being deemed unstable due to the presence of radiolucent lines in all zones and evidence of migration 15 mm (although the constrained mechanism itself was intact) which required further surgery (Figure 4).

A Summary Highlighting the Complications Seen in 3 Patients in Our Study. Complications were seen in 7% of all cases (n = 3) as follows.

Postoperative infection and Girdlestone's procedure.

Loosening and migration of uncemented cup.

Pelvic detachment of cemented cup.

The first patient had delayed postoperative wound healing and a staphylococcus aureus infection was diagnosed from serial microbiological swabs. She subsequently underwent a debridement and Girdlestone's procedure and required input from the plastic surgeons to assist in closing her wound. She recovered well and was keen to pursue another total hip arthroplasty in order to improve her mobility and was then referred to a tertiary centre for further revision surgery.

The second case involved a patient who underwent a primary total hip arthroplasty following a native hip joint

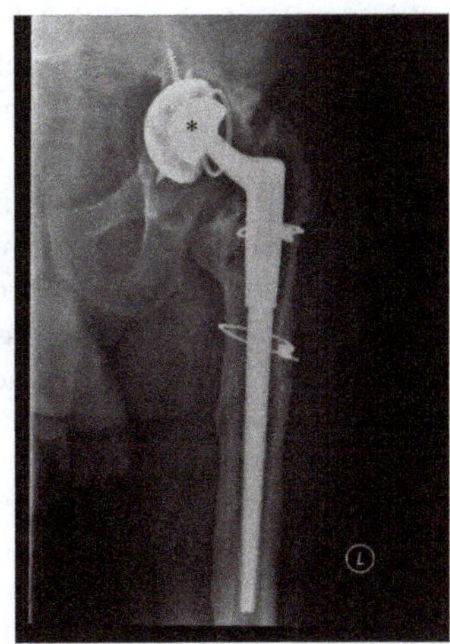

FIGURE 4: Radiograph demonstrating the failure of an uncemented acetabular shell for the left hip*.

septic arthritis 10 years before. He developed aseptic loosening (negative microbiology of aspirates and tissue samples) and thus a revision arthroplasty was done. This too failed due to aseptic loosening and thus a cementless constrained tripolar device was fitted. After 6 months, a similar picture was seen with the cup having migrated by approximately and no conclusive evidence to suggest infection. He was referred to a tertiary centre for further evaluation and treatment.

Our final case was a cemented cup done for a frail 86-year-old lady following recurrent dislocations. Unfortunately, the device became detached from the pelvis and revised capture/captive cup was done. However, given her frailty and comorbidities, the patient did not survive more than 6 months and thus for the purpose of this study further assessment was not possible. Most importantly, no redislocations have been evident from our series.

4. Discussion

Recurrent instability is often multifactorial and is frequently not associated with a clearly identifiable cause. For those affected, they are often old and frail undergoing rapid deterioration of their systems and as such the loss of skeletal muscle mass coupled with polyethylene wear and dementia may be some of the contributory factors leading to dislocation.

By locking or capturing the femoral head within the acetabular component, the constrained device can be a short to medium term solution when deployed by the revision hip surgeon in treating a particular group of patients who have significant comorbidities and recurrent dislocations. The constrained design is successful in reducing dislocations in such patient groups though it can lead to increasing levels of loosening. The variety in designs allows different head sizes, offset, and rim elevation which manifests in different ranges of motion. Impingement is seen once the limit is reached and thus forces are dissipated between the bone-shell and shell liner boundaries [24]. In a revision series, the devices have shown to reduce the dislocation rate to 6% but after a decade the loosening risk was noted to be at 9% [21].

On the other hand, the dual mobility device (tripolar unconstrained acetabular cup) aims to not only reduce dislocation risk but also lower loosening by increasing the functional diameter of the head and thus reducing impingement, wear, and dissociation. Since their development (Novae-1®, Serf, Décines, France) in the 1970s, they have provided a reliable solution in the revision setting for older low-demand patients as supported by midterm data with rates of dislocation at 1.1% and loosening at 2.2%, although there is a lack of significant evidence to support their use in the younger high demand patient [31–34]. The aim is to allow a greater range of motion through the use of a large diameter head before it impinges against the polyethylene liner hence preventing intraprosthetic dislocation [34]. Apart from their use in revision surgery, dual mobility cups have been implanted in primary surgery as well as in treating neck of femur fractures, tumour resection, and spastic disorders with dislocation rates varying between 0 and 14% and survivorship rates between 80 and 98% ranging from a period of 5 to 15 years [35–37].

Despite a survival rate of 30% in our cohort (representing the mixed nature of the population of a peripheral unit over a period of 8 years) which is unlikely to lead to any concrete conclusions, we believe the use of a capture/captive cup is an effective short to medium term tool in dealing with recurrent dislocation. With our monoblock femoral components, not using the dual mobility method but instead a capture/captive cup saved performing a femoral revision. The use of a constrained cup rather than a dual mobility device is likely to be of greater benefit also in patients with neuromuscular disorders, dementia, and low demand or patients without functional abductors. From our experience, it is clinically significant in reducing pain and over two-thirds of patients return to some form of mobility which, in a group of people of a certain demographic and medical status, of whom only less than 50% will survive at 2 years, may be considered as a significant result in terms of improving quality of life.

From our series, the use of cemented components was favourable and less likely to lead to complications although the numbers of uncemented cups were small, thus negating any significant conclusion. Previous studies on constrained acetabular components have quoted loosening/complication rates requiring revision to be between 4% and 11.8% [22, 24, 25]. Our experiences are well within such parameters. Furthermore, in our cohort, no redislocations were evident as supported by Shrader et al. [23]; however, rates of redislocation between 2.4% and 29% have been reported [22, 38]. Failure due to pull-off from the acetabular side wall or separation can occur (5% in total cohort and 8% in alive patients), thus highlighting a potential problem with the use of this technique; therefore all our patients are counselled regarding this complication.

A constrained acetabular component provides durable protection against additional dislocations without substantial deleterious effects on component fixation. Such components should be considered when a correctable cause of instability cannot be identified. Although we acknowledge that there are limitations to our data in terms of the follow-up period being short and the sample numbers being small, from our experience, the use of such a device should be considered to treat recurrent dislocation in comparison with other modalities which may be less effective especially in a group of patients with comorbidities or those who are fragile, elderly, and low-demand in nature.

Conflict of Interests

The authors declare that there is no conflict of interests regarding the publication of this paper.

References

[1] R. Y. G. Woo and B. F. Morrey, "Dislocations after total hip arthroplasty," *The Journal of Bone & Joint Surgery—American Volume*, vol. 64, no. 9, pp. 1295–1306, 1982.

[2] C. D. Fackler and R. Poss, "Dislocation in total hip arthroplasties," *Clinical Orthopaedics and Related Research*, vol. 151, pp. 169–178, 1980.

[3] S. A. Paterno, P. F. Lachiewicz, and S. S. Kelley, "The influence of patient-related factors and the position of the acetabular component on the rate of dislocation after total hip replacement," *The Journal of Bone & Joint Surgery—American Volume*, vol. 79, no. 8, pp. 1202–1210, 1997.

[4] A. Ekelund, N. Rydell, and O. S. Nilsson, "Total hip arthroplasty in patients 80 years of age and older," *Clinical Orthopaedics and Related Research*, vol. 281, pp. 101–106, 1992.

[5] R. S. Turner, "Postoperative total hip prosthetic femoral head dislocations. Incidence, etiologic factors, and management," *Clinical Orthopaedics and Related Research*, no. 301, pp. 196–204, 1994.

[6] D. Fender, W. M. Harper, and P. J. Gregg, "Outcome of Charnley total hip replacement across a single health region in England: the results at five years from a regional hip register," *The Journal of Bone and Joint Surgery—British Volume*, vol. 81, no. 4, pp. 577–581, 1999.

[7] J. Charnley, "The long-term results of low-friction arthroplasty of the hip performed as a primary intervention," *The Journal of Bone & Joint Surgery—British Volume*, vol. 54, no. 1, pp. 61–76, 1972.

[8] D. P. Newington, G. C. Bannister, and M. Fordyce, "Primary total hip replacement in patients over 80 years of age," *The Journal of Bone & Joint Surgery—British Volume*, vol. 72, no. 3, pp. 450–452, 1990.

[9] M. D. Earll, T. K. Fehring, W. L. Griffin, J. B. Mason, T. McCoy, and S. Odum, "Success rate of modular component exchange for the treatment of an unstable total hip arthroplasty," *Journal of Arthroplasty*, vol. 17, no. 7, pp. 864–869, 2002.

[10] S. T. Woolson and Z. O. Rahimtoola, "Risk factors for dislocation during the first 3 months after primary total hip replacement," *The Journal of Arthroplasty*, vol. 14, no. 6, pp. 662–668, 1999.

[11] G. M. Alberton, W. A. High, and B. F. Morrey, "Dislocation after revision total hip arthroplasty: an analysis of risk factors and treatment options," *The Journal of Bone & Joint Surgery—American Volume*, vol. 84, no. 10, pp. 1788–1792, 2002.

[12] L. D. Dorr, A. W. Wolf, R. Chandler, and J. P. Conaty, "Classification and treatment of dislocations of total hip arthroplasty," *Clinical Orthopaedics and Related Research*, vol. 173, pp. 151–158, 1983.

[13] P. J. Daly and B. F. Morrey, "Operative correction of an unstable total hip arthroplasty," *The Journal of Bone & Joint Surgery—American Volume*, vol. 74, no. 9, pp. 1334–1343, 1992.

[14] A. P. Charlwood, N. W. Thompson, N. S. Thompson, D. E. Beverland, and J. R. Nixon, "Recurrent hip arthroplasty dislocation: good outcome after cup augmentation in 20 patients followed for 2 years," *Acta Orthopaedica Scandinavica*, vol. 73, no. 5, pp. 502–505, 2002.

[15] P. E. Beaulé, T. P. Schmalzried, P. Udomkiat, and H. C. Amstutz, "Jumbo femoral head for the treatment of recurrent dislocation following total hip replacement," *The Journal of Bone & Joint Surgery—American Volume*, vol. 84, no. 2, pp. 256–263, 2002.

[16] S. Byström, B. Espehaug, O. Furnes, and L. I. Havelin, "Femoral head size is a risk factor for total hip luxation: a study of 42,987 primary hip arthroplasties from the Norwegian Arthroplasty Register," *Acta Orthopaedica Scandinavica*, vol. 74, no. 5, pp. 514–524, 2003.

[17] J. Parvizi and B. F. Morrey, "Bipolar hip arthroplasty as a salvage treatment for instability of the hip," *The Journal of Bone & Joint Surgery—American Volume*, vol. 82, no. 8, pp. 1132–1139, 2000.

[18] S. J. Kaplan, W. H. Thomas, and R. Poss, "Trochanteric advancement for recurrent dislocation after total hip arthroplasty," *The Journal of Arthroplasty*, vol. 2, no. 2, pp. 119–124, 1987.

[19] K. Strømsøe and K. Eikvar, "Fascia lata plasty in recurrent posterior dislocation after total hip arthroplasty," *Archives of Orthopaedic and Trauma Surgery*, vol. 114, no. 5, pp. 292–294, 1995.

[20] T. Fujishiro, T. Nishikawa, S. Takikawa, Y. Saegusa, S. Yoshiya, and M. Kurosaka, "Reconstruction of the iliofemoral ligament with an artificial ligament for recurrent anterior dislocation of total hip arthroplasty," *Journal of Arthroplasty*, vol. 18, no. 4, pp. 524–527, 2003.

[21] B. R. B. Bremner, D. D. Goetz, J. J. Callaghan, W. N. Capello, and R. C. Johnston, "Use of constrained acetabular components for hip instability: an average 10-year follow-up study," *Journal of Arthroplasty*, vol. 18, no. 7, pp. 131–137, 2003.

[22] G. S. Shapiro, D. E. Weiland, D. C. Markel, D. E. Padgett, T. P. Sculco, and P. M. Pellicci, "The use of a constrained acetabular component for recurrent dislocation," *The Journal of Arthroplasty*, vol. 18, no. 3, pp. 250–258, 2003.

[23] M. W. Shrader, J. Parvizi, and D. G. Lewallen, "The use of a constrained acetabular component to treat instability after total hip arthroplasty," *The Journal of Bone & Joint Surgery—American Volume*, vol. 85, no. 11, pp. 2179–2183, 2003.

[24] R. J. K. Khan, D. Fick, R. Alakeson et al., "A constrained acetabular component for recurrent dislocation," *The Journal of Bone and Joint Surgery—British Volume*, vol. 88, no. 7, pp. 870–876, 2006.

[25] E. Bigsby, M. R. Whitehouse, G. C. Bannister, and A. W. Blom, "The medium term outcome of the Omnifit constrained acetabular cup," *HIP International*, vol. 22, no. 5, pp. 505–510, 2012.

[26] K. R. Berend, A. V. Lombardi Jr., T. H. Mallory, J. B. Adams, J. H. Russell, and K. L. Groseth, "The long-term outcome of 755 consecutive constrained acetabular components in total hip arthroplasty: examining the successes and failures," *Journal of Arthroplasty*, vol. 20, supplement 3, no. 3, pp. 93–102, 2005.

[27] W. H. Harris, "Traumatic arthritis of the hip after dislocation and acetabular fractures: treatment by mold arthroplasty. An end-result study using a new method of result evaluation," *The Journal of Bone and Joint Surgery—American Volume*, vol. 51, no. 4, pp. 737–755, 1969.

[28] P. Marchetti, R. Binazzi, V. Vaccari et al., "Long-term results with cementless Fitek (or Fitmore) cups," *Journal of Arthroplasty*, vol. 20, no. 6, pp. 730–737, 2005.

[29] J. G. DeLee and J. Charnley, "Radiological demarcation of cemented sockets in total hip replacement," *Clinical Orthopaedics and Related Research*, vol. 121, pp. 20–32, 1976.

[30] G. S. Tompkins, J. J. Jacobs, L. R. Kull, A. G. Rosenberg, and J. O. Galante, "Primary total hip arthroplasty with a porous-coated acetabular component: seven-to-ten-year results," *The Journal of Bone & Joint Surgery—American Volume*, vol. 79, no. 2, pp. 169–176, 1997.

[31] F. Leiber-Wackenheim, B. Brunschweiler, M. Ehlinger, A. Gabrion, and P. Mertl, "Treatment of recurrent THR dislocation using of a cementless dual-mobility cup: a 59 cases series with a mean 8 years' follow-up," *Orthopaedics and Traumatology: Surgery and Research*, vol. 97, no. 1, pp. 8–13, 2011.

[32] M. Hamadouche, D. J. Biau, D. Huten, T. Musset, and F. Gaucher, "The use of a cemented dual mobility socket to treat recurrent dislocation," *Clinical Orthopaedics and Related Research*, vol. 468, no. 12, pp. 3248–3254, 2010.

[33] F. L. Langlais, M. Ropars, F. Gaucher, T. Musset, and O. Chaix, "Dual mobility cemented cups have low dislocation rates in THA revisions," *Clinical Orthopaedics and Related Research*, vol. 466, no. 2, pp. 389–395, 2008.

[34] O. Guyen, V. Pibarot, G. Vaz, C. Chevillotte, and J. Béjui-Hugues, "Use of a dual mobility socket to manage total hip arthroplasty instability," *Clinical Orthopaedics and Related Research*, vol. 467, no. 2, pp. 465–472, 2009.

[35] S. Tarasevicius, M. Busevicius, O. Robertsson, and H. Wingstrand, "Dual mobility cup reduces dislocation rate after arthroplasty for femoral neck fracture," *BMC Musculoskeletal Disorders*, vol. 11, article 175, 2010.

[36] J.-M. Philippeau, J.-M. Durand, J.-P. Carret, S. Leclercq, D. Waast, and F. Gouin, "Dual mobility design use in preventing total hip replacement dislocation following tumor resection," *Orthopaedics & Traumatology, Surgery & Research*, vol. 96, no. 1, pp. 2–8, 2010.

[37] R. J. M. Sanders, B. A. Swierstra, and J. H. M. Goosen, "The use of a dual-mobility concept in total hip arthroplasty patients with spastic disorders: no dislocations in a series of ten cases at midterm follow-up," *Archives of Orthopaedic and Trauma Surgery*, vol. 133, no. 7, pp. 1011–1016, 2013.

[38] M. J. Anderson, W. R. Murray, and H. B. Skinner, "Constrained acetabular components," *Journal of Arthroplasty*, vol. 9, no. 1, pp. 17–23, 1994.

19

Ultrastructure of Intervertebral Disc and Vertebra-Disc Junctions Zones as a Link in Etiopathogenesis of Idiopathic Scoliosis

Evalina L. Burger,[1] Andriy Noshchenko,[1] Vikas V. Patel,[1] Emily M. Lindley,[1] and Andrew P. Bradford[2]

[1] *The Spine Center, Department of Orthopaedics, University of Colorado Denver, Aurora, CO 80045, USA*
[2] *Division of Basic Reproductive Sciences, Department of Obstetrics & Gynecology, University of Colorado Denver, Aurora, CO 80045, USA*

Correspondence should be addressed to Andriy Noshchenko; andriy.noshchenko@ucdenver.edu

Academic Editor: Chan S. Shim

Background Context. There is no general accepted theory on the etiology of idiopathic scoliosis (IS). An important role of the vertebrae endplate physes (VEPh) and intervertebral discs (IVD) in spinal curve progression is acknowledged, but ultrastructural mechanisms are not well understood. *Purpose.* To analyze the current literature on ultrastructural characteristics of VEPh and IVD in the context of IS etiology. *Study Design/Setting.* A literature review. *Results.* There is strong evidence for multifactorial etiology of IS. Early wedging of vertebra bodies is likely due to laterally directed appositional bone growth at the concave side, caused by a combination of increased cell proliferation at the vertebrae endplate and altered mechanical properties of the outer annulus fibrosus of the adjacent IVD. Genetic defects in bending proteins necessary for IVD lamellar organization underlie altered mechanical properties. Asymmetrical ligaments, muscular stretch, and spine instability may also play roles in curve formation. *Conclusions.* Development of a reliable, cost effective method for identifying patients at high risk for curve progression is needed and could lead to a paradigm shift in treatment options. Unnecessary anxiety, bracing, and radiation could potentially be minimized and high risk patient could receive surgery earlier, rendering better outcomes with fewer fused segments needed to mitigate curve progression.

1. Introduction

There is no generally accepted scientific theory for the etiology of idiopathic scoliosis (IS). Treatment of this disease remains pragmatic with an incomplete scientific basis [1]. The current strategy of treatment depends on a patient's age [2]. In children, scoliotic deformity causes a persistent stress in the motion segments, which induces a progressive elastoplastic strain that modifies the geometry of the motion segment, which in turn worsens the excessive strain [2, 3]. Thus, in the pediatric spine the aim of treatment is to prevent the motion segment deformity. In adult scoliosis, significant deformation of the intervertebral disc (IVD) and the capsuloligamentous structures produce instability of the motion segments and slow deformation of the vertebrae through remodeling with disc herniation and neural compression. Hence in adult scoliosis a stable balance is necessary to prevent further deformation of the spine [3–5].

IS may be observed in the infantile, juvenile, or adolescent period, but the trigger factor for curve onset is unknown. There is evidence that the spinal growth spurt plays a significant role in the onset and progression of spinal deformation, especially in the adolescent period. It has been shown that spinal growth can be attributed to increases in the vertebrae height, while the height of discs does not increase [1, 6]. This is likely modulated by loading, according to the Hueter-Volkmann principle [2, 7]. Human vertebrae grow longitudinally by ossification of the vertebral endplate physes

(VEPh). VEPh adjacent to the discs produce longitudinal growth, while appositional growth enlarges the vertebrae in diameter [1, 8]. Theoretically, axial compression can diminish axial growth by reducing the number of proliferating chondrocytes in the hypertrophic zone [9]. Wedging of discs in scoliosis may be caused by asymmetric tissue remodeling or selective concave side degeneration [10]. As scoliosis tends to progress during the growth spurt, it is possible that the growth plate plays an important role in the development of the deformity [9–11]. The interaction between VEPh and adjoined IVD could play a significant role in the initiation and progression of the spinal deformation, especially at the apical zone. Stokes and Aronsson [12] noted that while the IVD does not appear to be the primary factor in the etiology of IS, the IVD contributes to the progression of the scoliosis curve when it becomes significantly wedged. The IVD interface under load shows characteristics of dysplasia which can be associated with changes in discal properties [1]. Despite many studies on the etiology and pathogenesis of scoliosis, the interaction between VEPh and IVD both morphologically and ultrastructurally has not been studied well.

The purpose of the present paper is to review current literature on the morphological and ultrastructural characteristics of the IVD and the VEPh in relation to the clinical manifestation of IS, with an emphasis on the etiology and pathogenesis of this disease. We below present a review of: (a) clinical manifestation of IS; (b) etiological and pathogenetic factors and concepts of IS; (c) morphological and ultrastructural features of the IVD and VEPh in IS. The following sources of information were used to collect the data: (1) electronic data bases: Ovid Medline and Embase till September 2013; (2) hand search using reference lists of reviews and book chapters; no restrictions concerning type of publication and language were used.

2. Clinical Manifestation of IS

IS was originally defined as a structural, lateral curvature of the spine of unknown etiology [13]. The Scoliosis Research Society then defined scoliosis as a lateral curvature of the spine which exceeds 10 degrees by the Cobb method on a standing radiograph [14]. Later it was noted that the presence of structural rotation at the apical segment is essential [15]. Currently, scoliosis is regarded as a three-dimensional curvature of the spine in the coronal and sagittal planes with rotation in the axial plane [12]. If the curvature is present before skeletal maturity and has no other diagnostic features that categorize it as neuromuscular, congenital, traumatic, infectious, postinfectious, or syndrome-related, then it is regarded as IS [15]. The age of onset is the basis of the classification. Infantile IS (IIS) idiopathic scoliosis (IIS) starts before age 3 (≈1% of cases), juvenile (JIS) occurs between 3 and 10 years (around 20% of cases), while adolescent IS (AIS) is defined, if curve onset is between 10 years and skeletal maturity [16]. There are also distinctions in the clinical appearance between different forms of IS. IIS often has spontaneous resolutions (20% and 80%), predominant in boys, and mostly has left thoracic curvature. The curve is seldom present at birth and mainly develops during the first 6 month of life. Resolved curves typically do not recur during the adolescent growth spurt. In adulthood very few patients have back pain or an increased disability score [13, 17, 18]. Thoracic and lumbar curves that reach between 50 and 80 degrees at skeletal maturity may continue to progress slowly in adult life [19]. IIS is also associated with plagiocephaly (100% of children with early onset of IIS), mental retardation, congenital heart disease, and congenital dislocation of the hip [20]. Congenital inguinal hernia and generalized joint laxity have been found among relatives of diseased children [20]. Using magnetic resonance imaging (MRI) demonstrated that the incidence of neural axis abnormalities in children with IIS and JIS is around 20% including Arnold-Chiari malformation, associated cervicothoracic syringx, syringomyelia, and low-lying conus [21, 22]. Wynne Davies [20] suggested that the etiology of IIS must be multifactorial, with a genetic tendency to the deformity which can then be "triggered off" in different individuals by different factors, some medical, some themselves genetic, and some social. JIS is prevalent in boys between ages four and six and in girls between ages seven and nine [13, 23, 24]. Right sided curves are observed in 50–77.5% of cases, regardless of sex or age. A single thoracic curve is the most common (around 62%), followed by double thoracic and lumbar (22%) and thoracolumbar (15%). Curve progression is difficult to predict. Spontaneous resolutions are much less common than in IIS (around 7%) [23], and progression may occur in more than 50% of cases [24]. Associated diseases were observed in 29% of patients including mental deficiency (12%), spina bifida occulta (6%), inguinal hernia (3%), epilepsy (2%), pyloric stenosis (2%), congenital dislocation of hip (1%), dextrocardia (1%), metatarsus varus (1%), joint laxity (1%), hemimelia (1%), and absent thumb (1%) [23]. Around 13% of all patients with JIS have a history of family involvement [23]. Patients with JIS are at risk of curve progression during pubertal growth, especially if the curve exceeds 30° at the onset of the pubertal growth spurt [25]. AIS occurs in 2–4% of children during the pubertal growth spurt, mainly in females [14, 26, 27]. The ratio of girls to boys increases from 1.6 : 1 at 9-10 years of age to 6.4 : 1 at 11-12 years of age [28]. Thoracic curves are observed in 33%–48% [28–30], thoracolumbar/lumbar 21%–40% [28–30], double/triple curves 9%–38% [28–30], and lumbar curves around 8% [28, 29]. Data concerning rate of curve progression are heterogeneous and vary from 1.6% to 68% depending on the study and subjects enrolled [31]. Soucacos et al. [32] reported by results of 6-year prospective cohort study in Greek population that curve progression occurs in around 15% of children with AIS, while 27.4% demonstrate spontaneous improvement of at least 5 degrees. Xu et al. [30] suggested that in skeletally immature AIS patients (Risser sign 0–3) with initial curve magnitude ranging from 20 to 40 degrees rate of curve progression was 24%–32% depending on the type of spine deformity. Risk factors for curve progression include type of spine deformity, in particular, right thoracic and double curves in girls, and right lumbar curves in boys; age at onset of menses in girls (although data are contradictive); menarche status; skeletal maturity (Risser sign 0–3); and curve magnitude equal to or greater than 30° [32, 33]. An MRI study of the brainstem and spinal cord showed that 2% of children with presumed AIS had such abnormalities as hydrosyringomyelia, Arnold-Chiari malformation tethered spinal cord, tumor, and diastematomyelia [34]. This is approximately ten times less than in patients with infantile and juvenile IS. An epidemiological case-control study revealed evidence of a genetic component in the etiology of AIS [35].

The data above imply that genetic predisposition plays a significant role in the etiology of IS; however genetic determinants of the disease are likely multifactorial. These variations may determine clinical features such as age of clinical manifestation, gender, association with congenital malformations, type of scoliotic curve, severity of curve progression, or resolution.

3. Etiological and Pathogenetic Factors and Concepts of IS

Current etiologic research on IS focuses on biological and biomechanical factors and relates mainly to the growth of the central nervous system (CNS), disturbances of bilateral symmetry and development instability, hormonal regulation and intercellular signaling, platelet calmodulin, melatonin, muscles, bone density, elastic fibers, and the skeletal framework including vertebral disproportionate growth and genetics [11]. There are several hypotheses pointing to congenital disorders of the CNS as an important factor in scoliotic spine deformation. The following sections describe the primary hypotheses.

3.1. The Nottingham Concept. This concept was proposed by Burwell and coauthors in 1992 and focuses on the relationship between developmental abnormality in the CNS and rib-vertebra angle asymmetry, which leads to a cyclical failure of the mechanisms of rotational trunk control involving falls. This in turns leads to the initiation of the deformity with loss of lordosis. Curve progression occurs as a result of gravity acting on both the abnormal as well as the normal vertebral growth [36].

3.2. Neurodevelopmental Concept of Maturational Delay of the CNS Body Schema. This concept was proposed in 2006 [37] as a further development of the Nottingham concept and suggests that spine deformity in scoliosis is the result of a combination of different factors including left-right skeletal length asymmetries involving growth plates (physes) and probably vertebral body growth plates; periapical rib length asymmetry; neuromuscular asymmetry; the rapid spinal elongation in the adolescent growth spurt that results from growth principally of vertebral body growth plates under the influence of steroid hormones; a delay in CNS maturation leading to impaired neuromuscular adjustments on a rapidly elongating spine; and movement of the spine and trunk in the upright posture unique to humans which leads to the neuromuscular adjustment of the rapidly elongating spine.

The results of the experimental and clinical studies all confirm the association of the CNS disorders with scoliosis development [38–46]. Unfortunately it is difficult to conclude whether the CNS dysfunctions reflect a possible cause of scoliotic spine deformity, consequence, or whether they develop parallel to the curve formation.

According to the Neurodevelopmental concept, which regards dysfunction of the CNS as a primary factor of IS, changes in the vertebrae-disc interaction must be secondary and may be caused by the axial load asymmetry.

3.3. The Braking of Bilateral Symmetry in relation to Left-Right Asymmetry Initiated in Embryonic Life. It has been suggested that developmental instability may be the initial factor in scoliotic curve formations having genetic determinants [47–49]. This conclusion was based on the fact that children with AIS have increased left-right asymmetry including arm and leg length, trunk shape, breast size, skull and face, teeth, brain stem, femoral neck-shaft angles, dermatoglyphic characteristics, vibration sensitivity, and somatosensory perception [44, 47, 50–56].

If the concepts of braking of bilateral symmetry and developmental instability are true, we can expect existence of a primordial morphological asymmetry in the structure of the vertebrae endplates, annulus fibrosus of the discs, and the disc-vertebrae joints not only at the apical level, but also at other spine levels.

3.4. The Neuroendocrine Hypothesis. Initially this hypothesis suggested melatonin deficiency as a source for AIS, and stems from the fact that pinealectomized chickens and pinealectomized rats maintained in a bipedal mode developed spine deformities more often than controls [57–59]. The same result was obtained in melatonin-deficient mice without pinealectomy [60]. The spine deformity development in pinealectomized chickens correlated with delay of the cortical somatosensory evoked potentials, suggesting a conduction disturbance of brain stem function. It was suggested that these findings implicate neurotransmitters or neurohormonal systems in the pineal body as a major contributing factor in this type of experimental scoliosis [57]. Machida et al. [61] reported that the level of serum melatonin was significantly lower in patients who had progressive curves in comparison with those who had a stable curve. The level of melatonin appeared to be a useful predictor for progression of spine curvature in IS, but further experiments in nonhuman primates and other clinical trials have not confirmed this conclusion [62–67].

3.5. Impairment of Melatonin Signaling Transduction. Moreau et al. [68] have shown that melatonin signaling was impaired in cultured osteoblasts from AIS patients to different degrees allowing their classification in 3 distinct groups. The authors suggested the presence of distinct mutations, interfering with melatonin signal transduction. Their conclusion was that changes in G-proteins functioning which are an important link in the intracellular melatonin signaling can be considered a possible mechanism in the etiopathogenesis of AIS. A hypofunctionality of G-proteins may be caused by increased serine phosphorylation leading to their inactivation, which is provided by kinases and phosphatases. Protein kinase C delta (PKCδ) is one of them. Azeddine et al. [69] demonstrated the ability of PKCδ to compose a complex with melatonin receptors MT2 in osteoblast cells derived from AIS patients. Such complexes were not detected in control cells. Further studies have shown an asymmetric expression of melatonin receptor mRNA in bilateral paravertebral muscles in patients with AIS [70]. It has been also found that a polymorphism of the promoter of the melatonin receptor 1B (MTNR1B/MT2) gene is associated with AIS [71]. Such an association was not found for the melatonin receptor 1A (MT1) gene [72]. There is also evidence that the function of G-protein-coupled receptors may be modulated by estrogen. In particular, 17 beta estradiol may activate MT1 receptors, increase MT2 receptors density [73], and correct or diminish melatonin signaling dysfunction revealed in osteoblasts taken from patients with AIS [74].

Melatonin signaling affects cell processes on several levels by binding to two specific G-protein coupled receptors, MT1 and MT2. One or both of these receptors exist on a variety of cell types. Melatonin receptors are associated primarily with four G-protein subunits. Melatonin signaling is generally a negative regulator of cell function via reduction of intracellular messengers such as cAMP, Ca^{2+}, and cGMP (cyclic guanosine monophosphate) via G-protein subunits. Melatonin also regulates cell processes via nuclear signaling and transcription factors [75]. Melatonin may increase cAMP accumulation in the osteoblasts of patients with IS [68]. To note, cAMP is used for intracellular signaling transduction and is involved in the regulation of different cell functions, including synthesis and proliferative activity. There are some data that cAMP and G-proteins participate in the effects of mechanotransduction in different tissues, including bone and cartilage [76–79]. Changes in the melatonin transduction pathways may significantly modify cellular activity including osteoblasts and osteoclasts. Melatonin is an important regulator of bone modeling and remodeling and is synthesized by the pineal gland and bone marrow [80]. Data on the direct effect of melatonin on bone cells are contradictory. It was reported that melatonin promotes osteoblast cell differentiation and proliferation [81] and increases bone mass by suppression resorption through downregulation of osteoclast formation and activation [82]. However, other authors report on the suppressive effect of melatonin on osteoblastic and osteoclastic activities [83]. It was noted that an inhibitory effect of melatonin on osteoblastic cells was seen when incubated in the presence of osteoclastic cells [84]. If the inhibitory effect of melatonin on both the cell lines is true, we may suppose that a defect in melatonin transduction in combination with other factors contributes to the accelerated anterior vertebral endochondral bone overgrowth, which in turn correlates with scoliotic curve occurrence and more active longitudinal growth of patients with AIS in comparison with their peers [85–87]. Increased osteoclast activity may cause stimulation of bone remodeling leading to spine slenderness. It may also explain the fact that in patients with AIS the longitudinal growth of the spinal cord fails to keep up with the pace of the growth of the vertebral column (disproportionate neuroosseous growth) [88].

Based on these results it is possible to speculate on the features that we may find in the morphological structure of vertebrae endplates, intervertebral discs, and their junctions in patients with IS. In particular, we may expect to find increased proliferative activity different from the age related changes and effects of the axial load asymmetry.

3.6. Platelet Calmodulin as Predictor of Scoliotic Curve Severity. The role of platelets in the pathogenesis of IS has been discussed for many years. It was noted that platelets and muscle fibers share the same contractile proteins (actin and myosin). In scoliotic patients, both spinal and peripheral muscles showed frequent abnormalities when examined by light and electron microscopy [89, 90]. Patients with IS differed from patients with other types of scoliosis [89]. They had increased calcium content and decreased muscle spindles in their muscles. It was suggested that there is a specific neuromuscular disorder causing IS linked with a membrane defect—namely impaired calcium pump [91]. Structural and functional abnormalities of platelets attributed to a defect of calcium transport in the membrane and/or contractile protein metabolism were also reported in patients with AIS [90]. Later Kindsfater et al. [92] and Lowe et al. [93] showed that platelet calmodulin levels correlate with scoliotic curve progression. They even proposed to use this index as a predictor of the curve progression. The significant difficulty in this field was the lack of normal data and the large variability in baseline levels for platelet calmodulin [94]. It was suggested that changes in the platelet calmodulin are acquired and parallel to curve progression reflecting systemic defects of cell membranes [92].

3.7. Platelet/Skeletal Hypothesis. Burwell and Dangerfield [95] proposed the platelet/skeletal hypothesis, which involves morphological, mechanical, vascular, platelet, hormonal, and growth mechanisms. This hypothesis assumes that presence of a small scoliosis curve in the human upright position alters the vertebral body growth endplate physes, which lead to microinsults. These microinsults activate endothelial cells, which then results in dilated vessels and vascular "lakes" adjacent to the disc growth plates. Activated platelets circulate through vessels, particularly in the curve apex on the medullary aspect of endplate physes. The platelets are activated by the slowing of blood flow in the dilated vessels and vascular "lakes", repeated mechanical microinsults that lead to vascular damage with exposure of endothelial collagen, endothelial cells, and release of different intracellular signaling factors. Platelet activation is associated with a calcium-calmodulin complex formation. Vertebrae growth plates are stimulated by growth factors from platelets as well as mechanically. It promotes an overgrowth and a spine deformity progression. A molecular predisposition to platelet activation may involve hormones and genetic polymorphisms.

We would like to point out another possible mechanism, which may explain the increase of platelet calmodulin levels in some patients with IS. As described above, a defect in melatonin signaling transduction associated with the impaired of G-protein cAMP inhibition was revealed in the osteoblasts of patients with IS [68]. This finding is consistent with the polymorphism of the promoter of melatonin receptor 1B gene, which was later reported [71]. It should be noted that human platelets use the same melatonin signaling mechanisms as in the osteoblasts, including melatonin receptors and G-protein-cAMP inhibition system [96]. Besides, melatonin inhibits several physiological intracellular processes [97], including the activity of Ca^{2+}/calmodulin-dependent protein kinase II (CaM-kinase II), and acts as a universal calmodulin antagonist in cells inhibiting Ca^{2+} influx [98]. If melatonin signaling is impaired in platelets, then platelet activation may be associated with an increase in cAMP generation, increase in the calmodulin and Ca^{2+} levels, and inhibition of aggregation. Inhibition of platelet aggregation is used as a marker of decreased G-protein activity and increased cAMP generation [99]. Thus, if impaired melatonin signaling is involved in IS, than platelet aggregation must be decreased in patients with IS. Unfortunately, the results of clinical studies are contradictory. Se Il Suk et al. [100] tested bleeding time, platelet aggregation, and titer of platelet plasminogen activator inhibitors in 52 patients with IS and in 49 controls. Statistically significant differences were not found. However, a more recent study performed by Ho et al. [101] showed that among 32 patients with IS who underwent preoperative coagulation screening tests, 8 had prolonged activated partial thromboplastin time and 5 were diagnosed with a specific coagulation abnormality potentially associated with increased bleeding. It was concluded that in the tested group of patients with IS, the risk of specific inherited haemostatic disorders was higher (around 10 times) than in the general population. Theoretically, an increase in platelet calmodulin levels and other changes in platelet functions and morphology observed in IS may be a cell specific secondary effect of such systemic disorder as melatonin signaling defect, which is genetically predisposed and linked with melatonin receptors and G-protein dysfunction. It is known that G-protein signaling defects in platelets are mainly subclinical [102]. Also, it has been known for years that certain cellular functions of platelets and in neurosecretory cells are very similar [102, 103]. Thus, some neurological dysfunctions in IS may also be explained by the melatonin signaling defect.

3.8. The Elastic Fiber System Role in the Pathogenesis of Idiopathic Scoliosis. Hadley-Miller et al. [104] studied the elastic fiber system using fresh-frozen histological specimens of ligamentum flavum removed from 23 patients with scoliosis and 5 age-matched controls at the time of an operation. Abnormalities on immunohistochemical staining including a marker for disarrangement of the fibers and differences in density of staining were found in 18 of the scoliotic specimens. It was also noted that in 4 scoliotic cases the amount of secreted fibrillin was normal, but the fibrillin failed to bind to other macromolecules, to form a sedimentable complex and to incorporate into the extracellular matrix. It was assumed that mutations in the gene encoding for fibrillin caused the production of abnormal fibrillin, such as in Marfan's syndrome. Research in this field is very important not only because ligaments play a significant role in spine stability, but also because fibrillins take part in embryonic development, in particular, skeletal elements, and skeletal muscle [105, 106]. In addition, some cells in the annulus fibrosus of IVD have been described as fibroblast-like [107]. There is evidence that melatonin may significantly modify the activity of fibroblasts. For instance, strong expression of basic fibroblast growth factor (bFGF) was found in the epineurium of rats that underwent pinealectomy in comparison with control and melatonin treated animals [108]. The role of these mechanisms in the etiopathogenesis of IS has not yet been investigated.

3.9. Changes of the Hormonal Regulation. Clinical observations have revealed a tendency for increased thoracolumbar spine height and slenderness in children with IS [86–88, 109]. Skogland and Miller [110] showed that girls with IS had a significantly higher response to the growth hormone stimulation test than controls. Higher growth hormone secretion was also found by Ahl et al. [111] among girls with IS in the pubertal stage. Interestingly, the level of serum somatomedin A (insulin-like growth factor-2) in girls with IS was lower than in controls [112]. Some authors report an increased risk of scoliosis progression in patients treated with growth hormone [113, 114], while another did not confirm this finding [115]. Growth hormone (somatotropin) is synthesized and secreted by the anterior pituitary gland. It stimulates growth and cell reproduction and stimulates cellular division in cartilage by acting through both systemic and local insulin-like growth factors (IGF) [116]. Several genetic studies have not shown a significant association between AIS and the single-nucleotide polymorphism of the growth hormone receptor and IGF-1 gene [117, 118]. However, an association between IGF-1 polymorphism and type of AIS spine deformity was found in Korean population [119]. Serum concentration of IGF1 significantly correlates with curve acceleration [120]. It should be noted that melatonin modulates secretion of growth hormone and IGF in culture, inhibits pituitary cAMP accumulation, and reduces growth hormone release [121]. Significant modulation of function of growth hormone function by melatonin was shown in rats [122]. In particular, melatonin inhibits endogenous production of IGF1 [123]. Thus, a defect in melatonin signaling may provoke secondary changes in the function of growth hormone-IGF1 axis and cause bone growth stimulation effects.

Published data concerning serum content of testosterone in AIS are contradictive. Skogland and Miller [110] revealed significantly increased mean serum levels of testosterone in girls with AIS, whose skeletal age was between 9 and 12 years. Raczkowski [124] also reported on the relative increased level of testosterone in girls aged 12–17 years with moderate and severe right thoracic curves (AIS) in comparison with girls of the same age with mild left lumbar scoliosis, while Esposito et al. [125] revealed decrease serum testosterone in

AIS, but types of spine deformity were not taken into consideration. Theoretically, increased levels of testosterone may contribute to vertebrae overgrowth and scoliosis progression. Androgens stimulate trabecular and cortical bone modeling independently from systemic or local IFG1 production in males [126]. Testosterone metabolism in the growth zone chondrocytes of females has some differences causing specificity of the response [127]. Interestingly, nocturnal melatonin secretion is increased in patients with hypogonadotropic hypogonadism and testosterone administration normalizes melatonin concentrations in these patients [128]. Thus, it is possible to assume that an increased level of testosterone in girls with AIS may be associated with a defect in melatonin signaling.

Estrogen levels in AIS also appear to be important, but the data are conflicting. Skogland and Miller [110] did not find significant differences in blood levels of estradiol, prolactin, follicle stimulating hormone, or luteinizing hormone between girls with AIS and controls, aged 7–17 years. Raczkowski [124] also reported on the absence of statistically significant differences in estrogen levels during the follicular and luteal phase between girls, aged 12–17 years, with right thoracic scoliosis and slight lumbar functional scoliosis. However, Kulis et al. [129, 130] have found a significantly lower level of estradiol and parathormone in girls with IS aged 11–14 in comparison with healthy controls. Esposito et al. [125] also reported on lower blood content of 17β-estradiol and progesterone in AIS girls with respect to control. Decreased level of estradiol observed at the earlier pubertal period may reflect a maturity delay. On the contrary, Goldberg et al. [131] reported that menarche in girls with IS in the Irish population was 0.39 years earlier than the national mean. Those diagnosed at a younger age were generally taller than their peers, indicating that the growth spurt in girls with IS was earlier. A study in Scandinavian girls found that menarche occurs significantly later in girls with a thoracolumbar or a double primary curve than in the control group. At the time of menarche, the girls with a thoracolumbar or double primary curve were significantly taller than those in the control group [132].

A decreased estrogen level corresponds with a decrease in bone mineral content (BMC), bone mineral density (BMD), lower osteocyte count, and lower trabecular thickness in the trabecular bone in girls with IS [133, 134]. Estrogen deficiency leads to an increase in bone remodeling in which resorption overtakes formation through an increase in immune function, which culminates in an increased production of tumor necrosis factor (TNF) by activated T cells. TNF increases osteoclast formation and bone resorption both directly and by augmenting the sensitivity of maturing osteoclasts to the essential osteoclastogenic factor RANKL [135]. The mechanism by which estrogen plays a role in IS may be linked with calmodulin. There is evidence that calmodulin decreases the estrogen binding capacity of estrogen receptors [136]. It is possible that increased intracellular levels of calmodulin that result from impaired melatonin signaling may contribute to decreased effects of estrogen while the estrogen level in blood is normal in patients with IS. Decreases in parathormone in patients with IS [130] require further research and explanation. Current experimental data suggest that vitamin D3 and melatonin modulate the secretory activity of parathyroid gland [137–139].

It has been found that blood leptin levels are significantly decreased in girls with AIS [140, 141]. It was suggested that leptin plays an important role in the lower body mass, growth parameters, and bone mineral density in AIS girls. Causes of the reduced levels of circulating leptin in AIS have not been studied yet. Leptin is an adipose derived hormone that plays a key role in regulating energy intake and expenditure. It was shown in experiments that leptin may stimulate osteoblastic differentiation *in vitro*, likely promoting the expression of osteoblastic related genes [142]. Leptin can also act through hypothalamus augmenting signals that enhance osteocalcin excretion from osteoblasts that modulate glucose-insulin and weight homeostasis [143]. On the other hand, leptin is able to stimulate sympathetic neurons in the hypothalamus and indirectly inhibit bone formation. This effect may be diminished by administration of beta-adrenoblockers [144]. To note, melatonin interacting with insulin upregulates leptin expression by adipose cells [145]. Thus, it is possible to assume that a decreased level of circulating leptin may be associated with an impairment of melatonin signaling in adipocytes. Burwell et al. [146] proposed a "double neuroosseous theory" of pathogenesis of AIS in girls, which postulates that developmental disharmony expressed in spine and trunk between autonomic and somatic nervous systems leads to AIS. The important component of this theory is increased sensitivity of the hypothalamus to circulating leptin with bilateral asymmetry of the sympathetic nervous system response, which causes an asymmetry in axial skeletal growth and initiates the scoliotic spine deformity. A growth hormone-IGF axis plays a role as a modulator of these processes. The developmental abnormalities are accompanied by osteopenia, intervertebral disc degeneration, and platelet calmodulin dysfunction. However, the author noted that this double neuroosseous theory requires testing [146].

Thus, some features of hormonal regulation observed in patients with IS may be initiated by different predominant factors, the changes in hormonal regulation play a significant role in the morphological structure of bones, vertebrae endplates, and intervertebral discs contributing to a faster growth spurt, increased bone remodeling, decreased bone mineral density, and spine slenderness. Therefore, corresponding attributes may be observed in the vertebrae endplates and IVD structure at the different levels of the scoliotic spine.

3.10. Genetic Factors. Study of AIS in twins demonstrated that monozygous twins have a significantly higher rate of concordance and correlation between curve development and progression than dizygous twins [35, 147], suggesting a genetic predisposition to the disease [148]. Potential candidate genes have been previously identified [149–151]. Single nucleotide polymorphisms (SNPs) of different genes have been defined as having association with susceptibility or progression of AIS during last decade, Table 1. These include

TABLE 1: Genes showed an association with AIS.

#	Identified Genes	Population tested	Published by
1	Genes potentially associated with IS: 2p15-13, 6q13, 15q12	Analysis of the Human Cytogenetics Database	Brewer et al., 1998 [149]
2	Genes associated with IS: 6p, distal 10q, 18q	A genome-wide search in one large family (7 affected members).	Wise et al., 2000 [151]
3	Genes associated with IS: 19p13.3 (D19S216; D19S894; D19S1034) D2S160-D2S347-D2S112 No linkage was found with markers on the X chromosome	Seven families with AIS consisting of 25 affected members were studied.	Chan et al., 2002 [165]
4	Genes associated with IS: Xq23 (GATA172D05) in 15% of studied families stratified for genetic heterogeneity	202 families with at least 2 individuals with IS (total of 1198 individuals were studied).	Justice et al., 2003 [164]
5	Genes associated with IS: Matrilin-1 (MATN1) gene polymorphism, 1p35	Population of 81 trios (daughter/son affected by IS and both parents).	Montanaro et al., 2006 [155]
6	Genes associated with IS: Matrilin-1 (MATN1), rs1149048, 1p35 Association with AIS susceptability	222 cases (90% female) 750 controls (88% female) adolescents Chinese population	Chen et al., 2009 [156]
7	Genes associated with IS: Matrilin-1 (MATN1), rs 1065755, 1p35 Association with curve type	166 cases (80% female) 126 controls (100% female) Adolescents Korean population	Bae et al., 2012 [158]
8	Genes associated with IS: Matrilin-1 (MATN1) Association with curve severity and decrease of plasma mtrilin-1 level	25 cases (AIS) 25 controls Chinese population	Wang et al. 2009 [157]
9	Genes associated with IS: G-protein-coupled receptor 126 (GPR126), rs6570507, 6q24.1	1819 cases (AIS) 25934 controls Japanese population, 743 cases (AIS) 1209 controls Chinese Han population, 447 cases (AIS) 437 controls European ancestry population	Kou et al., 2013 [162]
10	Genes associated with IS: CHD7 gene polymorphism, 8q12	Genome-wide scan follow-up study of 52 families with history of IS (130 affected individuals).	Gao et al., 2007 [154]
11	Genes associated with IS: Melatonin receptor 1B gene (MTNR1B), rs4753426, 11q21-q22	Initial screening (472 cases and 304 controls), and separate replication test (342 cases and 347 controls)	Qui et al., 2007 [71]
12	Genes associated with IS: Estrogen receptor α gene XbaI, 6q25.1 (association with curve severity)	304 girls with IS were tested.	Inoue et al., 2002 [167]
13	Genes associated with IS: Estrogen receptor α (ERα) gene XbaI, 6q25.1 (may be associated with a risk of AIS)	202 cases 174 controls	Wu et al., 2006 [168]
14	Genes associated with IS: 21 candidate genes on chromosomes 6 and 10	5 families with triple IS spine deformities	Marosy et al., 2010 [180]
15	Genes associated with IS: Estrogen receptor α (ERα) gene, 6q25.1	147 cases (53% AIS, 47% unaffected sisters) 104 controls (no AIS) Age 13–19 years	Esposito et al., 2009 [125]

TABLE 1: Continued.

#	Identified Genes	Population tested	Published by
16	Genes associated with IS: Calmodulin 1 (CALM1) gene Melatonin receptor 1B (MTNR1B) gene, rs1562444, 11q14.3	30 AIS cases (6 male, 24 female) 30 controls (age- and gender-matched) Chinese population	Zhuang et al., 2007 [201]
17	Genes associated with IS: Estrogen receptor 1 (ESR1) gene rs2234693, 6q25.1;	67 cases (double curve patients) 100 nonscoliotic controls	Zhao et al., 2008 [170]
18	Calmodulin 1 (CALM1) gene: rs12885713, rs5871, 14q24-q31	67 cases (double curve patients) 100 nonscoliotic controls 100 AIS cases 100 Controls	Zhao et al., 2008 [170] Zhao et al., 2009 [171]
19	Genes associated with IS: Estrogen receptor β gene −458T>C site polymorphisms of 14q23.2. Association with AIS in females and with curve severity.	218 cases (176 female; 42 male) with AIS 140 healthy controls.	Zhang et al., 2009 [172]
20	Genes associated with IS: G-protein coupled estrogen receptor 1 (GPER1), rs3808351, rs10269151, 426655s3, 7p22.3 Association with curve severity	389 cases (336 female; 53 male) 338 controls (289 female; 49 male) Age: 10–19 years Chinese Han population	Peng et al., 2012 [174]
21	Genes associated with IS: D17S947–D17S798 17p11	A three-generation family of Italian ancestry that included 11 members affected by IS Genome scanning was performed with 358 microsatellite markers.	Baghernajad Salehi et al., 2002 [181]
22	Genes associated with IS: The osteoprotegerin gene 1181 G → C polymorphism was associated with the bone mineral density of the lumbar spine in females with AIS, 8q24.	198 females with AIS were tested.	Eun et al., 2009 [182]
23	Genes associated with IS: The tryptophan hydroxylase (TPH1) rs10488682, 11p15.1. Association with susceptibility to AIS	103 AIS patients (Cobb angle > 30°), and 107 nonscoliotic controls. All subjects were Han Chinese 10–20 years of age.	Wang et al., 2008 [183]
24	Genes associated with IS: The tryptophan hydroxylase (TPH1), rs10488682, 11p15.1. The estrogen receptor α (ERα) rs9340799, 6q25.1 Association with cure progression and success of brace treatment	312 AIS cases (90 progressive, and 222 no progression) Brace treatment Chinese population	Xu et al., 2011 [30]
25	Gene associated with IS: 5-hydroxytryptamine (serotonin) receptor A (HTR1A), rs6294, 5q12.3	103 AIS cases 108 controls (age- and gender-matched) Chinese population	Wang et al., 2010 [199]
26	Genes associated with IS: Fibrillin 3 (FBN3), rs35579498, rs7257948 19p13 Association with curve occurrence and progression in AIS	273 AIS patients, aged 10–18 years 287 control-healthy age-matched female adolescents.	Cao et al., 2008 [166]
27	Gene associated with IS: Metalloproteinase-3 (MMP3) promoter gene 11q22.3	53 patients with AIS and 206 nonscoliotic controls. Age was not specified.	Aulisa et al., 2007 [184]
28	Gene associated with IS: Metalloproteinase-9 (MMP9), rs2250889, 20q13.12	190 AIS cases 190 controls Female Chinese Han population	Huang et al., 2011 [198]
29	Gene associated with IS: Interleukin-6 (IL6) promoter gene 7p21-p15	53 patients with AIS and 206 nonscoliotic controls. Age was not specified.	Aulisa et al., 2007 [184]

Table 1: Continued.

#	Identified Genes	Population tested	Published by
30	Gene associated with IS: Interleukin-6 (IL6) Association with bone mineral density in AIS	198 AIS cases (female) 120 controls (female) Age: 11–14 years Korean population	Lee et al., 2010 [186]
31	Gene associated with IS: Inrleukin-17 receptor C (IL-17RC) gene, rs708567, 3p.25.3.	529 cases (AIS, female 100%) 512 controls (female 100%) Age: 11 to 18 years Chinese Han population	Zhou et al., 2012 [187]
32	Gene associated with IS: Neural adhesion molecules CHL1, rs1400180, 3p26.3	419 AIS families	Sharma et al., 2011 [195]
33	Gene associated with IS: Ladybird homeobox 1 (LBX1) rs11190870, 10q24.31	1376 cases (AIS, female 100%) 11297 controls (female 100%) Japanese population; 300 cases (AIS, Cobb > 30 degree) 780 controls Southern Chinese population; 513 cases (AIS) 440 controls Chinese Han population	Takahashi et al., 2011 [192] Fan et al., 2012 [194] Gao et al., 2013 [193]
34	Gene associated with IS: Vitamin D3 receptor gene polymorphism (VDR Bsml), 12q13-14. Associated with low bone mass and low bone mineral density at the lumbar spine in girls with AIS	198 Korean girls 11–13 years of age with AIS, and 120 age-matched healthy girls (control). 164 females 9–20 years of age with AIS, and 122 age-matched healthy girls (control)	Suh et al., 2010 [189] Xia et al., 2007 [190]
35	Gene associated with IS: Histone methyltransferase (DOT1L), rs12459350, 19p13.3;	500 cases (AIS) 497 controls	Mao et al., 2013 [196]
36	Gene associated with IS: Chromosome 17 open reading frame 67 (C17orf67), rs4794665, 17q22.	500 cases (AIS) 497 controls	Mao et al., 2013 [196]
37	Gene associated with IS: Neurotrophin 3 (NTF3) gene, rs11063714, 12p13 Association with curve severity	362 cases 377 controls Chinese Han population	Qiu et al., 2013 [175]
38	Gene associated with IS: SH3GL1 protein-coding gene, 19p13.3	214 IS cases (68 male, 146 female)	Yang et al., 2012 [197]
39	Gene associated with IS: Lysosomal protein transmembrane 4 beta (LAPTM4B), rs2449539, 8q22.1 Insulin-like growth factor 1 (IFG1), rs5742612, 12q23.2 Association with susceptibility to AIS and curve severity	68 AIS cases 35 controls (age- and sex-matched) Korean population	Moon et al., 2013 [119]

a polymorphism of the promoter of melatonin receptor 1B gene (MTNR1B) that was revealed in Chinese population [71] corresponding with previously revealed impairment of the melatonin transduction pathway [68]. However, this result was not replicated in Japanese [152] and Caucasian [153] populations. An association of AIS was also found with the CHD7 gene (chromodomain helicase DNA-binding protein 7 gene) [154]. Splicing mutations within coding exons of CHD7 have been identified in a majority of patients with CHARGE syndrome (coloboma of eye, heart defects, atresia of the choane, retardation of growth and/or development, genital, and/or urinary abnormalities, and ear abnormalities and deafness). It was hypothesized that milder variants of the CHD7 polymorphism could underlie IS susceptibility [154]. A link between matrilin-1 gene polymorphism (MATN1) and AIS has been found in European [155], Chinese [156, 157], and Korean [158] populations but was not replicated in Japanize population [159]. Wang et al. [157] noted that MATN1 polymorphism in AIS corresponds with decrease of plasma matrilin-1 levels. Matrilin-1 was previously named cartilage matrix protein (CMP) and is mostly found in cartilage. CMP is a bridging molecule that connects matrix components in cartilage to form an integrated matrix filamentous network [160]. Biglycan/matrilin-1 or decorin/matrilin-1 complex acts as a linkage between collagen VI microfibrils and aggrecan or alternatively collagen II [161]. Thus, a defect of CMP/matrilin-1 molecules may cause a significant impairment of the cartilage ultrastructure. Genetic variants of GPR126 gene showed association with AIS in Japanese, Chinese Han, and European-ancestry populations [162]. This gene encodes G-protein-coupled receptor 126 required for normal differentiation of promyelinating Schwann cells and axons myelination [163]. This gene is highly expressed in cartilage [162] and probably is involved in regulation of the cAMP level in cells [163] and development of spinal cord [162]. Data on the role of X chromosome in the pathogenesis of IS are contradictory. Justice et al. [164] reported on the association between familial IS and a polymorphism of X chromosome particularly GATA172D05. This region includes several loci whose functions have been related to cellular interactions within the extracellular matrix of neural tissue and a chordin-like protein, which is known to be essential to the correct patterning of the zebrafish axial skeleton through bone morphogenetic proteins signaling. The genes that encode two of the collagen type IV alpha chains have also been mapped to this region. However, evidence of the X chromosome polymorphism was only found in 15% of the studied families, which had X-linked dominant inheritance. Chan et al. [165] did not find any link between the X-chromosome polymorphism and IS but revealed a significant association between the abnormal phenotype of the distal short arm of chromosome 19p13.3 and AIS. Within this region, there are more than 70 possible genes expressed in chondrocytes, osteoclasts, muscles, or tendon that could be potential candidate genes for IS. In particular, fibrillin-3 gene is in this region. Polymorphisms of this gene may be associated with body height of the AIS patients, or occurrence and progression of AIS [166]. Data on the association of the estrogen receptor gene polymorphism with susceptibility to IS are contradictory. Inoue et al. [167] reported on the association between estrogen receptor α (ERα) gene polymorphism and curve severity. Wu et al. [168] confirmed the association between the ERα gene polymorphism and AIS. Xu et al. [30] suggested that the ERα SNP is associated with curve progression. These findings could not be replicated by Tang et al. [169]. However, Zhao et al. [170] reported on statistically significant associations between polymorphism of the ERα and calmodulin-1 (CALM1) [171] genes with susceptibility to AIS and the type of scoliotic curvature. Esposito et al. [125] identified four ERα gene polymorphisms in AIS. In addition, Zhang et al. [172] reported an association between SNP of the estrogen receptor β (ERβ) gene with AIS susceptibility and curve type and severity in females. On the contrary, Takahashi et al. [173] did not find any association between these estrogen receptor genes and susceptibility to AIS or curve severity in the Japanese population. It was reported that polymorphism of G-protein-coupled estrogen receptor (GPER) [174] and neurotropin 3 (NTF3) [175] genes has significant association with curve severity in AIS in Chinese Han population. These findings were not replicated in Japanese population [176]. It has been proposed that a disturbance in proteoglycan (PG) synthesis and formation in the vertebral growth plate is a basic cause of IS. It was suggested that aggrecan gene expression was significantly decreased in cultivated chondroblasts from patents with IS [177]. However, Marosy et al. [178] showed the lack of an association between the aggrecan gene and familial IS, but other potential candidate genes were revealed on 15q25-26. To note, fibrillin-1 (FBN1) gene, which is associated with Marfan syndrome, is located nearby (at15q21.1). Nevertheless, an association between a polymorphism of the FBN1 gene and AIS was not found [179]. Twenty-one candidate genes on chromosomes 6 and 10 were found in families with triple IS spine deformities [180]. Salehi et al. [181] reported on the link between familial IS and 17p11 (D17S947-D17S798) gene polymorphism. These protein genes play a role in glycoproteoglycan sulfation, the process that is important for the organization of osteoligamentous structures. A significant association was found between the osteoprotegerin (OPG) gene polymorphism and bone mineral density of the lumbar spine in female with AIS [182]. OPG is a cytokine that is a member of the tumor necrotic factor superfamily, which inhibits the production of osteoclasts and thus indirectly stimulates bone modeling. The OPG gene polymorphisms may indirectly stimulate osteoclastogenesis and bone remodeling. Wang et al. [183] have found a significant association between a tryptophan hydroxylase (TPH1) gene polymorphism and susceptibility to AIS in Chinese population. Xu et al. [30] suggested that the TPH1 gene SNP is associated with the risk of curve progression. The TPH1 is involved in the synthesis of the neurotransmitter serotonin from tryptophan, which then can be transformed to melatonin. Thus a polymorphism of this gene can contribute to reduced synthesis of both serotonin and melatonin. However, this SNP was not replicated in Japanese [159] and Caucasian [153] populations. It was shown that a MMP-3 promoter gene polymorphism is significantly associated with AIS [184]. But this finding was not replicated in Chinese population [185]. The MMP-3 relates to the matrix metalloproteinase family that is involved in the breakdown of extracellular matrix, in particular degrading of fibronectin, collagens III, IV, IX, and X, and cartilage proteoglycans and tissue remodeling, as well as in disease processes, such as arthritis and metastasis. An IL-6 (interleukin 6) promoter gene polymorphism was also reported as having association with AIS [184], in particular, bone mineral density in AIS patients [186]. The IL-6 is a cytokine with a wide variety of biological functions. It plays an essential role in the final differentiation of B-cells into Ig-secreting cells. This protein is primarily produced at sites of acute and chronic inflammation, where it induces a transcriptional inflammatory response through corresponding receptors. This suggests an involvement of the immune system and inflammatory processes in the pathogenesis of AIS. However, no link between IL-6 and AIS was found in Chinese population [185]. Instead, in Chinese population, an association between the interleukin-17 receptor C (IL-17RC) gene polymorphism and the susceptibility to AIS was shown [187]. The Il-17RC promotes the production of proinflammatory cytokines such as

TNFα, IL-1β, and IL-6 [187]. Mórocz et al. [188] demonstrated that SNP of such genes as BMP4, Il6, leptin, MMP3, and MTNR1B may not have significant association with AIS, if they were tested separately. However, combinations of these genes SNP have significant association with susceptibility to AIS in the Hungarian population. It was reported that a vitamin D receptor (VDR) gene SNP is associated with decreased bone mineral density, in particular of the lumbar spine in girls with AIS (Korean population) [189, 190]. The VDR are expressed in cells of different tissues, including bone and the parathyroid gland. Vitamin D is involved in the regulation of parathormone secretion [137]. Thus, this finding corresponds with decreased levels of parathormone revealed in girls with IS [130]. However, Chen et al. [191] did not find any association between the VDR gene polymorphism and bone mineral density in Chinese AIS girls. Variants near LBX1 gene encoding ladybird homeobox-1 have significant link with AIS in Japanese [192] and Chinese populations [193, 194]. The LBX1 encodes transcription factor required for the development of interneurons in the dorsal horn of the spinal cord and migration and development of muscle precursor cells for limb muscles, diaphragm, and hypoglossal cord [163]. The CHL1 gene was recognized as a candidate gene linked with susceptibility to AIS [195]. This gene encodes family of neural cell adhesion molecules that may be involved in signal transduction pathways [163]. Polymorphism of other two genes DOT1L encoding histone methyltransferase and C17orf67 (chromosome 17 open reading frame 67) are shown as linked with susceptibility to AIS [196]. The histone methyltransferase DOT1L plays a complex role in cartilage biology and may be associated with osteoarthritis [163, 196]. Characteristics of the protein that is encoded by C17orf67 are not studied well [196]. Other genes SNPs that have been reported as having association with AIS are SH3GL1 [197], LAPTM4B [119], IFG1 [119], MMP9 [198], HTR1A [199], and TIMP2 [200].

Axial Biotech Inc. [202] has developed a test to identify patients with low risk of scoliotic curve progression using 53 genetic markers. Published results suggested that the test has high negative predictive value (97%–100%), but low positive predictive value (8%–25%) [203]. It means that cases with high risk of scoliotic deformity progression can be underdiagnosed by this test. The test showed lack of predictive value in Japanese population [162].

In summary, published data concerning association between gene polymorphism and AIS are heterogeneous and have limited replicability. We may assume that AIS may have different patterns of genetic determinants depending on the ethnic population. Combinations of these determinants probably predispose individuals to the disease. Defects in the molecular structure of different proteins, caused by genetic polymorphism, may lead to different ultrastructural features at different systems and tissues of the body, including the CNS, hormonal regulation, the immune system, connective tissue, bone, cartilage, ligaments, and muscles, which form specific conditions for the spine curve triggering and progression.

3.11. Biomechanical Factors. Biomechanical factors play a significant role in the progression of scoliosis. A vicious cycle of asymmetrical loading has been hypothesized to explain this effect. It was suggested that increased compression on the concave side of the curve decelerates growth, while reduced loading on the convex side accelerates growth according to the Hueter-Volkmann's law and creates a larger deformity [1–3, 204, 205]. Today, these phenomena may be explained by the effects of mechanotransduction, which include intracellular and extracellular signaling factors such as mechanosomes, corresponding genes, nitric oxide (NO), cAMP, gene encoding enzymes, bone morphogenic proteins (BMP) 1 and 4, and growth factors such as IGF-1, IGF-2, vascular endothelial growth factor (VEGF), and transforming growth factor-β_1 (TGF-β_1), which act via autocrine and paracrine mechanisms [206–208]. Signal transduction pathways such as IGF-1 may interact with estrogen in the proliferative response to mechanical strain [209]. An interaction between different anabolic intracellular pathways may enhance the upregulation of these signaling pathways, ultimately leading to the cellular response on mechanical loading [209]. Experimental studies show that for normal bone modeling, bone strain should not exceed 2 MPa (MPa-megapascal = 10^6 newtons/m^2). If mechanical strain exceeds 60 MPa, then microscopic fatigue damage and a decrease in bone growth may occur [210]. Unfortunately, there is a paucity of data related directly to the quantitative *in vivo* assessment of strain at the surface of the human vertebrae endplates and the association between strain and the morphological and ultrastructural characteristics of the vertebrae endplates and discs in patients with IS, especially in the upright position [211, 212]. Meir et al. [213] reported results of hydrostatic pressure measured across the IVD in recumbent anaesthetized scoliotic patients during surgery. It was shown that intradiscal pressure and stress in scoliotic discs are abnormal and have higher hydrostatic pressure (0.25 MPa) than those measured in nonscoliotic discs (<0.07 MPa). Stress in the concave annulus was greater than in the convex annulus, indicating asymmetric loading. The authors noted that without the presence of muscle activity and horizontal positioning of the patients, it is difficult to explain this finding from the point of view of the "vicious cycle" hypothesis.

4. Morphological and Ultrastructural Features of Scoliotic IVD and VEPh

4.1. Disc Cells and Extracellular Matrix Features. It was suggested that asymmetry in mechanical loading is the main factor that leads to morphological changes in scoliotic IVD and VEPh. The effects of mechanotransduction are important components in the response of bone and cartilage to mechanical load. Mechanotransduction pathways involve specific cytoskeletal components, such as vimentin and actin. Johnson and Roberts [214] compared the presence of such cytoskeletal components as phalloidin-labeled filamentous actin (F-actin) and vimentin in the disc cells of patients with scoliosis, in subjects without disc pathology, and in subjects with degenerative disc diseases. F-actin-positive cells appearing stellate or dendritic were observed in the outer annulus of scoliotic discs. Such cells were not seen in the outer annulus fibrosus of nonscoliotic or degenerative discs. F-actin appeared more prominent on the convex side of the scoliotic curve than on the concave side, not corresponding with the putative response. The authors suggested that cells in scoliotic discs tend to change phenotype in comparison with nonscoliotic discs. This study had considerable limitations (see Table 2) necessitating further investigation. Ford et al. [215] used transmission electron microscopy and immunostaining markers and revealed that cells of scoliotic discs exhibited a healthy appearance and abundant endoplasmic reticulum, which indicated a high level of secretory activity, while proliferative activity was decreased. Specimens for this study were taken from the anterior annulus of the discs, thus asymmetrical load probably did not impact the results.

Bertram et al. [216] demonstrated that chondrocyte-typical extracellular-matrix gene expression was higher in scoliotic IVDs than in the normal spine. Histological analysis showed mild degeneration of the IVDs, including minor granular changes, clefts and tears, and mucoid matrix degeneration that was accompanied with accelerated anabolic matrix metabolism, which included higher extracellular matrix gene expression of collagen type II, biglican, collagen type XI, collagen type XII, aggrecan, lumican, chondromodulin-I precursor, and decorin. Antoniou et al. [217] revealed a decrease in the total collagen content in the scoliotic annulus and endplate regions. Glycosaminoglycan content was also decreased in the scoliotic endplates and nucleus regions. However, the total protein level was significantly elevated. Water content was considerably lower in the scoliotic annulus and endplate regions. Levels of marker for type II collagen synthesis were higher in the nucleus, annulus, and endplate regions of scoliotic discs than in the corresponding regions of normal discs. By contrast, the presence of total denaturated collagen was significantly elevated in the nucleus of normal tissue as compared to scoliotic tissue. The authors suggested that these scoliotic changes are due to an altered and ineffective synthetic response to a pathologic mechanical environment. These results correspond with the finding that proteoglycan molecules in patients with AIS contained more protein and less carbohydrates than the proteoglycans of normal tissue [223]. It was shown that a chondroadherin level was lower at the concave site of the scoliotic discs than at the convex side, suggesting changes in matrix homeostasis [222]. He et al. [224] showed that patients with AIS had significantly more type I and type II collagen on the convex side of IVDs compared with the concave side. Similar results had previously been obtained by Roberts et al. [221]. They also pointed out that staining patterns for collagen types III, VI, and IX were different in scoliotic IVDs in comparison with nonscoliotic IVDs [221]. Gene expression of type X collagen, which was associated with hypertrophic changes and cartilage mineralization, was revealed mainly at the concave side of the apical disc in patients with IS [225]. Yu et al. [219] showed that in scoliotic IVD (AIS and neuromuscular scoliosis), the elastic fibers were sparse, and collagen and elastic fiber networks were disorganized with a loss of lamellar structure. Cell clusters, a typical degenerative feature, were seen in scoliotic discs but not in age-matched controls. However, based on these data it is impossible to determine whether the finding of a sparse elastic fiber network in the IVD of patients with IS is a primary or secondary factor. Akhtar et al. [220] showed that in the degenerated regions of scoliotic IVDs there was a disruption of collagen and elastic fibers accompanied by losses of keratan sulfate (KS) proteoglycan, and degeneration of elastic fibers that was accompanied by the loss of α-elastin. KS-bearing proteoglycan (lumican or fibromodulin) is closely associated with the lamellar organization of collagen fibers and elastic fibers in the IVD. It was hypothesized that impaired cellular metabolism of lumican and/or fibromodulin can contribute to the development of scoliotic spine deformity. As specimens in this study were taken from the medial parts of the IVDs, asymmetrical axial load did not impact the results. Thus, this finding probably reflects systemic features of scoliotic cells. Stern et al. [218] demonstrated significantly higher synthesis of deoxyribonucleic acid, proteoglycan, and hydroxyproline in cells from scoliotic disks in comparison with cells taken from osteochondrotic and herniated discs. There was no evidence of enhanced senescence (physiologic aging) [226] or apoptosis [227] of IVD cells in patients with IS in comparison to those with neuromuscular scoliosis or disc degenerative diseases. Unfortunately, a comparison between IS disc cells and normal age-matched disc cells was not performed in these studies. IVD degeneration correlated with the level of matrix metalloproteinases (MMP), which contribute to extracellular matrix degrading and tissue remodeling and are involved in inflammatory reactions [228]. The MMP level was asymmetric and prevailed at the convex site of IVDs in patients with AIS [228].

In summary, the most important features of the IVD in IS are as follows: (1) increased synthetic and decreased proliferative cells activity; (2) changes and asymmetry of collagen synthesis and degrading; (3) increased synthesis of proteins; (4) impairment of collagen turnover that results in failure of the synthesized extracellular matrix components to organize into a normal lamellar structure; (5) decreased water content and increased hydrostatic pressure. Initial genetic determinants probably comprise the basis of these IVD features, which may then be significantly modulated by the mechanical environment and other factors during disease manifestation. Overall these microstructural features decrease the ability of scoliotic discs to tolerate load and contribute to disc wedging and Schmorl's nodes occurrence. This is more evident at the apex of the lumbar curvature where load is higher, while wedging of the vertebral body prevails at the apex of the thoracic curvature [204, 205, 229].

4.2. Vertebrae Endplate Features. Roberts et al. [221] pointed out that the prevalence and extent of calcification in the cartilage endplate of the scoliotic specimens were the most striking finding of their study. Calcification appeared to start at one or both ends of the individual cells before it encompassed the cell and became more widespread throughout the matrix. It was prominent in the cartilage endplate nearest the anterior rim. Calcification may also expand into the IVD.

Table 2: Morphological and ultrastructural studies.

#	Findings	Objects/Materials	Method	The main limitations of the study	Authors
1	F-actin-positive cells were observed in the outer anulus of scoliotic discs and appeared stellate or dendritic, rather than bipolar and fibroblastic. F-actin appeared more prominent on the convex side of the scoliotic curve than on the concave side	Specimens of 13 human intervertebral discs: Normal—3; Low back pain—4; Spondylolisthesis—3; Scoliosis—3	Morphology of IVD cells was examined using confocal microscopy and labeling of such cytoskeleton components as F-actin and vimentin.	(1) Small amount of specimens. (2) Statistical analysis was not performed (3) Studied subjects were not matched by age and gender. (4) Specimens were not matched by the spine level. (5) Type of scoliosis was not specified	Johnson and Roberts, 2003 [214]
2	Cells from anterior anulus of scoliotic discs had increased secretory activity and decreased proliferative activity.	The anterior annulus tissue of discs: Scoliotic—5 (aged 16–26); Degenerative—5 (aged 43–56); Prolapsed discs—5 (aged 33–52)	Histology and transmission electron microscopy with immunostaining markers.	(1) Subjects gender was not taken into consideration. (2) Statistical analysis was not performed.	Ford et al., 2002 [215]
3	Morphologic disc degeneration in IS was associated with stronger anabolic matrix metabolism. Higher mRNA expression of extracellular matrix molecules like collagen II, aggrecan, biglican, decorin, lumical, and chondromodulin was revealed.	Study groups: Idiopathic scoliosis (11 female and 5 male aged 10–22 years); Patients with acute trauma (2 female, and 5 male aged 28–55); Autopsy control adolescents (4 male and 4 female aged 8 to 17 years); Autopsy control adults (7 male and 3 female aged 47–77 years)	Histological examination. Gene expression analysis.	(1) Studied subjects were not matched by age and gender.	Bertram et al., 2006 [216]
4	Higher collagen Type II synthetic levels and increased total protein content with no matrix turnover. Scoliotic changes are due to an altered and ineffective synthetic response to a pathologic mechanical environment.	Specimens of IVD and vertebrae endplates: (i) 15 scoliotic (female) aged 11–15 years; (ii) 17 normal control subjects (no details)	Discs and endplates were analyzed for their water, collagen, proteoglycan, and protein content. Biochemical methods were used.	(1) The scoliotic tissue was analyzed mainly at the convex and central side of the disc where the tissue is experiencing tension and not compressive force (2) Control group was not clearly identified.	Antoniou et al., 2001 [217]
5	Cells obtained from scoliotic discs showed higher synthetic activity than cells from degenerative and herniated discs.	Studied subjects: IS—6 patients (mean age—24.4 years); Osteochondrosis—6 patients (mean age 42.8 years); Disc herniation—6 patients (mean age 35.2 years)	Cultures of disc cells were studied. Deoxyribonucleic acid content, hydroxyproline content, and proteoglycan synthesis were determined.	(1) Gender of the studied subjects was not taken into consideration. (2) Studied subjects were not matched by age.	Stern et al., 2004 [218]
6	In scoliotic discs, elastic fibers were sparse, and the collagen and elastic fiber networks were disorganized with loss of lamellar structure. Cell clusters (degenerative feature) were seen in scoliotic discs but not in age-matched control discs.	Studied subjects: IS—3 female (age 12–22 years); Neuromuscular—3 female (age 14–16 years); Control—2 (1 female with spinal tumor aged 12 years; 1 male with trauma aged 17 years)	Micrographs of the sections of IVDs were examined by polarized light to visualize collagen organization. The elastic fiber network was visualized immunohistechemically or by histochemical staining with orcein.	(1) Small amount of cases and controls. (2) Statistical analysis was not performed.	Yu et al., 2005 [219]

Table 2: Continued.

#	Findings	Objects/materials	Method	The main limitations of the study	Authors
7	In scoliosis, impaired regulation of collagen fibrillogenesis by lumican or fibromodulin may result in lamellar structure.	Studied subjects: IS—3 female patients (13, 15, and 17 years old); Normal control—2 male (20, 24 years old)	Specimens from medial (anterior, central and posterior) parts of L1–L3 discs were studied. Ultrastructural relations among keratan sulfate proteoglycan, α-elastin, collagen fibers, and elastic fibers were studied.	(1) Small case and control groups. (2) Cases and controls were not matched by gender and age. (3) Statistical analysis was not performed.	Akhtar et al., 2005 [220]
8	Proteoglycan and water content were reduced in scoliotic discs, particularly toward concavity of the curve. The distribution of some collagen types differed in scoliotic discs. Calcification of the cartilage endplates and adjacent discs was revealed in scoliosis.	Studied subjects: Scoliosis—20 patients including 15 with IS, 4 with congenital, and 1 with unknown type. Age: 3–42 years (mean—14.4). Gender was not indicated. Control—12 subjects. Age 17–83 (mean—58.1). Gender was not identified.	The morphology and composition of the IVD and vertebrae cartilage endplates were studied	(1) Case and controls were not matched by age and gender. (2) Cases with IS and congenital scoliosis were not analyzed separately. (3) Specimens were not matched by the spine level (T6–T10 for scoliosis; L1–L5 for controls). (4) Statistical analysis was not performed.	Roberts et al., 1993 [221]
9	A chondroadherin level decreased at the concave site of scoliotic discs	Studied subjects: Scoliosis (AIS)—7 patients (5 female and 2 male), age 14–17 years. Control—2 nonscoliotic subjects aged 29 and 87 years. Gender was not specified.	Specimens from scoliotic subjects were taken during surgery (1 T9/T10, 3 T12/L1, and 3 L1/L2 discs). Control specimens were obtained during autopsy (2-L4/L5 discs)	(1) Small amount of cases and controls (2) Cases and controls were not matched by age (3) Cases and control specimens were not matched by the spine level (4) Statistical analysis was not performed.	Haglund et al., 2009 [222]

The author noted that most studied patients with scoliosis had not reached skeletal maturity at the time of the study. Therefore, endochondral ossification should be ongoing in epiphyseal regions, such as the cartilage endplate. Calcification of the IVD has also been described in healthy children, which resolved later in life. To note, cases and controls were not matched by age and gender in that study.

There was evidence that the proliferative and hypertrophic chondrocytes in the anterior column of AIS patients were more active than those on the posterior column [230, 231]. These features seem to be more evident in patients with AIS than those with congenital scoliosis. It has also been shown that in AIS the proliferative potential and apoptosis ratios of chondrocytes in the proliferative and hypertrophic zone in the convex side were significantly higher than in the concave side, particularly in the apical vertebral growth plate [232]. Changes in proliferative activity of chondrocytes correlated with the radiographic data of the spine deformity. However, it was unclear whether these differences in proliferation were the primary cause or were due to secondary changes. The authors suggested that these findings may be secondary and result from mechanical causes.

Expression of cell signaling factors is an important marker of cell activity. It was found that expression of transforming growth factor β1 (TGF β1) and basic fibroblast growth factor (bFGF) was higher on the concave side in patients with AIS, while expression of the core protein of proteoglycan was higher on the convex side [233, 234]. TGFβ relates to the family of bone morphogenetic proteins and regulates growth and proliferation of cells. TGFβ1 acts through corresponding receptors and mediates a transcriptional activation. In particular, it regulates collagen type II gene expression which suggests an important role in the repair process during early IVD degeneration. However, this effect depends on whether the cells are fully differentiated or undergoing phenotype loss [235]. To note, melatonin stimulates TGFβ1 activity [236], thus, an impairment in melatonin signaling may modify this effect in patients with IS. FGFs are a family of growth factors involved in wound healing and embryonic development. One of the most important functions of bFGF is the promotion of endothelial proliferation and angiogenesis [237]. But it is also known that excessive release of bFGF during loading and/or injury of the cartilage matrix may contribute to the onset or progression of osteoarthritis. This pathological role may be related to the ability of bFGF to decrease proteoglycan synthesis and to antagonize the activity of anabolic growth factors in cartilage such as IGF-1 and BMP-7 and stimulate matrix metalloproteinase-13, which is a matrix catabolic cartilage-degenerative enzyme [238].

Experimental data suggest that melatonin modulates the effects of bFGF and inhibits bFGF gene expression [239]. Administration of melatonin reduced the cartilage endplate vascularity of degenerated intervertebral discs. It may have a stimulative effect on bone formation. However, bFGF and TGFβ1 are involved in the mechanisms of mechanotransduction. Thus, the effects of mechanotransduction and impairment of melatonin signaling pathways may overlap, making endplate cells more sensitive to mechanical impact. Increases in (bFGF) correspond to the results of inflammatory endplate changes, which are present at the concave apex in patients with AIS [229].

The majority of published data in the field of morphology and ultrastructure of IVD and VEPh in IS have serious limitations that make interpretation of the results difficult. Some of these limitations are summarized in Table 2. There is also a lack of data on the morphological and ultrastructural appearance of in infantile and juvenile IS.

5. Discussion

Our literature review supports the theory of a multifactorial etiology for IS. The different hypotheses highlight the diverse aspects of the etiopathogenetic mechanisms. Some of these mechanisms may be regarded as risk factors with different contributions in each disease case. This approach allows us to explain the wide variability of the clinical appearance in IS and hopefully predict disease occurrence and progression in future. Combinations of different genetic determinants are likely the main etiologic factor, which can be classified in two main groups. First, polymorphism of genes that may cause cell signaling impairments in different tissues, including bone and cartilage, and changes in hormonal regulation. Theoretically, combinations of these genetic features may contribute to such clinical appearances as skeletal and spinal overgrowth, decrease in bone mineral density, delay of skeletal maturity and spine slenderness, and dysfunction of the central and autonomic nervous systems which predispose occurrence and progression of the scoliotic spine curvature. The second groups of genetic determinants are likely associated with systemic defects in the structure of connective tissue and cartilage and may be with changes in embryogenesis. They may be linked with such clinical appearances as instability of spine, body asymmetry, and some concomitant congenital abnormalities. There is a high probability that polymorphisms of other genes that are associated with IS will be identified in the future. We may expect that the profile of IS genetic determinants significantly varies in different ethnic populations.

Serum content of such hormones as IGF1, testosterone, estradiol, leptin, and parathormone as well as matrilin-1 can be used as additional prognostic markers during earlier pubertal period, especially in cases with spine curvature $<30^\circ$, which are the most difficult to predict. The melatonin signaling in AIS should be further studied, as this may allow for the development of new diagnostic criteria for predicting curvature onset or progression. The correlation found between the appearance of melatonin signaling impairments in osteoblasts and lymphocytes allows a wider use of this approach for predicting curve onset and progression, especially during earliest stages of the disease [240]. Another intriguing finding is polymorphism of estrogen receptors genes, which suggests defects in estrogen signaling. The role of calmodulin signaling mechanisms in IS requires further clarification. The immune system, including T and B cells, may also play a role in pathogenesis of AIS.

The data suggest that progressive, in particular, double spine scoliotic deformity, should be associated with abnormal IVD structure. IVD wedging in AIS begins or enhances at adolescent growth spurt when body weight increases dramatically. The IVD wedging is most prominent in the lumbar spine where axial loading is maximal. Markers of VEPh cell activity at the concave and convex sides suggest that strain at the concave side is probably not enough to reduce cell proliferation during the beginning of curve progression. Thus, earlier wedging of vertebrae may be explained by the prevalence of a laterally directed appositional bone growth at the concave side. If appositional bone growth is also directed anteriorly or posteriorly, it may cause a rotational component of the deformity. This appositional growth results from the interaction of the vertebrae endplate with the outer annulus fibrosus of the adjacent IVD, which is also wedged. This IVD wedging is probably caused by changes in the disc's mechanical properties associated with sparse extracellular matrix and impaired lamellar structure. These are caused by defects in bending proteins, which are synthesized by cells in the IVD and involved in spatial organization of cartilage molecules. A genetic predisposition for increased metalloproteinase activity may also play role in accelerated disc degeneration. Asymmetrical ligament and muscular stretch are also involved in the curve formation and particularly in spine instability [4]. Biomechanical factors modulate the curve formation by gradually forming the "vicious cycle" effect.

We hypothesize that earlier treatment aimed at abnormal intervertebral discs in combination with reasonable spine stabilization may help prevent adjacent vertebrae wedging and curve progression in those patients who are predisposed to severe curve development. The ability to predict curve onset and progression using risk factors assessment could significantly individualize and improve diagnosis and treatment outcomes in patients with IS. The first steps in this field have already been taken, but further research is necessary to develop accurate and sensitive tools for risk assessment.

Conflict of Interests

The authors declare that there is no conflict of interests regarding the publication of this paper.

References

[1] I. A. F. Stokes, R. G. Burwell, and P. H. Dangerfield, "Biomechanical spinal growth modulation and progressive adolescent scoliosis—a test of the 'vicious cycle' pathogenetic hypothesis:

summary of an electronic focus group debate of the IBSE," *Scoliosis*, vol. 1, no. 1, article 16, 2006.

[2] I. A. F. Stokes, H. Spence, D. D. Aronsson, and N. Kilmer, "Mechanical modulation of vertebral body growth: implications for scoliosis progression," *Spine*, vol. 21, no. 10, pp. 1162–1167, 1996.

[3] S. Lupparelli, E. Pola, L. Pitta, O. Mazza, V. de Santis, and L. Aulisa, "Biomechanical factors affecting progression of structural scoliotic curves of the spine," *Studies in Health Technology and Informatics*, vol. 91, pp. 81–85, 2002.

[4] D. Fabris, S. Costantini, U. Nene, V. Lo Scalzo, and F. Finocchiaro, "The surgical treatment of adult lumbar scoliosis," *Chirurgia Narzadow Ruchu i Ortopedia Polska*, vol. 69, no. 4, pp. 279–285, 2004.

[5] J. F. Fraser, R. C. Huang, F. P. Girardi, and F. P. Cammisa Jr., "Pathogenesis, presentation, and treatment of lumbar spinal stenosis associated with coronal or sagittal spinal deformities," *Neurosurgical Focus*, vol. 14, no. 1, article e6, 2003.

[6] I. A. F. Stokes and L. Windisch, "Vertebral height growth predominates over intervertebral disc height growth in adolescents with scoliosis," *Spine*, vol. 31, no. 14, pp. 1600–1604, 2006.

[7] C. T. Mehlman, A. Araghi, and D. R. Roy, "Hyphenated history: the Hueter-Volkmann law," *The American Journal of Orthopedics*, vol. 26, no. 11, pp. 798–800, 1997.

[8] S. L. Weinstein, *The Pediatric Spine: Principles and Practice*, Lippincott Williams & Wilkins, Philadelphia, Pa, USA, 2nd edition, 2001.

[9] I. A. Stokes, J. Gwadera, A. Dimock, C. E. Farnum, and D. D. Aronsson, "Modulation of vertebral and tibial growth by compression loading: diurnal versus full-time loading," *Journal of Orthopaedic Research*, vol. 23, no. 1, pp. 188–195, 2005.

[10] M. R. Urban, J. C. T. Fairbank, S. R. S. Bibby, and J. P. G. Urban, "Intervertebral disc composition in neuromuscular scoliosis: changes in cell density and glycosaminoglycan concentration at the curve apex," *Spine*, vol. 26, no. 6, pp. 610–617, 2001.

[11] R. G. Burwell, "Aetiology of idiopathic scoliosis: current concepts," *Pediatric Rehabilitation*, vol. 6, no. 3-4, pp. 137–170, 2003.

[12] I. A. F. Stokes and D. D. Aronsson, "Disc and vertebral wedging in patients with progressive scoliosis," *Journal of Spinal Disorders*, vol. 14, no. 4, pp. 317–322, 2001.

[13] P. Fernandes and S. L. Weinstein, "Natural history of early onset scoliosis," *Journal of Bone and Joint Surgery A*, vol. 89, supplement 1, pp. 21–33, 2007.

[14] B. V. Reamy and J. B. Slakey, "Adolescent idiopathic scoliosis: review and current concepts," *The American Family Physician*, vol. 64, no. 1, pp. 111–116, 2001.

[15] J. W. Ogilvie, "Adult scoliosis: evaluation and nonsurgical treatment," *Instructional Course Lectures*, vol. 41, pp. 251–255, 1992.

[16] M. B. Dobbs and S. L. Weinstein, "Infantile and juvenile scoliosis," *Orthopedic Clinics of North America*, vol. 30, no. 3, pp. 331–341, 1999.

[17] R. Wynne-Davies, "Familial (idiopathic) scoliosis. A family survey," *Journal of Bone and Joint Surgery B*, vol. 50, no. 1, pp. 24–30, 1968.

[18] O. Diedrich, A. von Strempel, M. Schloz, O. Schmitt, and C. N. Kraft, "Long-term observation and management of resolving infantile idiopathic scoliosis. A 25-year follow-up," *Journal of Bone and Joint Surgery B*, vol. 84, no. 7, pp. 1030–1035, 2002.

[19] S. L. Weinstein, D. C. Zavala, and I. V. Ponseti, "Idiopathic scoliosis. Long-term follow-up and prognosis in untreated patients," *Journal of Bone and Joint Surgery A*, vol. 63, no. 5, pp. 702–712, 1981.

[20] R. Wynne Davies, "Infantile idiopathic scoliosis. Causative factors, particularly in the first six months of life," *Journal of Bone and Joint Surgery B*, vol. 57, no. 2, pp. 138–141, 1975.

[21] P. Gupta, L. G. Lenke, and K. H. Bridwell, "Incidence of neural axis abnormalities in infantile and juvenile patients with spinal deformity: is a magnetic resonance image screening necessary?" *Spine*, vol. 23, no. 2, pp. 206–210, 1998.

[22] M. B. Dobbs, L. G. Lenke, D. A. Szymanski et al., "Prevelance of neural axis abnormalities in patients with infantile idiopathic scoliosis," *Journal of Bone and Joint Surgery A*, vol. 84, no. 12, pp. 2230–2234, 2002.

[23] U. M. Figueiredo and J. I. P. James, "Juvenile idiopathic scoliosis," *Journal of Bone and Joint Surgery B*, vol. 63, no. 1, pp. 61–66, 1981.

[24] V. T. Tolo and R. Gillespie, "The characteristics of juvenile idiopathic scoliosis and results of its treatment," *Journal of Bone and Joint Surgery B*, vol. 60, no. 2, pp. 181–188, 1978.

[25] Y. P. Charles, J.-P. Daures, V. de Rosa, and A. Diméglio, "Progression risk of idiopathic juvenile scoliosis during pubertal growth," *Spine*, vol. 31, no. 17, pp. 1933–1942, 2006.

[26] W. J. Kane, "Scoliosis Prevalence: a call for a statement of terms," *Clinical Orthopaedics and Related Research*, vol. 126, pp. 43–46, 1977.

[27] T. B. Grivas, E. Vasiliadis, V. Mouzakis, C. Mihas, and G. Koufopoulos, "Association between adolescent idiopathic scoliosis prevalence and age at menarche in different geographic latitudes," *Scoliosis*, vol. 1, no. 1, article 9, 2006.

[28] H.-K. Wong, J. H. P. Hui, U. Rajan, and H.-P. Chia, "Idiopathic scoliosis in Singapore schoolchildren: a prevalence study 15 years into the screening program," *Spine*, vol. 30, no. 10, pp. 1188–1196, 2005.

[29] S.-W. Suh, H. N. Modi, J.-H. Yang, and J.-Y. Hong, "Idiopathic scoliosis in Korean schoolchildren: a prospective screening study of over 1 million children," *European Spine Journal*, vol. 20, no. 7, pp. 1087–1094, 2011.

[30] L. Xu, X. Qiu, X. Sun et al., "Potential genetic markers predicting the outcome of brace treatment in patients with adolescent idiopathic scoliosis," *European Spine Journal*, vol. 20, no. 10, pp. 1757–1764, 2011.

[31] H.-K. Wong and K.-J. Tan, "The natural history of adolescent idiopathic scoliosis," *Indian Journal of Orthopaedics*, vol. 44, no. 1, pp. 9–13, 2010.

[32] P. N. Soucacos, K. Zacharis, K. Soultanis, J. Gelalis, T. Xenakis, and A. E. Beris, "Risk factors for idiopathic scoliosis: review of a 6-year prospective study," *Orthopedics*, vol. 23, no. 8, pp. 833–838, 2000.

[33] L.-E. Peterson, A. L. Nachemson, D. S. Bradford et al., "Prediction of progression of the curve in girls who have adolescent idiopathic scoliosis of moderate severity. Logistic regression analysis based on data from the Brace Study of the Scoliosis Research Society," *Journal of Bone and Joint Surgery A*, vol. 77, no. 6, pp. 823–827, 1995.

[34] J. R. Davids, E. Chamberlin, and D. W. Blackhurst, "Indications for magnetic resonance imaging in presumed adolescent idiopathic scoliosis," *Journal of Bone and Joint Surgery A*, vol. 86, no. 10, pp. 2187–2195, 2004.

[35] M. O. Andersen, K. Thomsen, and K. O. Kyvik, "Adolescent idiopathic scoliosis in twins: a population-based survey," *Spine*, vol. 32, no. 8, pp. 927–930, 2007.

[36] R. G. Burwell, A. A. Cole, T. A. Cook et al., "Pathogenesis of idiopathic scoliosis. The Nottingham concept," *Acta Orthopaedica Belgica*, vol. 58, supplement 1, pp. 33–58, 1992.

[37] R. G. Burwell, B. J. Freeman, P. H. Dangerfield et al., "Etiologic theories of idiopathic scoliosis: neurodevelopmental concept of maturational delay of the CNS body schema ("body-in-the-brain")," *Studies in Health Technology and Informatics*, vol. 123, pp. 72–79, 2006.

[38] J. A. Sevastik, "Dysfunction of the autonomic nerve system (ANS) in the aetiopathogenesis of adolescent idiopathic scoliosis," *Studies in Health Technology and Informatics*, vol. 88, pp. 20–23, 2002.

[39] C. Barrios and J. I. Arrotegui, "Experimental kyphoscoliosis induced in rats by selective brain stem damage," *International Orthopaedics*, vol. 16, no. 2, pp. 146–151, 1992.

[40] R. Herman, J. Mixon, and A. Fisher, "Idiopathic scoliosis and the central nervous system: a motor control problem. The Harrington Lecture, 1983. Scoliosis Research Society," *Spine*, vol. 10, no. 1, pp. 1–14, 1985.

[41] X. Sun, Y. Qiu, and Z. Zhu, "Variations of the position of the cerebellar tonsil in adolescent idiopathic scoliosis with severe curves: a MRI study," *Studies in Health Technology and Informatics*, vol. 123, pp. 565–570, 2006.

[42] Í. T. Benli, O. Üzümcügil, E. Aydin, B. Ateş, L. Gürses, and B. Hekimoğlu, "Magnetic resonance imaging abnormalities of neural axis in Lenke type 1 idiopathic scoliosis," *Spine*, vol. 31, no. 16, pp. 1828–1833, 2006.

[43] A. E. Oestreich, L. W. Young, and T. Y. Poussaint, "Scoliosis circa 2000: radiologic imaging perspective. I. Diagnosis and pretreatment evaluation," *Skeletal Radiology*, vol. 27, no. 11, pp. 591–605, 1998.

[44] X. Guo, W. W. Chau, C. W. Y. Hui-Chan, C. S. K. Cheung, W. W. N. Tsang, and J. C. Y. Cheng, "Balance control in adolescents with idiopathic scoliosis and disturbed somatosensory function," *Spine*, vol. 31, no. 14, pp. E437–E440, 2006.

[45] M. L. M. Lao, D. H. K. Chow, X. Guo, J. C. Y. Cheng, and A. D. Holmes, "Impaired dynamic balance control in adolescents with idiopathic scoliosis and abnormal somatosensory evoked potentials," *Journal of Pediatric Orthopaedics*, vol. 28, no. 8, pp. 846–849, 2008.

[46] M. Beaulieu, C. Toulotte, L. Gatto et al., "Postural imbalance in non-treated adolescent idiopathic scoliosis at different periods of progression," *European Spine Journal*, vol. 18, no. 1, pp. 38–44, 2009.

[47] R. G. Burwell, P. H. Dangerfield, B. J. Freeman et al., "Etiologic theories of idiopathic scoliosis: the breaking of bilateral symmetry in relation to left-right asymmetry of internal organs, right thoracic adolescent idiopathic scoliosis (AIS) and vertebrate evolution," *Studies in Health Technology and Informatics*, vol. 123, pp. 385–390, 2006.

[48] C. J. Goldberg, F. E. Dowling, E. E. Fogarty, and D. P. Moore, "Adolescent idiopathic scoliosis as developmental instability," *Genetica*, vol. 96, no. 3, pp. 247–255, 1995.

[49] C. J. Goldberg, E. E. Fogarty, D. P. Moore, and F. E. Dowling, "Scoliosis and developmental theory: adolescent idiopathic scoliosis," *Spine*, vol. 22, no. 19, pp. 2228–2238, 1997.

[50] R. G. Burwell, N. J. James, and F. Johnson, "Standardised trunk asymmetry scores. A study of back contour in healthy schoolchildren," *Journal of Bone and Joint Surgery B*, vol. 65, no. 4, pp. 452–463, 1983.

[51] A. E. Geissele, M. J. Kransdorf, C. A. Geyer, J. S. Jelinek, and B. E. van Dam, "Magnetic resonance imaging of the brain stem in adolescent idiopathic scoliosis," *Spine*, vol. 16, no. 7, pp. 761–763, 1991.

[52] M. Nissinen, M. Heliovaara, J. Seitsamo, and M. Poussa, "Trunk asymmetry, posture, growth, and risk of scoliosis: a three-year follow-up of Finnish prepubertal school children," *Spine*, vol. 18, no. 1, pp. 8–13, 1993.

[53] H. Normelli, J. A. Sevastik, G. Ljung, and A.-M. Jonsson-Soderstrom, "The symmetry of the breasts in normal and scoliotic girls," *Spine*, vol. 11, no. 7, pp. 749–752, 1986.

[54] M. Pecina, O. Lulic-Dukic, and A. Pecina-Hrncevic, "Hereditary orthodontic anomalies and idiopathic scoliosis," *International Orthopaedics*, vol. 15, no. 1, pp. 57–59, 1991.

[55] M. J. Saji, S. S. Upadhyay, and J. C. Y. Leong, "Increased femoral neck-shaft angles in adolescent idiopathic scoliosis," *Spine*, vol. 20, no. 3, pp. 303–311, 1995.

[56] M. P. Wyatt, R. L. Barrack, and S. J. Mubarak, "Vibratory response in idiopathic scoliosis," *Journal of Bone and Joint Surgery B*, vol. 68, no. 5, pp. 714–718, 1986.

[57] M. Machida, J. Dubousset, Y. Imamura, T. Iwaya, T. Yamada, and J. Kimura, "An experimental study in chickens for the pathogenesis of idiopathic scoliosis," *Spine*, vol. 18, no. 12, pp. 1609–1615, 1993.

[58] M. Machida, J. Dubousset, Y. Imamura, Y. Iwaya, T. Yamada, and J. Kimura, "Role of melatonin deficiency in the development of scoliosis in pinealectomised chickens," *Journal of Bone and Joint Surgery B*, vol. 77, no. 1, pp. 134–138, 1995.

[59] J. Dubousset and M. Machida, "Possible role of pineal gland in pathogenesis of idiopathic scoliosis. Experimental and clinical studies," *Bulletin de l'Academie Nationale de Medecine*, vol. 185, no. 3, pp. 593–604, 2001.

[60] M. Machida, J. Dubousset, T. Yamada et al., "Experimental scoliosis in melatonin-deficient C57BL/6J mice without pinealectomy," *Journal of Pineal Research*, vol. 41, no. 1, pp. 1–7, 2006.

[61] M. Machida, J. Dubousset, Y. Imamura, Y. Miyashita, T. Yamada, and J. Kimura, "Melatonin: a possible role in pathogenesis of adolescent idiopathic scoliosis," *Spine*, vol. 21, no. 10, pp. 1147–1152, 1996.

[62] K. M. C. Cheung, T. Wang, A. M. S. Poon et al., "The effect of pinealectomy on scoliosis development in young nonhuman primates," *Spine*, vol. 30, no. 18, pp. 2009–2013, 2005.

[63] K. M. Bagnall, V. J. Raso, D. L. Hill et al., "Melatonin levels in idiopathic scoliosis: diurnal and nocturnal serum melatonin levels in girls with adolescent idiopathic scoliosis," *Spine*, vol. 21, no. 17, pp. 1974–1978, 1996.

[64] A. S. Hilibrand, L. C. Blakemore, R. T. Loder et al., "The role of melatonin in the pathogenesis of adolescent idiopathic scoliosis," *Spine*, vol. 21, no. 10, pp. 1140–1146, 1996.

[65] A. B. Fagan, D. J. Kennaway, and A. D. Sutherland, "Total 24-hour melatonin secretion in adolescent idiopathic scoliosis: a case-control study," *Spine*, vol. 23, no. 1, pp. 41–46, 1998.

[66] W. Brodner, P. Krepler, M. Nicolakis et al., "Melatonin and adolescent idiopathic scoliosis," *Journal of Bone and Joint Surgery B*, vol. 82, no. 3, pp. 399–403, 2000.

[67] K. T. Suh, S. S. Lee, S. J. Kim, Y. K. Kim, and J. S. Lee, "Pineal gland metabolism in patients with adolescent idiopathic scoliosis," *Journal of Bone and Joint Surgery B*, vol. 89, no. 1, pp. 66–71, 2007.

[68] A. Moreau, D. S. Wang, S. Forget et al., "Melatonin signaling dysfunction in adolescent idiopathic scoliosis," *Spine*, vol. 29, no. 16, pp. 1772–1781, 2004.

[69] B. Azeddine, K. Letellier, D. S. Wang, F. Moldovan, and A. Moreau, "Molecular determinants of melatonin signaling dysfunction in adolescent idiopathic scoliosis," *Clinical Orthopaedics and Related Research*, no. 462, pp. 45–52, 2007.

[70] L. H. S. Sekhon, N. Duggal, J. J. Lynch et al., "Magnetic resonance imaging clarity of the Bryan, Prodisc-C, Prestige LP, and PCM cervical arthroplasty devices," *Spine*, vol. 32, no. 6, pp. 673–680, 2007.

[71] X. S. Qiu, N. L. S. Tang, H. Y. Yeung et al., "Melatonin receptor 1B (MTNR1B) gene polymorphism is associated with the occurrence of adolescent idiopathic scoliosis," *Spine*, vol. 32, no. 16, pp. 1748–1753, 2007.

[72] J. A. Morcuende, R. Minhas, L. Dolan et al., "Allelic variants of human melatonin 1A receptor in patients with familial adolescent idiopathic scoliosis," *Spine*, vol. 28, no. 17, pp. 2025–2028, 2003.

[73] M. I. Masana, J. M. Soares Jr., and M. L. Dubocovich, "17β-Estradiol modulates hMT1 melatonin receptor function," *Neuroendocrinology*, vol. 81, no. 2, pp. 87–95, 2005.

[74] K. Letellier, B. Azeddine, S. Parent et al., "Estrogen cross-talk with the melatonin signaling pathway in human osteoblasts derived from adolescent idiopathic scoliosis patients," *Journal of Pineal Research*, vol. 45, no. 4, pp. 383–393, 2008.

[75] J. Vanecek, "Cellular mechanisms of melatonin action," *Physiological Reviews*, vol. 78, no. 3, pp. 687–721, 1998.

[76] P. Das, D. J. Schurman, and R. L. Smith, "Nitric oxide and G proteins mediate the response of bovine articular chondrocytes to fluid-induced shear," *Journal of Orthopaedic Research*, vol. 15, no. 1, pp. 87–93, 1997.

[77] A. J. El Haj, L. M. Walker, M. R. Preston, and S. J. Publicover, "Mechanotransduction pathways in bone: calcium fluxes and the role of voltage-operated calcium channels," *Medical and Biological Engineering and Computing*, vol. 37, no. 3, pp. 403–409, 1999.

[78] G. R. Erickson, L. G. Alexopoulos, and F. Guilak, "Hyper-osmotic stress induces volume change and calcium transients in chondrocytes by transmembrane, phospholipid, and G-protein pathways," *Journal of Biomechanics*, vol. 34, no. 12, pp. 1527–1535, 2001.

[79] F. M. Pavalko, S. M. Norvell, D. B. Burr, C. H. Turner, R. L. Duncan, and J. P. Bidwell, "A model for mechanotransduction in bone cells: the load-bearing mechanosomes," *Journal of Cellular Biochemistry*, vol. 88, no. 1, pp. 104–112, 2003.

[80] A. Conti, S. Conconi, E. Hertens, K. Skwarlo-Sonta, M. Markowska, and G. J. M. Maestroni, "Evidence for melatonin synthesis in mouse and human bone marrow cells," *Journal of Pineal Research*, vol. 28, no. 4, pp. 193–202, 2000.

[81] J. A. Roth, B.-G. Kim, F. Song, W.-L. Lin, and M.-I. Cho, "Melatonin promotes osteoblast differentiation and bone formation," *Journal of Biological Chemistry*, vol. 274, no. 31, pp. 22041–22047, 1999.

[82] H. Koyama, O. Nakade, Y. Takada, T. Kaku, and K.-H. W. Lau, "Melatonin at pharmacologic doses increases bone mass by suppressing resorption through down-regulation of the RANKL-mediated osteoclast formation and activation," *Journal of Bone and Mineral Research*, vol. 17, no. 7, pp. 1219–1229, 2002.

[83] N. Suzuki and A. Hattori, "Melatonin suppresses osteoclastic and osteoblastic activities in the scales of goldfish," *Journal of Pineal Research*, vol. 33, no. 4, pp. 253–258, 2002.

[84] D. P. Cardinali, M. G. Ladizesky, V. Boggio, R. A. Cutrera, and C. Mautalen, "Melatonin effects on bone: experimental facts and clinical perspectives," *Journal of Pineal Research*, vol. 34, no. 2, pp. 81–87, 2003.

[85] M. Ylikoski, "Growth and progression of adolescent idiopathic scoliosis in girls," *Journal of Pediatric Orthopaedics Part B*, vol. 14, no. 5, pp. 320–324, 2005.

[86] X. Guo, W.-W. Chau, Y.-L. Chan, and J. C.-Y. Cheng, "Relative anterior spinal overgrowth in adolescent idiopathic scoliosis," *Journal of Bone and Joint Surgery B*, vol. 85, no. 7, pp. 1026–1031, 2003.

[87] X. Guo, W.-W. Chau, Y.-L. Chan, J.-C.-Y. Cheng, R. G. Burwell, and P. H. Dangerfield, "Relative anterior spinal overgrowth in adolescent idiopathic scoliosis—result of disproportionate endochondral-membranous bone growth? Summary of an electronic focus group debate of the IBSE," *European Spine Journal*, vol. 14, no. 9, pp. 862–873, 2005.

[88] R. W. Porter, "The pathogenesis of idiopathic scoliosis: uncoupled neuro-osseous growth?" *European Spine Journal*, vol. 10, no. 6, pp. 473–481, 2001.

[89] R. Yarom and G. C. Robin, "Studies on spinal and peripheral muscles from patients with scoliosis," *Spine*, vol. 4, no. 1, pp. 12–21, 1979.

[90] R. Yarom, A. Muhlrad, S. Hodges, and G. C. Robin, "Platelet pathology in patients with idiopathic scoliosis. Ultrastructural morphometry, aggregations, X-ray spectrometry, and biochemical analysis," *Laboratory Investigation*, vol. 43, no. 3, pp. 208–216, 1980.

[91] T. G. Lowe, M. Edgar, J. Y. Margulies et al., "Etiology of idiopathic scoliosis: current trends in research," *Journal of Bone and Joint Surgery A*, vol. 82, no. 8, pp. 1157–1168, 2000.

[92] K. Kindsfater, T. Lowe, D. Lawellin, D. Weinstein, and J. Akmakjian, "Levels of platelet calmodulin for the prediction of progression and severity of adolescent idiopathic scoliosis," *Journal of Bone and Joint Surgery A*, vol. 76, no. 8, pp. 1186–1192, 1994.

[93] T. Lowe, D. Lawellin, D. Smith et al., "Platelet calmodulin levels in adolescent idiopathic scoliosis: do the levels correlate with curve progression and severity?" *Spine*, vol. 27, no. 7, pp. 768–775, 2002.

[94] T. G. Lowe, R. G. Burwell, and P. H. Dangerfield, "Platelet calmodulin levels in adolescent idiopathic scoliosis (AIS): can they predict curve progression and severity? Summary of an electronic focus group debate of the IBSE," *European Spine Journal*, vol. 13, no. 3, pp. 257–265, 2004.

[95] R. G. Burwell and P. H. Dangerfield, "Pathogenesis of progressive adolescent idiopathic scoliosis platelet activation and vascular biology in immature vertebrae: an alternative molecular hypothesis," *Acta Orthopaedica Belgica*, vol. 72, no. 3, pp. 247–260, 2006.

[96] M. I. Vacas, M. M. de las del Zar, M. Martinuzzo, and D. P. Cardinali, "Binding sites for [3H]-melatonin in human platelets," *Journal of Pineal Research*, vol. 13, no. 2, pp. 60–65, 1992.

[97] D. P. Cardinali, M. M. del Zar, and M. I. Vacas, "The effects of melatonin in human platelets," *Acta Physiologica Pharmacologica et Therapeutica Latinoamericana*, vol. 43, no. 1-2, pp. 1–13, 1993.

[98] D. P. Cardinali, D. A. Golombek, R. E. Rosenstein, R. A. Cutrera, and A. I. Esquifino, "Melatonin site and mechanism of action: single or multiple?" *Journal of Pineal Research*, vol. 23, no. 1, pp. 32–39, 1997.

[99] J. Yang, J. Wu, M. Anna Kowalska et al., "Loss of signaling through the G protein, G(z), results in abnormal platelet activation and altered responses to psychoactive drugs," *Proceedings of the National Academy of Sciences of the United States of America*, vol. 97, no. 18, pp. 9984–9989, 2000.

[100] S. I. S. Se Il Suk, I. K. K. In Kwon Kim, C. K. L. Choon Ki Lee, Y. D. K. Young Do Koh, and J. S. Y. Jin Sup Yeom, "A study on platelet function in idiopathic scoliosis," *Orthopedics*, vol. 14, no. 10, pp. 1079–1083, 1991.

[101] W. K. Ho, M. Baccala, J. Thom, and J. W. Eikelboom, "High prevalence of abnormal preoperative coagulation tests in patients with adolescent idiopathic scoliosis," *Journal of Thrombosis and Haemostasis*, vol. 3, no. 5, pp. 1094–1095, 2005.

[102] K. Freson, V. Labarque, C. Thys, C. Wittevrongel, and C. V. Geet, "What's new in using platelet research? To unravel thrombopathies and other human disorders," *European Journal of Pediatrics*, vol. 166, no. 12, pp. 1203–1210, 2007.

[103] A. Pletscher, "Blood platelets as neuronal models: use and limitations," *Clinical Neuropharmacology*, vol. 9, pp. 344–346, 1986.

[104] N. Hadley-Miller, B. Mims, and D. M. Milewicz, "The potential role of the elastic fiber system in adolescent idiopathic scoliosis," *Journal of Bone and Joint Surgery A*, vol. 76, no. 8, pp. 1193–1206, 1994.

[105] G. M. Corson, N. L. Charbonneau, D. R. Keene, and L. Y. Sakai, "Differential expression of fibrillin-3 adds to microfibril variety in human and avian, but not rodent, connective tissues," *Genomics*, vol. 83, no. 3, pp. 461–472, 2004.

[106] E. G. Cleary and M. A. Gibson, "Elastin-associated microfibrils and microfibrillar proteins," *International Review of Connective Tissue Research*, vol. 10, pp. 97–209, 1983.

[107] M. K. Chelberg, G. M. Banks, D. F. Geiger, and T. R. Oegema Jr., "Identification of heterogeneous cell populations in normal human intervertebral disc," *Journal of Anatomy*, vol. 186, part 1, pp. 43–53, 1995.

[108] M. Turgut, G. Öktem, A. Uysal, and M. E. Yurtseven, "Immunohistochemical profile of transforming growth factor-β1 and basic fibroblast growth factor in sciatic nerve anastomosis following pinealectomy and exogenous melatonin administration in rats," *Journal of Clinical Neuroscience*, vol. 13, no. 7, pp. 753–758, 2006.

[109] L. B. Skogland and J. A. A. Miller, "The length and proportions of the thoracolumbar spine in children with idiopathic scoliosis," *Acta Orthopaedica Scandinavica*, vol. 52, no. 2, pp. 177–185, 1981.

[110] L. B. Skogland and J. A. A. Miller, "Growth related hormones in idiopathic scoliosis. An endocrine basis for accelerated growth," *Acta Orthopaedica Scandinavica*, vol. 51, no. 5, pp. 779–789, 1980.

[111] T. Ahl, K. Albertsson-Wikland, and R. Kalen, "Twenty-four-hour growth hormone profiles in pubertal girls with idiopathic scoliosis," *Spine*, vol. 13, no. 2, pp. 139–142, 1988.

[112] L. B. Skogland, J. A. A. Miller, A. Skottner, and L. Fryklund, "Serum somatomedin A and non-dialyzable urinary hydroxyproline in girls with idiopathic scoliosis," *Acta Orthopaedica Scandinavica*, vol. 52, no. 3, pp. 307–313, 1981.

[113] E. D. Wang, D. S. Drummond, J. P. Dormans, T. Moshang, R. S. Davidson, and D. Gruccio, "Scoliosis in patients treated with growth hormone," *Journal of Pediatric Orthopaedics*, vol. 17, no. 6, pp. 708–711, 1997.

[114] J. F. Dymling and S. Willner, "Progression of a structural scoliosis during treatment with growth hormone. A case report," *Acta Orthopaedica Scandinavica*, vol. 49, no. 3, pp. 264–268, 1978.

[115] G. A. Day, I. B. McPhee, J. Batch, and F. H. Tomlinson, "Growth rates and the prevalence and progression of scoliosis in short-statured children on Australian growth hormone treatment programmes," *Scoliosis*, vol. 2, no. 1, article 3, 2007.

[116] C. J. Rosen and L. R. Donahue, "Insulin-like growth factors and bone: the osteoporosis connection revisited," *Proceedings of the Society for Experimental Biology and Medicine*, vol. 219, no. 1, pp. 1–7, 1998.

[117] X. S. Qiu, N. L. S. Tang, H.-Y. Yeung, Y. Qiu, and J. C. Y. Cheng, "Genetic association study of growth hormone receptor and idiopathic scoliosis," *Clinical Orthopaedics and Related Research*, vol. 462, pp. 53–58, 2007.

[118] Y. Yang, Z. Wu, T. Zhao et al., "Adolescent idiopathic scoliosis and the single-nucleotide polymorphism of the growth hormone receptor and IGF-1 genes," *Orthopedics*, vol. 32, no. 6, article 411, 2009.

[119] E. S. Moon, H. S. Kim, V. Sharma et al., "Analysis of single nucleotide polymorphism in adolescent idiopathic scoliosis in Korea: for personalized treatment," *Yonsei Medical Journal*, vol. 54, no. 2, pp. 500–509, 2013.

[120] J. Falcón, L. Besseau, D. Fazzari et al., "Melatonin modulates secretion of growth hormone and prolactin by trout pituitary glands and cells in culture," *Endocrinology*, vol. 144, no. 10, pp. 4648–4658, 2003.

[121] Z. Ostrowska, B. Kos-Kudla, E. Swietochowska, B. Marek, D. Kajdaniuk, and N. Ciesielska-Kopacz, "Influence of pinealectomy and long-term melatonin administration on GH-IGF-I axis function in male rats," *Neuroendocrinology Letters*, vol. 22, no. 4, pp. 255–262, 2001.

[122] P. Lissoni, M. Cazzaniga, G. Tancini et al., "Reversal of clinical resistance to LHRH analogue in metastatic prostate cancer by the pineal hormone melatonin: efficacy of LHRH analogue plus melatonin in patients progressing on LHRH analogue alone," *European Urology*, vol. 31, no. 2, pp. 178–181, 1997.

[123] J. O. Sanders, R. H. Browne, S. J. McConnell, S. A. Margraf, T. E. Cooney, and D. N. Finegold, "Maturity assessment and curve progression in girls with idiopathic scoliosis," *Journal of Bone and Joint Surgery A*, vol. 89, no. 1, pp. 64–73, 2007.

[124] J. W. Raczkowski, "The concentrations of testosterone and estradiol in girls with adolescent idiopathic scoliosis," *Neuroendocrinology Letters*, vol. 28, no. 3, pp. 302–304, 2007.

[125] T. Esposito, R. Uccello, R. Caliendo et al., "Estrogen receptor polymorphism, estrogen content and idiopathic scoliosis in human: a possible genetic linkage," *Journal of Steroid Biochemistry and Molecular Biology*, vol. 116, no. 1-2, pp. 56–60, 2009.

[126] K. Venken, S. Movérare-Skrtic, J. J. Kopchick et al., "Impact of androgens, growth hormone, and IGF-I on bone and muscle in male mice during puberty," *Journal of Bone and Mineral Research*, vol. 22, no. 1, pp. 72–82, 2007.

[127] P. Raz, E. Nasatzky, B. D. Boyan, A. Ornoy, and Z. Schwartz, "Sexual dimorphism of growth plate prehypertrophic and hypertrophic chondrocytes in response to testosterone requires metabolism to dihydrotestosterone (DHT) by steroid 5-alpha reductase type 1," *Journal of Cellular Biochemistry*, vol. 95, no. 1, pp. 108–119, 2005.

[128] R. Luboshitzky, O. Wagner, S. Lavi, P. Herer, and P. Lavie, "Abnormal melatonin secretion in hypogonadal men: the effect of testosterone treatment," *Clinical Endocrinology*, vol. 47, no. 4, pp. 463–469, 1997.

[129] A. Kulis, D. Zarzycki, and J. Jaśkiewicz, "Concentration of estradiol in girls with idiophatic scoliosis," *Ortopedia Traumatologia Rehabilitacja*, vol. 8, no. 4, pp. 455–459, 2006.

[130] A. Kulis and J. Jaśkiewicz, "Concentration of selected regulators of calciumphosphate balance in girls with idiopathic scoliosis," *Ortopedia Traumatologia Rehabilitacja*, vol. 11, no. 5, pp. 438–447, 2009.

[131] C. J. Goldberg, F. E. Dowling, and E. E. Fogarty, "Adolescent idiopathic scoliosis—early menarche, normal growth," *Spine*, vol. 18, no. 5, pp. 529–535, 1993.

[132] H. Normelli, J. Sevastik, and G. Ljung, "Anthropometric data relating to normal and scoliotic Scandinavian girls," *Spine*, vol. 10, no. 2, pp. 123–126, 1985.

[133] W. T. K. Lee, C. S. K. Cheung, Y. K. Tse et al., "Association of osteopenia with curve severity in adolescent idiopathic scoliosis: a study of 919 girls," *Osteoporosis International*, vol. 16, no. 12, pp. 1924–1932, 2005.

[134] J. C. Cheng, S. P. Tang, X. Guo, C. W. Chan, and L. Qin, "Osteopenia in adolescent idiopathic scoliosis: a histomorphometric study," *Spine*, vol. 26, no. 3, pp. E19–E23, 2001.

[135] M. N. Weitzmann and R. Pacifici, "Estrogen regulation of immune cell bone interactions," *Annals of the New York Academy of Sciences*, vol. 1068, no. 1, pp. 256–274, 2006.

[136] A. Bouhoute and G. Leclercq, "Calmodulin decreases the estrogen binding capacity of the estrogen receptor," *Biochemical and Biophysical Research Communications*, vol. 227, no. 3, pp. 651–657, 1996.

[137] A. S. Dusso and A. J. Brown, "Mechanism of vitamin D action and its regulation," *The American Journal of Kidney Diseases*, vol. 32, supplement 2, pp. S13–S24, 1998.

[138] H. Chen, S. Shoumura, S. Emura, M. Utsumi, T. Yamahira, and H. Isono, "Effects of melatonin on the ultrastructure of the golden hamster parathyroid gland," *Histology and Histopathology*, vol. 6, no. 1, pp. 1–7, 1991.

[139] S. Shoumura, H. Chen, S. Emura et al., "An in vitro study on the effects of melatonin on the ultrastructure of the hamster parathyroid gland," *Histology and Histopathology*, vol. 7, no. 4, pp. 715–718, 1992.

[140] Y. Qiu, X. Sun, X. Qiu et al., "Decreased circulating leptin level and its association with body and bone mass in girls with adolescent idiopathic scoliosis," *Spine*, vol. 32, no. 24, pp. 2703–2710, 2007.

[141] X. Sun, Y. Qiu, X.-S. Qiu, Z.-Z. Zhu, F. Zhu, and C.-W. Xia, "Association between circulating leptin level and anthropometric parameters in girls with adolescent idiopathic scoliosis," *National Medical Journal of China*, vol. 87, no. 9, pp. 594–598, 2007.

[142] J. Xu, T. Wu, Z. Zhong, C. Zhao, Y. Tang, and J. Chen, "Effect and mechanism of leptin on osteoblastic differentiation of hBMSCs," *Zhongguo Xiu Fu Chong Jian Wai Ke Za Zhi*, vol. 23, no. 2, pp. 140–144, 2009.

[143] S. P. Kalra, M. G. Dube, and U. T. Iwaniec, "Leptin increases osteoblast-specific osteocalcin release through a hypothalamic relay," *Peptides*, vol. 30, no. 5, pp. 967–973, 2009.

[144] K. Wlodarski and P. Wlodarski, "Leptin as a modulator of osteogenesis," *Ortopedia Traumatologia Rehabilitacja*, vol. 11, no. 1, pp. 1–6, 2009.

[145] M. I. C. Alonso-Vale, S. Andreotti, S. B. Peres et al., "Melatonin enhances leptin expression by rat adipocytes in the presence of insulin," *The American Journal of Physiology—Endocrinology and Metabolism*, vol. 288, no. 4, pp. E805–E812, 2005.

[146] R. G. Burwell, R. K. Aujla, M. P. Grevitt et al., "Pathogenesis of adolescent idiopathic scoliosis in girls—a double neuro-osseous theory involving disharmony between two nervous systems, somatic and autonomic expressed in the spine and trunk: possible dependency on sympathetic nervous system and hormones with implications for medical therapy," *Scoliosis*, vol. 4, article 24, 2009.

[147] K. L. Kesling and K. A. Reinker, "Scoliosis in twins: a meta-analysis of the literature and report of six cases," *Spine*, vol. 22, no. 17, pp. 2009–2015, 1997.

[148] L. M. Kruse, J. G. Buchan, C. A. Gurnett, and M. B. Dobbs, "Polygenic threshold model with sex dimorphism in adolescent idiopathic scoliosis: the Carter effect," *Journal of Bone and Joint Surgery*, vol. 94, no. 16, pp. 1485–1491, 2012.

[149] C. Brewer, S. Holloway, P. Zawalnyski, A. Schinzel, and D. Fitzpatrick, "A chromosomal deletion map of human malformations," *The American Journal of Human Genetics*, vol. 63, no. 4, pp. 1153–1159, 1998.

[150] P. F. Giampietro, R. D. Blank, C. L. Raggio et al., "Congenital and idiopathic scoliosis: clinical and genetic aspects," *Clinical Medicine & Research*, vol. 1, no. 2, pp. 125–136, 2003.

[151] C. A. Wise, R. Barnes, J. Gillum, J. A. Herring, A. M. Bowcock, and M. Lovett, "Localization of susceptibility to familial idiopathic scoliosis," *Spine*, vol. 25, no. 18, pp. 2372–2380, 2000.

[152] Y. Takahashi, M. Matsumoto, T. Karasugi et al., "Lack of association between adolescent idiopathic scoliosis and previously reported single nucleotide polymorphisms in MATN1, MTNR1B, TPH1, and IGF1 in a Japanese population," *Journal of Orthopaedic Research*, vol. 29, no. 7, pp. 1055–1058, 2011.

[153] L. M. Nelson, K. Ward, and J. W. Ogilvie, "Genetic variants in melatonin synthesis and signaling pathway are not associated with adolescent idiopathic scoliosis," *Spine*, vol. 36, no. 1, pp. 37–40, 2011.

[154] X. Gao, D. Gordon, D. Zhang et al., "CHD7 gene polymorphisms are associated with susceptibility to idiopathic scoliosis," *The American Journal of Human Genetics*, vol. 80, no. 5, pp. 957–965, 2007.

[155] L. Montanaro, P. Parisini, T. Greggi et al., "Evidence of a linkage between matrilin-1 gene (MATN1) and idiopathic scoliosis," *Scoliosis*, vol. 1, no. 1, article 21, 2006.

[156] Z. Chen, N.-L. Tang, X. Cao et al., "Promoter polymorphism of matrilin-1 gene predisposes to adolescent idiopathic scoliosis in a Chinese population," *European Journal of Human Genetics*, vol. 17, no. 4, pp. 525–532, 2009.

[157] B. Wang, Z.-J. Chen, Y. Qiu, and W.-J. Liu, "Decreased circulating matrilin-1 levels in adolescent idiopathic scoliosis," *Zhonghua Wai Ke Za Zhi*, vol. 47, no. 21, pp. 1638–1641, 2009.

[158] J. W. Bae, C.-H. Cho, W.-K. Min, and U.-K. Kim, "Associations between matrilin-1 gene polymorphisms and adolescent idiopathic scoliosis curve patterns in a Korean population," *Molecular Biology Reports*, vol. 39, no. 5, pp. 5561–5567, 2012, Erratum in *Molecular Biology Reports*, vol. 39, no. 9, p. 9275, 2012.

[159] S. Ohtori, T. Koshi, M. Yamashita et al., "Surgical versus nonsurgical treatment of selected patients with discogenic low back pain: a small-sized randomized trial," *Spine*, vol. 36, no. 5, pp. 347–354, 2011.

[160] Q. Chen, Y. Zhang, D. M. Johnson, and P. F. Goetinck, "Assembly of a novel cartilage matrix protein filamentous network: molecular basis of differential requirement of von Willebrand factor A domains," *Molecular Biology of the Cell*, vol. 10, no. 7, pp. 2149–2162, 1999.

[161] C. Wiberg, A. R. Klatt, R. Wagener et al., "Complexes of matrilin-1 and biglycan or decorin connect collagen VI microfibrils to both collagen II and aggrecan," *Journal of Biological Chemistry*, vol. 278, no. 39, pp. 37698–37704, 2003.

[162] I. Kou, Y. Takahashi, T. A. Johnson et al., "Genetic variants in GPR126 are associated with adolescent idiopathic scoliosis," *Nature Genetics*, vol. 45, no. 6, pp. 676–679, 2013.

[163] Weizman Institute of Science, "Gene Card. The human gene compendium," 2013, http://www.genecards.org/cgi-bin/carddisp.pl?gene=LBX1&search=LBX1 .

[164] C. M. Justice, N. H. Miller, B. Marosy, J. Zhang, and A. F. Wilson, "Familial idiopathic scoliosis: evidence of an X-linked susceptibility locus," *Spine*, vol. 28, no. 6, pp. 589–594, 2003.

[165] V. Chan, G. C. Y. Fong, K. D. K. Luk et al., "A genetic locus for adolescent idiopathic scoliosis linked to chromosome 19p13.3," *The American Journal of Human Genetics*, vol. 71, no. 2, pp. 401–406, 2002.

[166] X.-B. Cao, Y. Qiu, and X.-S. Qiu, "FBN3 gene polymorphisms in adolescent idiopathic scoliosis patients," *Zhonghua Yi Xue Za Zhi*, vol. 88, no. 43, pp. 3053–3058, 2008.

[167] M. Inoue, S. Minami, Y. Nakata et al., "Association between estrogen receptor gene polymorphisms and curve severity of idiopathic scoliosis," *Spine*, vol. 27, no. 21, pp. 2357–2362, 2002.

[168] J. Wu, Y. Qiu, L. Zhang, Q. Sun, X. Qiu, and Y. He, "Association of estrogen receptor gene polymorphisms with susceptibility to adolescent idiopathic scoliosis," *Spine*, vol. 31, no. 10, pp. 1131–1136, 2006.

[169] N. L.-S. Tang, H.-Y. Yeung, K.-M. Lee et al., "A relook into the association of the estrogen receptor α gene (PvuII, XbaI) and adolescent idiopathic scoliosis: a study of 540 Chinese cases," *Spine*, vol. 31, no. 21, pp. 2463–2468, 2006.

[170] D. Zhao, G.-X. Qiu, and Y.-P. Wang, "Is calmodulin 1 gene/estrogen receptor-alpha gene polymorphisms correlated with double curve pattern of adolescent idiopathic scoliosis?" *Zhonghua Yi Xue Za Zhi*, vol. 88, no. 35, pp. 2452–2456, 2008.

[171] D. Zhao, G.-X. Qiu, Y.-P. Wang et al., "Association of calmodulin1 gene polymorphisms with susceptibility to adolescent idiopathic scoliosis," *Orthopaedic Surgery*, vol. 1, no. 1, pp. 58–65, 2009.

[172] H.-Q. Zhang, S.-J. Lu, M.-X. Tang et al., "Association of estrogen receptor β gene polymorphisms with susceptibility to adolescent idiopathic scoliosis," *Spine*, vol. 34, no. 8, pp. 760–764, 2009.

[173] Y. Takahashi, M. Matsumoto, T. Karasugi et al., "Replication study of the association between adolescent idiopathic scoliosis and two estrogen receptor genes," *Journal of Orthopaedic Research*, vol. 29, no. 6, pp. 834–837, 2011.

[174] Y. Peng, G. Liang, Y. Pei, W. Ye, A. Liang, and P. Su, "Genomic polymorphisms of G-Protein Estrogen Receptor 1 are associated with severity of adolescent idiopathic scoliosis," *International Orthopaedics*, vol. 36, no. 3, pp. 671–677, 2012.

[175] Y. Qiu, S.-H. Mao, B.-P. Qian et al., "A promoter polymorphism of neurotrophin 3 gene is associated with curve severity and bracing effectiveness in adolescent idiopathic scoliosis," *Spine*, vol. 37, no. 2, pp. 127–133, 2012.

[176] Y. Ogura, Y. Takahashi, I. Kou et al., "A replication study for association of 5 single nucleotide polymorphisms with curve progression of adolescent idiopathic scoliosis in Japanese patients," *Spine*, vol. 38, no. 7, pp. 571–575, 2013.

[177] A. M. Zaidman, M. N. Zaidman, A. V. Korel, M. A. Mikhailovsky, T. Y. Eshchenko, and E. V. Grigorjeva, "Aggrecan gene expression disorder as aetiologic factor of idiopathic scoliosis," *Studies in Health Technology and Informatics*, vol. 123, pp. 14–17, 2006.

[178] B. Marosy, C. M. Justice, N. Nzegwu, G. Kumar, A. F. Wilson, and N. H. Miller, "Lack of association between the aggrecan gene and familial idiopathic scoliosis," *Spine*, vol. 31, no. 13, pp. 1420–1425, 2006.

[179] N. H. Miller, B. Mims, A. Child, D. M. Milewicz, P. Sponseller, and S. H. Blanton, "Genetic analysis of structural elastic fiber and collagen genes in familial adolescent idiopathic scoliosis," *Journal of Orthopaedic Research*, vol. 14, no. 6, pp. 994–999, 1996.

[180] B. Marosy, C. M. Justice, C. Vu et al., "Identification of susceptibility loci for scoliosis in FIS families with triple curves," *The American Journal of Medical Genetics A*, vol. 152, no. 4, pp. 846–855, 2010.

[181] L. Baghernajad Salehi, M. Mangino, S. de Serio et al., "Assignment of a locus for autosomal dominant idiopathic scoliosis (IS) to ohuman chromosome 17p11," *Human Genetics*, vol. 111, no. 4-5, pp. 401–404, 2002.

[182] I.-S. Eun, W. W. Park, K. T. Suh, J. I. Kim, and J. S. Lee, "Association between osteoprotegerin gene polymorphism and bone mineral density in patients with adolescent idiopathic scoliosis," *European Spine Journal*, vol. 18, no. 12, pp. 1936–1940, 2009.

[183] H. Wang, Z. Wu, Q. Zhuang et al., "Association study of tryptophan hydroxylase 1 and arylalkylamine n-acetyltransferase polymorphisms with adolescent idiopathic scoliosis in han chinese," *Spine*, vol. 33, no. 20, pp. 2199–2203, 2008.

[184] L. Aulisa, P. Papaleo, E. Pola et al., "Association between IL-6 and MMP-3 gene polymorphisms and adolescent idiopathic scoliosis: a case-control study," *Spine*, vol. 32, no. 24, pp. 2700–2702, 2007.

[185] Z. Liu, N. L. S. Tang, X.-B. Cao et al., "Lack of association between the promoter polymorphisms of MMP-3 and IL-6 genes and adolescent idiopathic scoliosis: a case-control study in a chinese han population," *Spine*, vol. 35, no. 18, pp. 1701–1705, 2010.

[186] J. S. Lee, K. T. Suh, and I. S. Eun, "Polymorphism in interleukin-6 gene is associated with bone mineral density in patients with adolescent idiopathic scoliosis," *Journal of Bone and Joint Surgery B*, vol. 92, no. 8, pp. 1118–1122, 2010.

[187] S. Zhou, X. S. Qiu, Z. Z. Zhu, W. F. Wu, Z. Liu, and Y. Qiu, "A single-nucleotide polymorphism rs708567 in the IL-17RC gene is associated with a susceptibility to and the curve severity of adolescent idiopathic scoliosis in a Chinese Han population: a case-control study," *Musculoskeletal Disorders*, vol. 13, article 181, 2012.

[188] M. Mórocz, Á. Czibula, Z. B. Grózer et al., "Association study of BMP4, IL6, Leptin, MMP3, and MTNR1B gene promoter polymorphisms and adolescent idiopathic scoliosis," *Spine*, vol. 36, no. 2, pp. E123–E130, 2011.

[189] K. T. Suh, I.-S. Eun, and J. S. Lee, "Polymorphism in vitamin D receptor is associated with bone mineral density in patients with adolescent idiopathic scoliosis," *European Spine Journal*, vol. 19, no. 9, pp. 1545–1550, 2010.

[190] C.-W. Xia, Y. Qiu, X. Sun et al., "Vitamin D receptor gene polymorphisms in female adolescent idiopathic scoliosis patients," *National Medical Journal of China*, vol. 87, no. 21, pp. 1465–1469, 2007.

[191] W.-J. Chen, Y. Qiu, F. Zhu et al., "Vitamin D receptor gene polymorphisms: no association with low bone mineral density

in adolescent idiopathic scoliosis girls," *Zhonghua Wai Ke Za Zhi*, vol. 46, no. 15, pp. 1183–1186, 2008.

[192] Y. Takahashi, I. Kou, A. Takahashi et al., "A genome-wide association study identifies common variants near LBX1 associated with adolescent idiopathic scoliosis," *Nature Genetics*, vol. 43, no. 12, pp. 1237–1240, 2011.

[193] W. Gao, Y. Peng, G. Liang et al., "Association between common variants near LBX1 and adolescent idiopathic scoliosis replicated in the Chinese Han population," *PLoS ONE*, vol. 8, no. 1, Article ID e53234, 2013.

[194] Y.-H. Fan, Y.-Q. Song, D. Chan et al., "SNP rs11190870 near LBX1 is associated with adolescent idiopathic scoliosis in southern Chinese," *Journal of Human Genetics*, vol. 57, no. 4, pp. 244–246, 2012.

[195] S. Sharma, X. Gao, D. Londono et al., "Genome-wide association studies of adolescent idiopathic scoliosis suggest candidate susceptibility genes," *Human Molecular Genetics*, vol. 20, no. 7, pp. 1456–1466, 2011.

[196] S. Mao, L. Xu, Z. Zhu et al., "Association between genetic determinants of peak height velocity during puberty and predisposition to adolescent idiopathic scoliosis," *Spine*, vol. 38, no. 12, pp. 1034–1039, 2013.

[197] T. Yang, Q. Jia, H. Guo et al., "Epidemiological survey of idiopathic scoliosis and sequence alignment analysis of multiple candidate genes," *International Orthopaedics*, vol. 36, no. 6, pp. 1307–1314, 2012.

[198] D.-S. Huang, G.-Y. Liang, and P.-Q. Su, "Association of matrix metalloproteinase 9 polymorphisms with adolescent idiopathic scoliosis in Chinese Han female," *Chinese Journal of Medical Genetics*, vol. 28, no. 5, pp. 532–535, 2011.

[199] H. Wang, Z.-H. Wu, Q.-Y. Zhuang, and G.-X. Qiu, "Association study of HTR1A and HTR1B with adolescent idiopathic scoliosis," *Zhonghua Wai Ke Za Zhi*, vol. 48, no. 4, pp. 296–299, 2010.

[200] J. Jiang, Y. Qiu, B.-P. Qian et al., "Association between tissue inhibitor of metalloproteinase-2 gene polymorphism and adolescent idiopathic thoracic scoliosis," *Zhonghua Wai Ke Za Zhi*, vol. 48, no. 6, pp. 423–426, 2010.

[201] Q.-Y. Zhuang, Z.-H. Wu, and G.-X. Qiu, "Is polymorphism of CALM1 gene or growth hormone receptor gene associated with susceptibility to adolescent idiopathic scoliosis?" *Chinese Medical Journal*, vol. 87, no. 31, pp. 2198–2202, 2007.

[202] Axial Biotech, "ScoliScore AIS Prognostic Test," Axial Biotech Inc., Salt Lake City, Utah, USA, 2010, http://www.axialbiotech.com/.

[203] K. Ward, J. W. Ogilvie, M. V. Singleton, R. Chettier, G. Engler, and L. M. Nelson, "Validation of DNA-based prognostic testing to predict spinal curve progression in adolescent idiopathic scoliosis," *Spine*, vol. 35, no. 25, pp. E1455–E1464, 2010.

[204] T. B. Grivas, E. Vasiliadis, M. Malakasis, V. Mouzakis, and D. Segos, "Intervertebral disc biomechanics in the pathogenesis of idiopathic scoliosis," *Studies in Health Technology and Informatics*, vol. 123, pp. 80–83, 2006.

[205] H. N. Modi, S. W. Suh, H.-R. Song, J.-H. Yang, H.-J. Kim, and C. H. Modi, "Differential wedging of vertebral body and intervertebral disc in thoracic and lumbar spine in adolescent idiopathic scoliosis—a cross sectional study in 150 patients," *Scoliosis*, vol. 3, no. 1, article 11, 2008.

[206] S. Nomura and T. Takano-Yamamoto, "Molecular events caused by mechanical stress in bone," *Matrix Biology*, vol. 19, no. 2, pp. 91–96, 2000.

[207] A. Liedert, D. Kaspar, R. Blakytny, L. Claes, and A. Ignatius, "Signal transduction pathways involved in mechanotransduction in bone cells," *Biochemical and Biophysical Research Communications*, vol. 349, no. 1, pp. 1–5, 2006.

[208] D. J. Papachristou, K. K. Papachroni, E. K. Basdra, and A. G. Papavassiliou, "Signaling networks and transcription factors regulating mechanotransduction in bone," *BioEssays*, vol. 31, no. 7, pp. 794–804, 2009.

[209] K.-H. W. Lau, S. Kapur, C. Kesavan, and D. J. Baylink, "Up-regulation of the Wnt, estrogen receptor, insulin-like growth factor-I, and bone morphogenetic protein pathways in C57BL/6J osteoblasts as opposed to C3H/HeJ osteoblasts in part contributes to the differential anabolic response to fluid shear," *Journal of Biological Chemistry*, vol. 281, no. 14, pp. 9576–9588, 2006.

[210] H. M. Frost, "A 2003 update of bone physiology and Wolff s law for clinicians," *Angle Orthodontist*, vol. 74, no. 1, pp. 3–15, 2004.

[211] J. Sarwark and C.-É. Aubin, "Growth considerations of the immature spine," *Journal of Bone and Joint Surgery A*, vol. 89, supplement 1, pp. 8–13, 2007.

[212] A. Meir, D. S. McNally, J. C. Fairbank, D. Jones, and J. P. Urban, "The internal pressure and stress environment of the scoliotic intervertebral disc—a review," *Proceedings of the Institution of Mechanical Engineers H*, vol. 222, no. 2, pp. 209–219, 2008.

[213] A. R. Meir, J. C. T. Fairbank, D. A. Jones, D. S. McNally, and J. P. G. Urban, "High pressures and asymmetrical stresses in the scoliotic disc in the absence of muscle loading," *Scoliosis*, vol. 2, no. 1, article 4, 2007.

[214] W. E. B. Johnson and S. Roberts, "Human intervertebral disc cell morphology and cytoskeletal composition: a preliminary study of regional variations in health and disease," *Journal of Anatomy*, vol. 203, no. 6, pp. 605–612, 2003.

[215] J. L. Ford, P. Jones, and S. Downes, "Cellularity of human annulus tissue: an investigation into the cellularity of tissue of different pathologies," *Histopathology*, vol. 41, no. 6, pp. 531–537, 2002.

[216] H. Bertram, E. Steck, G. Zimmermann et al., "Accelerated intervertebral disc degeneration in scoliosis versus physiological ageing develops against a background of enhanced anabolic gene expression," *Biochemical and Biophysical Research Communications*, vol. 342, no. 3, pp. 963–972, 2006.

[217] J. Antoniou, V. Arlet, T. Goswami, M. Aebi, and M. Alini, "Elevated synthetic activity in the convex side of scoliotic intervertebral discs and endplates compared with normal tissues," *Spine*, vol. 26, no. 10, pp. E198–206, 2001.

[218] S. Stern, K. Lindenhayn, and C. Perka, "Human intervertebral disc cell culture for disc disorders," *Clinical Orthopaedics and Related Research*, no. 419, pp. 238–244, 2004.

[219] J. Yu, J. C. T. Fairbank, S. Roberts, and J. P. G. Urban, "The elastic fiber network of the anulus fibrosus of the normal and scoliotic human intervertebral disc," *Spine*, vol. 30, no. 16, pp. 1815–1820, 2005.

[220] S. Akhtar, J. R. Davies, and B. Caterson, "Ultrastructural immunolocalization of α-elastin and keratan sulfate proteoglycan in normal and scoliotic lumbar disc," *Spine*, vol. 30, no. 15, pp. 1762–1769, 2005.

[221] S. Roberts, J. Menage, and S. M. Eisenstein, "The cartilage end-plate and intervertebral disc in scoliosis: calcification and other sequelae," *Journal of Orthopaedic Research*, vol. 11, no. 5, pp. 747–757, 1993.

[222] L. Haglund, J. Ouellet, and P. Roughley, "Variation in chondroadherin abundance and fragmentation in the human scoliotic disc," *Spine*, vol. 34, no. 14, pp. 1513–1518, 2009.

[223] A. Pedrini Mille, V. A. Pedrini, and C. Tudisco, "Proteoglycans of human scoliotic intervertebral disc," *Journal of Bone and Joint Surgery A*, vol. 65, no. 6, pp. 815–823, 1983.

[224] Y. He, Y. Qiu, F. Zhu, and Z. Zhu, "Quantitative analysis of types I and II collagen in the disc annulus in adolescent idiopathic scoliosis," *Studies in Health Technology and Informatics*, vol. 123, pp. 123–128, 2006.

[225] Q. Lin, Z.-H. Wu, Y. Liu et al., "Gene expression of type X collagen in the intervertebral disc of idiopathic scoliosis patients," *Zhongguo Yi Xue Ke Xue Yuan Xue Bao*, vol. 26, no. 6, pp. 696–699, 2004.

[226] S. Roberts, E. H. Evans, D. Kletsas, D. C. Jaffray, and S. M. Eisenstein, "Senescence in human intervertebral discs," *European Spine Journal*, vol. 15, supplement 3, pp. S312–S316, 2006.

[227] B. Chen, J. Fellenberg, H. Wang, C. Carstens, and W. Richter, "Occurrence and regional distribution of apoptosis in scoliotic discs," *Spine*, vol. 30, no. 5, pp. 519–524, 2005.

[228] J. K. G. Crean, S. Roberts, D. C. Jaffray, S. M. Eisenstein, and V. C. Duance, "Matrix metalloproteinases in the human intervertebral disc: role in disc degeneration and scoliosis," *Spine*, vol. 22, no. 24, pp. 2877–2884, 1997.

[229] G. R. Buttermann and W. J. Mullin, "Pain and disability correlated with disc degeneration via magnetic resonance imaging in scoliosis patients," *European Spine Journal*, vol. 17, no. 2, pp. 240–249, 2008.

[230] Y. Qiu and F. Zhu, "Anterior and posterior spinal growth plates in adolescent idiopathic scoliosis: a histological study," *Zhongguo Yi Xue Ke Xue Yuan Xue Bao*, vol. 27, no. 2, pp. 148–152, 2005.

[231] F. Zhu, Y. Qiu, H. Y. Yeung, K. M. Lee, and J. C.-Y. Cheng, "Histomorphometric study of the spinal growth plates in idiopathic scoliosis and congenital scoliosis," *Pediatrics International*, vol. 48, no. 6, pp. 591–598, 2006.

[232] S. Wang, Y. Qiu, Z. Zhu, Z. Ma, C. Xia, and F. Zhu, "Histomorphological study of the spinal growth plates from the convex side and the concave side in adolescent idiopathic scoliosis," *Journal of Orthopaedic Surgery and Research*, vol. 2, no. 1, article 19, 2007.

[233] H. Xu, G. Qiu, Z. Wu et al., "Expression of transforming growth factor and basic fibroblast growth factor and core protein of proteoglycan in human vertebral cartilaginous endplate of adolescent idiopathic scoliosis," *Spine*, vol. 30, no. 17, pp. 1973–1978, 2005.

[234] G.-X. Qiu, Q.-Y. Li, Y. Liu et al., "Expression of transforming growth factor-β1 and basic fibroblast growth factor in articular process cartilages of adolescent idiopathic scoliosis," *National Medical Journal of China*, vol. 86, no. 21, pp. 1478–1483, 2006.

[235] Y. Chen, Y. Hu, and Z. Lü, "Regulating effects of transforming growth factor-beta (TGF-beta) on gene expression of collagen type II in human intervertebral discs," *Zhonghua Wai Ke Za Zhi*, vol. 38, no. 9, pp. 703–706, 2000.

[236] M. Turgut, G. Öktem, S. Uslu, M. E. Yurtseven, H. Aktuğ, and A. Uysal, "The effect of exogenous melatonin administration on trabecular width, ligament thickness and TGF-β1 expression in degenerated intervertebral disk tissue in the rat," *Journal of Clinical Neuroscience*, vol. 13, no. 3, pp. 357–363, 2006.

[237] E. Solheim, "Growth factors in bone," *International Orthopaedics*, vol. 22, no. 6, pp. 410–416, 1998.

[238] H.-J. Im, P. Muddasani, V. Natarajan et al., "Basic fibroblast growth factor stimulates matrix metalloproteinase-13 via the molecular cross-talk between the mitogen-activated protein kinases and protein kinase Cδ pathways in human adult articular chondrocytes," *Journal of Biological Chemistry*, vol. 282, no. 15, pp. 11110–11121, 2007.

[239] E. Scott Graham, D. G. Hazlerigg, and P. J. Morgan, "Evidence for regulation of basic fibroblast growth factor gene expression by photoperiod and melatonin in the ovine pars tuberalis," *Molecular and Cellular Endocrinology*, vol. 156, no. 1-2, pp. 45–53, 1999.

[240] M.-Y. Akoume, B. Azeddine, I. Turgeon et al., "Cell-based screening test for idiopathic scoliosis using cellular dielectric spectroscopy," *Spine*, vol. 35, no. 13, pp. E601–E608, 2010.

20

Arthrodesis of the Trapeziometacarpal Joint Using a Chevron Osteotomy and Plate Fixation

G. Shyamalan,[1] R. W. Jordan,[1] and A. Jarvis[2]

[1] *Birmingham Heartlands Hospital, Bordesley Green East, Birmingham, West Midlands B9 5SS, UK*
[2] *Worthing Hospital, Lyndhurst Road, Worthing, West Sussex BN11 2DH, UK*

Correspondence should be addressed to R. W. Jordan; robert.jordan@doctors.org.uk

Academic Editor: Padhraig O'Loughlin

Introduction. Trapeziometacarpal (TM) osteoarthritis is common. Despite the availability of numerous surgical options, none has been definitively proven to be superior. This study aims to determine the union rate and key strength following arthrodesis using a chevron osteotomy and plate fixation. *Methods.* 32 consecutive cases of TM joint arthrodesis performed between 2001 and 2006 were retrospectively identified. A chevron osteotomy was used to resect joint surfaces and fixation obtained using an AO mini T-plate. The patients were followed up for a mean of 65 months. Outcomes included visual analogue pain score, patient satisfaction, pinch strength, radiographic union, radiographic signs of scaphotrapezial arthritis, and complications. *Results.* The 32 cases included 16 females and 8 males with an average age of 56 years. Overall there was a 90% patient satisfaction rate. Average key pinch strength was 8.4 kg and pain score was 2.5. The union rate was 94%, and the two patients with nonunion underwent successful revision surgery. Only one case of radiographic progression of scaphotrapezoid arthritis was identified during followup. *Conclusion.* TM joint arthrodesis using a chevron osteotomy and plate fixation has high patient satisfaction and low nonunion rates. The authors endorse this technique in the management of TM joint osteoarthritis.

1. Introduction

Osteoarthritis of the thumb is common affecting 16% to 25% of postmenopausal women [1]. Typically it presents with pain, weakness, and deformity and can result in significant disability. The severity of the disease can be described using the Eaton et al. classification shown in Table 1 [2, 3]. The majority of the disease in the early stages can be managed with nonoperative treatments such as activity modification, hand therapy with splinting, analgesia, and the use of corticosteroid injections. When symptoms are refractory to nonoperative measures, surgery may be required. Patients commonly request surgery when everyday tasks become impossible, by which time the trapeziometacarpal (TM) joint is usually stiff and deformed. The primary goal of surgery is pain relief whilst providing stability, strength, and mobility of the thumb.

Uncertainty is present regarding the best choice of surgical procedure for osteoarthritis of the TM joint [4, 5]. The surgical treatment options include reconstruction of the volar beak ligament [6], metacarpal osteotomy [7], arthroscopy [8], partial trapeziectomy [9], and excision of the trapezium alone [10], with interposed tendon [11], plus ligament reconstruction [12, 13], arthrodesis [14–17], silicone arthroplasty [18], and joint replacement [19]. Systematic and Cochrane reviews have concluded that the available evidence is insufficient to conclude that any treatment is superior [20–22].

Arthrodesis has been reported to provide good pain relief, functional improvement, and high satisfaction rate [14, 17, 23, 24]. The technique has been proposed to improve grip [25] resulting in its use in young patients with posttraumatic osteoarthritis. Arthrodesis is contraindicated in pantrapezial arthritis [26, 27] and hence its use is limited to patients with stage II and III osteoarthritis [28, 29]. Comparative studies of arthrodesis have shown no difference between treatments in terms of pain, function, and patient satisfaction with trapeziectomy [28], silicon arthroplasty [29], resection arthroplasty [28], joint arthroplasty [30], and ligament reconstruction and tendon interposition [25, 29, 31]. Critics of arthrodesis cite limited function, reduced movement,

Table 1: Eaton and Littler classification of trapeziometacarpal arthritis.

Stage	Description
I	Slight joint space widening (due to effusion)
II	Slight narrowing of joint with sclerosis and small osteophytes < 2 m
III	Marked narrowing of joint with osteophytes > 2 mm
IV	Pantrapezial arthritis with involvement of scaphotrapezial joint

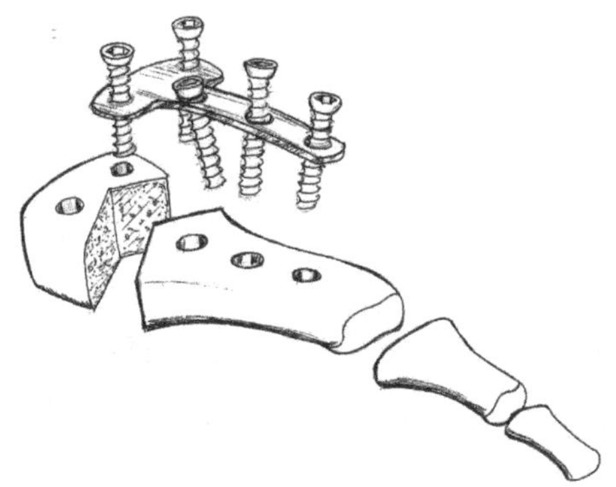

Figure 1: Chevron cuts and application of AO mini T-plate.

and subsequent development of adjacent joint arthrosis as disadvantages of the technique. However, reports have shown that function and movement are not significantly affected [14, 15, 17] and that subsequent osteoarthritis does not have a significant impact on pain or patient satisfaction [25].

Nonunion is a common complication after TM joint arthrodesis with the rate reported between 8% and 21% [25, 28, 29]. Arthrodesis must be performed by decorticating the eburnated cartilage surfaces, via a variety of bony cuts and end-to-end fixation. Flat surfaces or a cup and cone formation has been used but these configurations are difficult to hold in the optimal position. The chevron osteotomy was first described by Omer Jr. in 1969 [32] and the potential advantages of this configuration are the inherent stability and large contact area for union. The union rate following this procedure is reported at 83% for TM arthritis [33] and 100% for all digits of the hand [34]. Fixation options include multiple Kirschner wires, a tension band wire, power staples, compression screw(s), or a T-plate with multiple screws. The nonunion rate following arthrodesis with plate fixation has been reported to be lower (6%) than after all techniques combined (16%) [25]. The aim of this study is to determine the union rate and key strength following TM joint arthrodesis using a chevron osteotomy and plate fixation.

2. Methods

Consecutive cases of TM joint arthrodesis procedures performed at our centre by the senior author (A. Jarvis) between 2001 and 2006 were retrospectively collected. This procedure was offered to all patients regardless of age, sex, hand dominance, or occupation if nonoperative treatments had failed and stage II or III radiographic changes were present. The arthrodesis was the first surgical procedure in all cases. No other base of thumb operations were performed by the senior surgeon during this period for stage II or III disease.

The patients were positioned supine under general anesthesia, with the use of an arm table and a tourniquet. A dorsoradial three-leg zigzag incision was made, starting over the TM joint with care taken to avoid the superficial branches of the radial nerve. The TM joint was exposed through incising the joint capsule, respecting the superficial soft tissue structures. The joint surfaces were decorticated using chevron bone cuts with irrigation to prevent thermal bone necrosis. The apex of the chevron pointed proximally with the aim of achieving a 120-degree angle (see Figure 1). The apex of the distal cut was made perpendicular to the metacarpal but the proximal cut was altered to facilitate optimal flexion at the arthrodesis site. AlloMatrix was used until 2004 in 30% of cases, and after this the senior author introduced a low morbidity technique to take bone graft locally from the ipsilateral radial metaphysis. Thus several bone cores are obtained with an AO tap guide (see Figure 2) being used as a trephine via a small volar incision over the distal radius and these bone cores are impacted into the TM joint cavity. The metacarpal is reduced onto the trapezium and the position was checked clinically. The final position of the thumb must be truly functional, so that the thumb tip can reach the little finger tip. Once the position is trialed and accepted, it can be held with one or more 1.6 mm K-wires passed from the first metacarpal into the trapezium. This allows the surgeon to concentrate on plate application rather than reduction of the arthrodesis. The K-wire can be positioned through the wound but should not obstruct placement of the plate which is held by five screws. The wound is closed and a plaster incorporating the thumb is used to immobilise the thumb. Postoperatively, patients were usually discharged on the day of surgery, with followup arranged at two weeks for removal of sutures and change of the plaster slab. At the five-week visit, the plaster slab was removed, radiographs were taken (see Figure 3), and patients were provided with a removal thumb splint for further four weeks.

The patients were all called for review by the senior author, with mean followup of 64 months (range 36 to 84 months). There was no loss to followup. Patients were asked to score their pain according to the visual analogue score, one relating to no pain and 10 relating to severe pain. Pinch strength was measured using a pinch gauge dynamometer. Patients rated their overall satisfaction with the procedure as excellent, good, fair, or poor. Patients were also asked whether they felt their pain and function had improved and whether they could perform their activities of daily living following surgery.

Plain radiographs were assessed for union, defined as trabecular bridging on all views. The radiographs were also reviewed for the presence of arthrosis in the scaphotrapezial joint. Any complications postoperatively were also recorded.

FIGURE 2: AO tap guide.

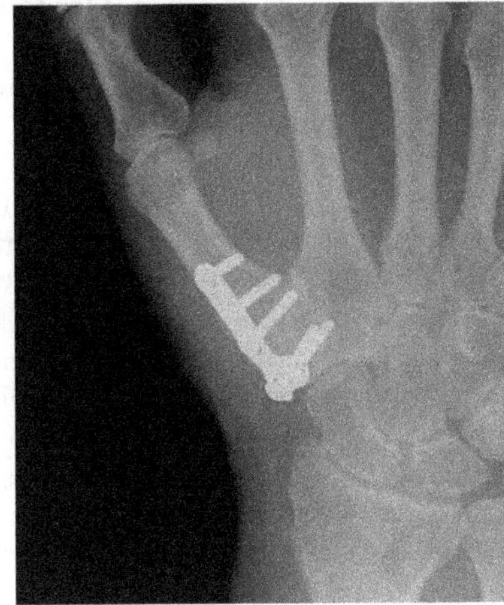

FIGURE 3: Postoperative plain radiographs of arthrodesis site.

3. Results

32 TM joint arthrodesis procedures were performed during the study period, 16 unilateral and 8 bilateral. Demographics included 20 females and 12 males, with an average age of 56 years (range: 42–70).

The average key pinch strength was 8.4 kg and the average visual analogue pain score was 2.5. All patients reported a subjective improvement in pain levels, hand function, and ability to perform activities of daily living. Overall there was a 90% satisfaction rate with the procedure, 60% rated excellent, 15% good, 15% fair, and 10% poor results.

The union rate of radiographs was 94%. Two patients required reoperation for clinical and radiographic nonunion involving further harvest of bone graft from the radial metaphysis and fixation with T-plate. Both patients reported a good result following the second procedure and went on to union. Only one case of radiographic progression of scaphotrapezial arthritis was identified at followup but the patient was asymptomatic.

Two patients reported transient radial nerve paraesthesia with symptoms settling in both patients at final followup. Six patients required removal of metalwork for local discomfort after union (19%).

4. Discussion

Recent systematic and Cochrane reviews have revealed that insufficient evidence is available to demonstrate superiority of any treatment option for TM joint osteoarthritis [20–22]. The results from this study show a 90% patient satisfaction rate and 94% union rate following Chevron osteotomies and T-plate fixation supporting this as an effective treatment method.

Previous studies have demonstrated similar satisfaction levels following various arthrodesis procedures [14, 17, 23, 24]. The average postoperative pinch strength of 8.4 kg is higher than the 5.9 kg reported in a previous study [23]. However, as preoperative measures were not available, it is not possible to comment on the improvement in pinch strength and this makes comparison between studies difficult. Previous studies have shown that key and chuck pinch grip are significantly better following arthrodesis than ligament reconstruction and tendon interposition [25] and the pinch strength achieved following arthrodesis in this study would support this.

The 6% nonunion rate is lower than previously reported in the literature where rates range from 8% to 21% [23–25, 28, 29]. This finding is supported by a retrospective review performed by Hartigan et al. who report a 16% nonunion rate following all types of arthrodesis but a lower rate of nonunion (6%) in cases where plate fixation was used [25]. The authors hypothesize two reasons for their low nonunion rate: the chevron configuration increases the contact area at the osteotomy site and the biomechanics of T-plate fixation improve chances of union. The senior author first started using the chevron bone cuts for TM joint arthrodesis in 1996. A variety of fixation techniques were used from Kirschner wires to single and double lag screws. Unfortunately there was a high failure rate and this contributed to a change in our practice to T-plate fixation from 2001.

It is widely believed that a fused TM joint accelerates arthritis in the adjacent joints, especially the scaphotrapezial joint. Our experience has been quite different with only one case of radiographic scaphotrapezoid arthritis identified during followup, leading us to conclude that TM joint arthrodesis does not accelerate arthritis in the adjacent thumb joints.

The authors recognise several limitations in the study design. The study involved a retrospective case series without a comparative group. The measurement of pinch strength and pain score was only performed postoperatively, and the addition of a preoperative measurement would highlight the amount of improvement seen following arthrodesis and facilitate comparisons to other studies. Subjective measures of outcome and satisfaction were obtained but the use of a validated outcome instrument would have the advantage of quantifying any improvement and again allow comparison with other studies.

5. Conclusion

Arthrodesis using a chevron osteotomy and plate fixation can give high patient satisfaction and union rates. This technique is safe and effective and is endorsed by the authors for the management of TM joint osteoarthritis.

Conflict of Interests

The authors declare that there is no conflict of interests regarding the publication of this paper.

References

[1] A. L. Armstrong, J. B. Hunter, and T. R. C. Davis, "The prevalence of degenerative arthritis of the base of the thumb in postmenopausal women," *Journal of Hand Surgery*, vol. 19, no. 3, pp. 340–341, 1994.

[2] R. G. Eaton, L. B. Lane, J. W. Littler, and J. J. Keyser, "Ligament reconstruction for the painful thumb carpometacarpal joint: a long-term assessment," *The Journal of Hand Surgery*, vol. 9, no. 5, pp. 692–699, 1984.

[3] R. G. Eaton, S. Z. Glickel, and J. W. Littler, "Tendon interposition arthroplasty for degenerative arthritis of the trapeziometacarpal joint of the thumb," *Journal of Hand Surgery*, vol. 10, no. 5, pp. 645–654, 1985.

[4] S. Dhar, I. C. M. Gray, W. A. Jones, and F. H. Beddow, "Simple excision of the trapezium for osteoarthritis of the carpometacarpal joint of the thumb," *Journal of Hand Surgery B*, vol. 19, no. 4, pp. 485–488, 1994.

[5] M. Lanzetta and G. Foucher, "A comparison of different surgical techniques in treating degenerative arthrosis of the carpometacarpal joint of the thumb. A retrospective study of 98 cases," *Journal of Hand Surgery*, vol. 20, no. 1, pp. 105–110, 1995.

[6] R. G. Eaton and J. W. Littler, "Ligament reconstruction for the painful thumb carpometacarpal joint," *Journal of Bone and Joint Surgery—Series A*, vol. 55, no. 8, pp. 1655–1666, 1973.

[7] M. M. Tomaino, "Treatment of Eaton stage I trapeziometacarpal disease with thumb metacarpal extension osteotomy," *Journal of Hand Surgery*, vol. 25, no. 6, pp. 1100–1106, 2000.

[8] R. W. Culp and M. S. Rekant, "The role of arthroscopy in evaluating and treating trapeziometacarpal disease," *Hand Clinics*, vol. 17, no. 2, pp. 315–319, 2001.

[9] R. García-Mas and X. Solé Molins, "Partial trapeziectomy with ligament reconstruction—tendon interposition in thumb carpo-metacarpal osteoarthritis. A study of 112 cases," *Chirurgie de la Main*, vol. 28, no. 4, pp. 230–238, 2009.

[10] W. H. GERVIS, "Excision of the trapezium for osteoarthritis of the trapezio-metacarpal joint," *The Journal of Bone and Joint Surgery B*, vol. 31, no. 4, pp. 537–539, 1949.

[11] A. I. Froimson, "Tendon interposition arthroplasty of carpometacarpal joint of the thumb," *Hand Clinics*, vol. 3, no. 4, pp. 489–503, 1988.

[12] R. I. Burton and V. D. Pellegrini Jr., "Surgical management of basal joint arthritis of the thumb. Part II. Ligament reconstruction with tendon interposition arthroplasty," *Journal of Hand Surgery*, vol. 11, no. 3, pp. 324–332, 1986.

[13] T. R. Davis and A. Pace, "Trapeziectomy for trapeziometacarpal joint osteoarthritis: Is ligament reconstruction and temporary stabilisation of the pseudarthrosis with a Kirschner wire important?" *Journal of Hand Surgery*, vol. 34, no. 3, pp. 312–321, 2009.

[14] H. B. Bamberger, P. J. Stern, T. R. Kiefhaber, J. J. McDonough, and R. M. Cantor, "Trapeziometacarpal joint arthrodesis: a functional evaluation," *Journal of Hand Surgery*, vol. 17, no. 4, pp. 605–611, 1992.

[15] R. E. Leach and P. E. Bolton, "Arthritis of the carpometacarpal joint of the thumb. Results of arthrodesis," *Journal of Bone and Joint Surgery Series A*, vol. 50, no. 6, pp. 1171–1177, 1968.

[16] R. E. Carroll, "Arthrodesis of the carpometacarpal joint of the thumb. A review of patients with a long postoperative period," *Clinical Orthopaedics and Related Research*, vol. 220, pp. 106–110, 1987.

[17] H. H. Stark, J. F. Moore, and C. R. J. H. Ashworth andBoyes, "Fusion of the first metacarpotrapezial joint for degenerative arthritis," *Journal of Bone and Joint Surgery—Series A*, vol. 59, no. 1, pp. 22–26, 1977.

[18] A. B. Swanson, "Disabling arthritis at the base of the thumb: treatment by resection of the trapezium and flexible (silicone) implant arthroplasty," *Journal of Bone and Joint Surgery A*, vol. 54, no. 3, pp. 456–471, 1972.

[19] J. Y. de La Caffiniere and P. Aucouturier, "Trapezio-metacarpal arthroplasty by total prosthesis," *Hand*, vol. 11, no. 1, pp. 41–46, 1979.

[20] G. Martou, K. Veltri, and A. Thoma, "Surgical treatment of osteoarthritis of the carpometacarpal joint of the thumb: a systematic review," *Plastic and Reconstructive Surgery*, vol. 114, no. 2, pp. 421–432, 2004.

[21] A. Wajon, E. Carr, I. Edmunds, and L. Ada, "Surgery for thumb (trapeziometacarpal joint) osteoarthritis," *Cochrane Database of Systematic Reviews*, no. 4, Article ID CD004631, 2009.

[22] G. M. Vermeulen, H. Slijper, R. Feitz, S. E. Hovius, T. M. Moojen, and R. W. Selles, "Surgical management of primary thumb carpometacarpal osteoarthritis: a systematic review," *The Journal of Hand Surgery*, vol. 36, no. 1, pp. 157–169, 2011.

[23] M. Rizzo, S. L. Moran, and A. Y. Shin, " Long-term outcomes of trapeziometacarpal arthrodesis in the management of trapeziometacarpal arthritis," *Journal of Hand Surgery*, vol. 34, no. 1, pp. 20–26, 2009.

[24] M. K. Karlsson, "Arthrodesis of the trapeziometacarpal joint," *Scandinavian Journal of Plastic and Reconstructive Surgery and Hand Surgery*, vol. 25, no. 2, pp. 167–171, 1991.

[25] B. J. Hartigan, P. J. Stern, and T. R. Kiefhaber, "Thumb carpometacarpal osteoarthritis: arthrodesis compared with ligament reconstruction and tendon interposition," *Journal of Bone and Joint Surgery*, vol. 83, no. 10, pp. 1470–1478, 2001.

[26] R. E. Carroll and N. A. Hill, "Arthrodesis of the carpo-metacarpal joint of the thumb," *The Journal of Bone and Joint Surgery*, vol. 55, no. 2, pp. 292–294, 1973.

[27] R. M. Cavallazzi and G. Spreafico, "Trapezio-metacarpal arthrodesis today why?" *Journal of Hand Surgery*, vol. 11, no. 2, pp. 250–254, 1986.

[28] E. E. J. Raven, G. M. M. J. Kerkhoffs, S. Rutten, A. J. W. Marsman, R. K. Marti, and G. H. R. Albers, "Long term results of surgical intervention for osteoarthritis of the trapeziometacarpal joint: comparison of resection arthroplasty, trapeziectomy with tendon interposition and trapezio-metacarpal arthrodesis," *International Orthopaedics*, vol. 31, no. 4, pp. 547–554, 2007.

[29] E. J. Taylor, K. Desari, J. C. D'Arcy, and A. V. Bonnici, "A comparison of fusion, trapeziectomy and silastic replacement for the treatment of osteoarthritis of the trapeziometacarpal joint," *Journal of Hand Surgery*, vol. 30, no. 1, pp. 45–49, 2005.

[30] P. C. Amadio and S. P. de Silva, "Comparison of the results of trapeziometacarpal arthrodesis and arthroplasty in men with osteoarthritis of the trapeziometacarpal joint," *Annales de Chirurgie de la Main et du Membre Superieur*, vol. 9, no. 5, pp. 358–363, 1990.

[31] R. Hart, M. Janeček, V. Šiška, B. Kučera, and V. Štipčák, "Interposition suspension arthroplasty according to Epping versus arthrodesis for trapeziometacarpal osteoarthritis," *European*

Surgery—Acta Chirurgica Austriaca, vol. 38, no. 6, pp. 433–438, 2006.

[32] G. E. Omer Jr., "Evaluation and reconstruction of the forearm and hand after acute traumatic peripheral nerve injuries," *Journal of Bone and Joint Surgery*, vol. 50, no. 7, pp. 1454–1478, 1968.

[33] J. K. Stanley, E. J. Smith, and A. G. Muirhead, "Arthrodesis of the metacarpo-phalangeal joint of the thumb: a review of 42 cases," *Journal of Hand Surgery*, vol. 14, no. 3, pp. 291–293, 1989.

[34] C. R. Pribyl, G. E. Omer Jr., and L. McGinty, "Effectiveness of the chevron arthrodesis in small joints of the hand," *Journal of Hand Surgery A*, vol. 21, no. 6, pp. 1052–1058, 1996.

21

Early Clinical Outcomes Associated with a Novel Osteochondral Allograft Transplantation System in the Knee

William J. Long,[1,2,3,4] **Joseph W. Greene,**[5,6] **and Fred D. Cushner**[7,8]

[1] *Insall Scott Kelly Institute, New York, NY 10065, USA*
[2] *New York University, New York, NY 10065, USA*
[3] *Hospital for Joint Disease, NYU, New York, NY 10065, USA*
[4] *St. Francis Hospital, Roslyn, NY 11548, USA*
[5] *Norton Healthcare, Louisville, KY 40207, USA*
[6] *Department of Orthopaedic Surgery, University of Louisville, Louisville, KY 40202, USA*
[7] *Southside Hospital, Bay Shore, NY 11706, USA*
[8] *Lenox Hill Hospital, Northwell Health System, New York, NY 10065, USA*

Correspondence should be addressed to William J. Long; doctor_long@hotmail.com

Academic Editor: Werner Kolb

Background. Osteochondral defects of the knee are a common finding at the time of arthroscopic intervention. *Purpose/Hypothesis.* To report our outcomes after utilizing a new technique of osteochondral allograft transplantation for focal cartilage defects. *Study Design.* Case series. *Methods.* All patients treated with osteochondral allograft transplantation with a Zimmer Chondrofix plug (Zimmer Inc., Warsaw, IN) for focal cartilage defects over a 12-month period were followed up at a minimum of 24 months. Failures were documented and radiographs were evaluated. *Results.* 61 knees (58 patients) underwent grafting. Three cases were lost to follow-up. In the remaining 58 cases the average age was 40 (range 18–59). At a mean follow-up of 28 months (range 24–36), there were 5 failures requiring further surgery. Mean KOOS scores in the Pain, Symptoms, ADL, Sports, and Quality of Life dimensions were 82, 79, 84, 66, and 58, respectively. Radiographs demonstrated maintenance of the subchondral bone without graft absorption or subsidence. *Conclusions.* Our observations suggest that osteochondral allograft transplantation leads to a satisfactory activity level and function at early follow-up while avoiding the inherent complexities associated with other cartilage restoration techniques. Longer follow-up is warranted to monitor the subchondral bone, articular surface, and patient outcome measures.

1. Introduction

Each year it is estimated that chondral defects of the knee affect more than 900,000 people in the United States and result in more than 200,000 procedures [1]. In 34% of all knee arthroscopies, one or more focal full-thickness or nearly full-thickness cartilage defects are seen [2–4]. It is also estimated that 36% of all athletes have a cartilage defect in the knee [5]. Human articular cartilage has limited ability to self-repair, so damage to the articular cartilage in the knee is a potential risk factor in the development of early-onset osteoarthritis and can result in loss of movement and pain [6–8].

Full-thickness articular cartilage defects, defined as Outerbridge grades III–IV [9], are likely to progress to early degenerative wear and become increasingly symptomatic [10]; thus surgical treatment is recommended [11]. A variety of surgical options exist for the treatment of full-thickness chondral defects in the knee such as debridement, microfracture, osteochondral autograft transfer (OAT), osteochondral allograft transplantation (OCA), and autologous chondrocyte implantation (ACI). Each of these techniques presents its own unique set of limitations.

Microfracture is the most common method employed for cartilage restoration in the knee [12]. It relies on marrow stimulation and the influx of marrow products into the cartilage defect. The mature fibrocartilage formed is less durable than native type II collagen, resulting in some degradation over time [13]. Some surgical algorithms use approximately 2 cm^2

as the upper threshold for microfracture and beyond this move onto more advanced cartilage restoration techniques [14–16].

OATS and mosaicplasty are techniques involving the transport of osteochondral plugs from another area of the knee to the defect. Disadvantages associated with these techniques include leaving an articular cartilage defect in another location of the knee, progression of osteoarthritic changes at the donor site, the relative size limitation of <20 mm^2 [17], and the fact that an arthrotomy may be required. As larger areas of OATs are required, more donor site complaints and symptoms occur [18].

OCA eliminates the donor site complications and size limitations of OATS by obtaining the donor tissue from a cadaver. It allows treatment of both cartilage and underlying bony defects to a greater degree than ACI. This technique has shown promising results at long-term follow-up [19]. Limitations to OCA involve the need for donor tissue and the timing of transplantation, which is best achieved between 14 and 28 days to allow testing of the tissue, without the significant loss of cell viability that occurs over time [20].

As first proposed in 1994 ACI allows the treatment of large cartilage defects in the knee. Unfortunately, it is expensive, costing approximately 66,000 dollars per case [21]. The technique requires a 2-stage procedure (harvesting and implantation) and is less successful with bone loss at the base of the lesion [22].

In an effort to avoid the individual complications and limitations associated with each of these techniques, we have been using a relatively new technique of osteochondral allograft transplantation, Chondrofix® Osteochondral Allograft (Zimmer Inc., Warsaw, IN). These allografts consist of decellularized hyaline cartilage and cancellous bone that maintain the mechanical properties of unprocessed osteochondral grafts.

Similar to OCA, Chondrofix transplantation is single-stage and guarantees an immediate reliable tissue transfer of an osteochondral unit; however the grafts are readily available on the shelf, thus eliminating the narrow timing aspects to OCA. The aim of this study was to evaluate the results of this technique retrospectively in a selected group of patients with the goal of analyzing patient outcomes and understanding which factors could influence the clinical outcome in order to clarify the correct indication of this treatment option.

2. Methods

This study was approved by our Health System Institutional Review Board. All patients between the ages of 18 and 60 who had received a Chondrofix plug in the twelve-month period between February 2012 and February 2013 were retrospectively included in the study.

The procedures were performed by one of two fellowship-trained, board-certified orthopaedic surgeons. Inclusion criteria included a symptomatic full-thickness cartilage lesion identified preoperatively by advanced imaging or prior arthroscopy, though the size of the lesion was consistently underestimated. Patients with inflammatory arthritis or significant uni- or tricompartmental arthritis were not considered candidates for transplantation.

Table 1: Primary diagnosis.

DJD	27
PF DJD	15
ACL tear	5
OCD lesion	4
PF instability	3

DJD: degenerative joint disease; PF: patellofemoral; ACL: anterior cruciate ligament; OCD: osteochondritis dissecans.

A tourniquet was used, and the knee was examined arthroscopically. Once the final decision to perform osteochondral allograft transplantation was taken, the lesion was sized, prepared, and grafted with instrumentation provided in the Chondrofix set. One or more plugs were placed depending on the size and shape of the lesion. The instrumentation was introduced through an appropriately sized accessory portal, and the procedure was visualized arthroscopically. An arthrotomy was employed only in the case of a patellar lesion, allowing the patella to be everted for perpendicular preparation and grafting of the defect.

Postoperatively all patients were allowed to weight-bear as tolerated and encouraged to progress to full range of motion. A brace was only used if required due to an associated procedure (e.g., cruciate ligament reconstruction). Patients were instructed to avoid high impact activities for 6 weeks. Follow-up visits occurred at 3 weeks, 6 weeks, 3 months, 6 months, and yearly thereafter. Radiographs of the knee were obtained (weight bearing anteroposterior, lateral, and skyline) at the 3-week, six-month, and yearly follow-ups.

Clinical evaluation included range of motion (ROM), presence of an effusion, and radiographic changes. They completed the Tegner score [23], and the Knee Injury and Osteoarthritis Outcome Score (KOOS) patient-derived outcome tool [24]. Patients who were unable to be evaluated in person completed the scores over the telephone.

3. Results

61 cases in 58 patients were eligible for inclusion. The average age was 40.0 (range 18–59) and 59% of cases were in male patients. The primary diagnoses (Table 1) were degenerative joint disease (DJD) in 27 cases, patellofemoral (PF) DJD in 15 cases, anterior cruciate ligament (ACL) tear and resultant instability in 5 cases, osteochondritis dissecans (OCD) lesion in 4 cases (Figures 1(a) and 1(b)), and PF instability and DJD in 3 cases.

Procedures performed concomitantly (Table 2) include arthroscopic partial meniscectomy in 18 cases, ACL reconstruction in 5 cases, open proximal realignment and lateral release in 4 cases, arthroscopic lateral release in 4 cases, microfracture in 2 cases, and lateral meniscus repair, patellofemoral arthroplasty in 1 case each. Four knees had undergone prior ACL reconstruction, 1 knee had prior arthroscopic lateral release, and 1 knee had previous open osteochondral allografting.

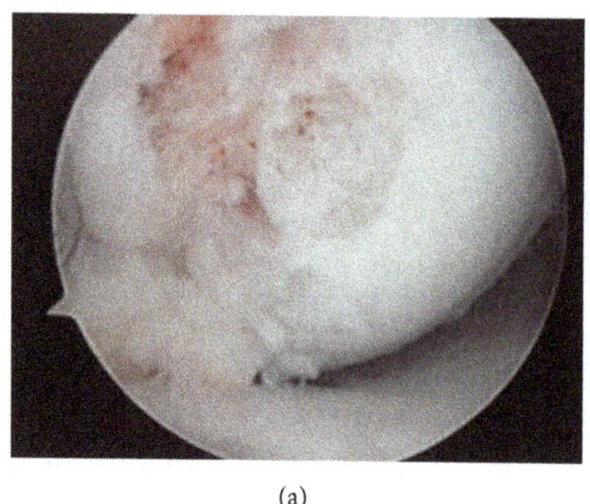
(a)

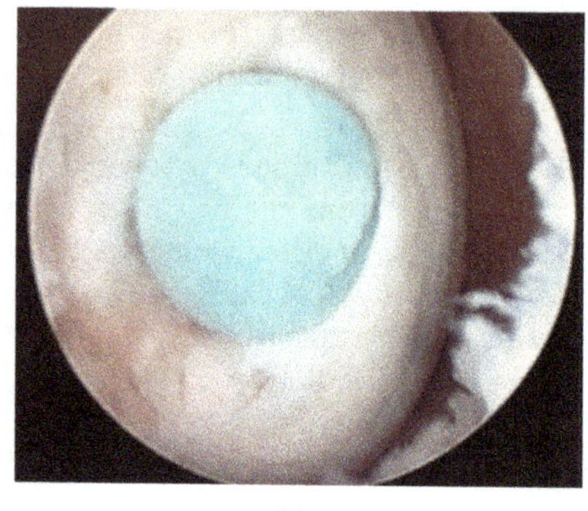
(b)

FIGURE 1: Failed OATS for a MFC OCD lesion revised to a Chondrofix plug.

TABLE 2: Other procedures.

Concomitant procedures	
Partial meniscectomy	18
ACLR	5
PRLR	4
Arthroscopic lateral release	4
Microfracture	2
Lateral meniscus repair	1
PFA	1
Prior procedures	
ACL	4
Arthroscopic lateral release	1
Open osteochondral allograft	1

ACLR: anterior cruciate ligament reconstruction; PRLR: proximal realignment and lateral release; PFA: patellofemoral arthroplasty.

Graft placement was in the medial femoral condyle (MFC) in 19 cases, the trochlea in 15 cases, the patella in 9 cases, the lateral femoral condyle in 4 cases, and multiple locations in 18 cases. Thirty-one of the cases utilized only one Chondrofix graft; 2 were used in 23 cases, 3 in 3 cases, and 4 in 4 cases. The sizes of the plugs used in the 31 cases with one plug are also listed, providing a reasonable estimate to the size of the lesions treated (Table 3).

Follow-up was achieved in 95% of cases (58 of 61). Mean follow-up was 28 months (range 24–36 months). Average Tegner activity level was 4 (range 1–7). The mean KOOS Pain, Symptom, Activities of Daily Living (ADL), Sports, and Quality of Life (QoL) domains were 82, 79, 84, 66, and 58, respectively (Table 4). Average ROM was 0 to 129 degrees. No patients were noted to have a persistent postoperative effusion. Radiographs demonstrated maintenance of the subchondral bone without any obvious graft absorption or subsidence.

Five clinical failures were noted to have gone on to subsequent surgery during the follow-up period. Three patients with DJD required conversion to arthroplasty, 1 required conversion to a total knee arthroplasty (TKA), 1 required conversion to a unicompartmental knee arthroplasty (UKA) (Figures 2(a) and 2(b)), and one patient who had a PFA at the same time as her grafting required conversion to a TKA. One 34-year-old patient with patellofemoral disease saw another surgeon and had a revision cartilage procedure, and another had a revision of one of two trochlear plugs. There were no infections. Three cases were lost to follow-up.

TABLE 3: Location, number, and size of graft plugs.

Location of lesions	
MFC	19
Multiple	18
Trochlea	15
Patella	9
LFC	4
Number of plugs	
1	31
2	23
3	3
4	4
Size of individual plugs (mm)	
7	2
9	11
11	11
15	7

MFC: medial femoral condyle; LFC: lateral femoral condyle.

TABLE 4: KOOS scores.

Domain	Mean	SD
Pain	82	±22
Symptoms	79	±18
ADLs	84	±21
Sports	66	±33
QoL	58	±29

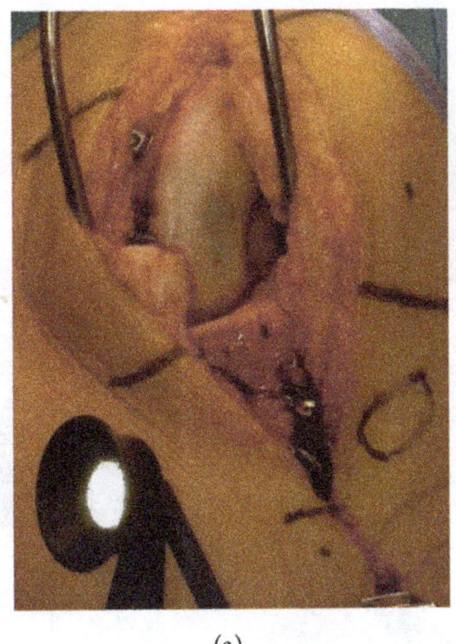
(a)

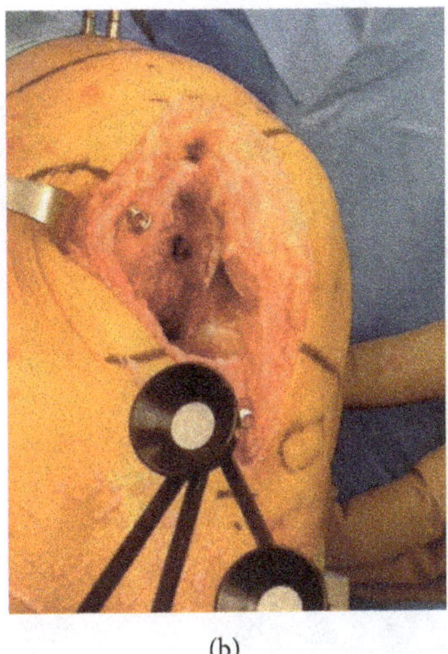
(b)

FIGURE 2: (a) Intact Chondrofix plugs in the MFC at the time of UKA. (b) Stable underlying bony integration of the bony portion of the plug for femoral component seating.

4. Discussion

A number of arthroscopic repair or reconstructive techniques can be performed in the setting of full-thickness cartilage defects in the knee. Various materials, such as allografts, autografts, synthetic polymers, and periosteal and perichondral flaps, have been proposed, but the 4 techniques that have gained widespread use and interest during the last decade in North America are microfracture, OCA, OATS, and ACI procedures.

Currently, the important step of determining the area of the defect is accomplished either by attempting to interpret radiographic images prior to surgery or by using mechanical instrumentation during an arthroscopic diagnostic examination. Unfortunately, the sensitivity of conventional magnetic resonance imaging (MRI) is still limited. Improved diagnostic performance has been seen with 3-Tesla (T) MRIs compared with 1.5 T protocols [25, 26]. In a study comparing 3 T MRI to arthroscopy, the ability of MRI to predict articular cartilage lesions was examined. When using the Outerbridge classification the values for sensitivity, specificity, and accuracy were 57%, 71%, and 63%, respectively [27]. It is particularly difficult to determine the depth of the lesion [28]. Therefore, surgeons cannot rely on preoperative imaging to accurately determine treatment choice, leaving much of the decision-making process to the arthroscopic evaluation of the defect grade and size.

Thus both the complexity of existing techniques and the difficulty in predicting the size of the lesion lead us to consider this novel Chondrofix option. We were fairly familiar with this technique, having used it with Tru-Fit plugs for the preceding five years [29]. With the Chondrofix system, multiple graft sizes (7–15 mm) are available for off-the-shelf use. Single-stage implantation using an arthroscopic approach with a small incision for graft insertion can be used for all lesions with the exception of the patella, where a miniarthrotomy is required for access.

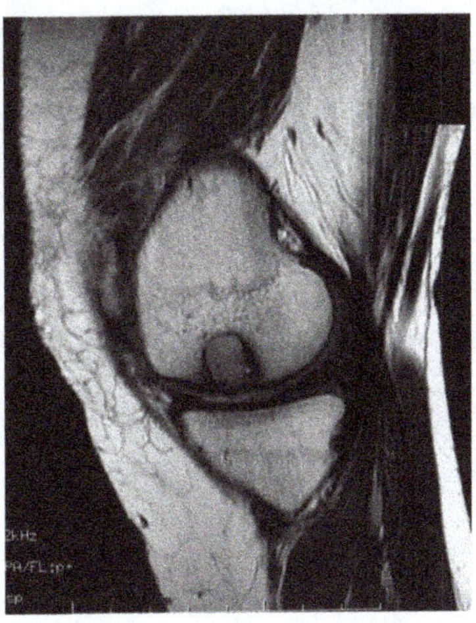

FIGURE 3: MRI evaluation of a Chondrofix plug at 3 months after implantation.

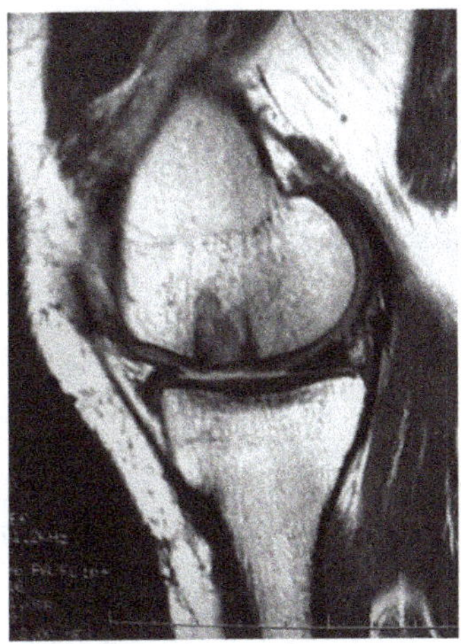

FIGURE 4: MRI evaluation of a plug at 8 months after implantation with further bony incorporation.

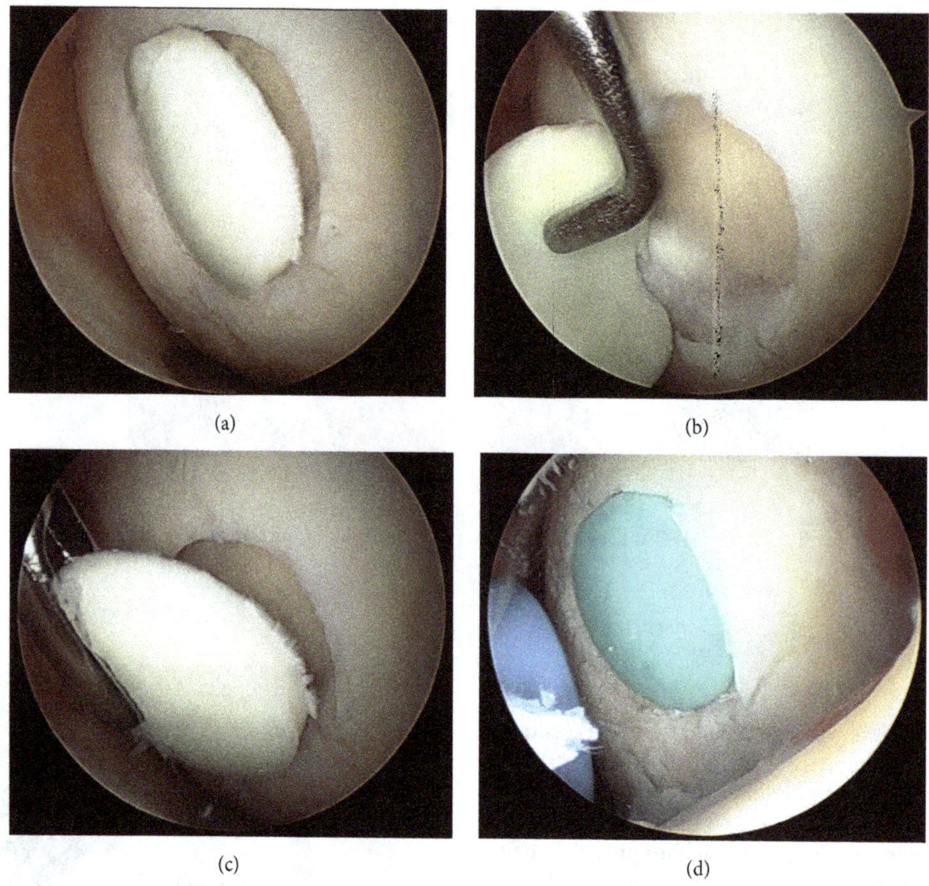

FIGURE 5: Cartilage surface delamination of a plug overlying a stable bony base with successful revision to a similarly sized plug.

Our primary concerns with this new graft option were with respect to its incorporation and durability as the grafts are acellular and treated in a novel fashion, prior to implantation. Our radiographic review did not demonstrate any significant changes. A more sensitive MRI evaluation was available for two cases that had follow-up imaging for new injuries to the knee. The first (Figure 3) was performed at 3 months and the second (Figure 4) at 8 months. They both demonstrate incorporation of the bony portion of the graft, with some changes to the overlying cartilage surface, which will have to be followed up carefully over the longer-term.

Outside the cohort in this paper, we have seen one novel failure mechanism. In this case the cartilage surface delaminated from the underlying bone on the plug. It occurred in a labourer during a squat at lift of a 100 lb piece of equipment. Arthroscopic evaluation demonstrated a well-incorporated bone base separated from the overlying cartilage (Figures 5(a)–5(d)). A successful revision to a new plug was performed, and the patient has done well to a year following revision.

The failures in this series were evaluated. Four of the five failures had two plugs in a single compartment. The plugs used were all at least 9 mm, consistent with larger defects. Thus the failure rate was 1/31 for single-plug cases and 4/23 for two-plug cases. Interestingly, none of the even larger 3- and 4-plug cases failed. Location of the lesion did not predict failure, with 3 failures in MFC lesions and 2 in trochlear lesions.

5. Conclusions

While it is generally accepted that focal chondral lesions often progress towards osteoarthritis, a review of the literature presents compelling evidence that between 10 and 40% of all patients aged <40 years undergoing arthroscopic surgery for other reasons have treatable chondral injuries that will remain unaddressed [2–4]. The current study demonstrates a simple, arthroscopic, off-the-shelf solution that appears to provide reasonable clinical outcomes at short-term follow-up.

There are a number of obvious limitations to this study: it is a short-term retrospective follow-up; preoperative scores were not obtained; there were a number of different diagnoses and concomitant procedures performed; and there was no comparative group. In the future, we are planning more comprehensive and rigorous prospective comparative studies involving both preoperative and postoperative evaluations with advanced imaging, to better compare outcomes with these cartilage lesions. Based on this study, Chondrofix plugs appear to be a reasonable on-demand option for addressing full-thickness cartilage lesions encountered at the time of arthroscopy, with acceptable short-term patient satisfaction and function.

Competing Interests

The authors declare that they have no competing interests.

References

[1] W. W. Curl, J. Krome, E. S. Gordon, J. Rushing, B. P. Smith, and G. G. Poehling, "Cartilage injuries: a review of 31,516 knee arthroscopies," *Arthroscopy*, vol. 13, no. 4, pp. 456–460, 1997.

[2] A. Årøen, S. Løken, S. Heir et al., "Articular cartilage lesions in 993 consecutive knee arthroscopies," *The American Journal of Sports Medicine*, vol. 32, no. 1, pp. 211–215, 2004.

[3] K. Hjelle, E. Solheim, T. Strand, R. Muri, and M. Brittberg, "Articular cartilage defects in 1,000 knee arthroscopies," *Arthroscopy*, vol. 18, no. 7, pp. 730–734, 2002.

[4] W. Widuchowski, J. Widuchowski, and T. Trzaska, "Articular cartilage defects: study of 25,124 knee arthroscopies," *Knee*, vol. 14, no. 3, pp. 177–182, 2007.

[5] D. C. Flanigan, J. D. Harris, T. Q. Trinh, R. A. Siston, and R. H. Brophy, "Prevalence of chondral defects in Athletes' Knees: a systematic review," *Medicine and Science in Sports and Exercise*, vol. 42, no. 10, pp. 1795–1801, 2010.

[6] E. Arendt and R. Dick, "Knee injury patterns among men and women in collegiate basketball and soccer. NCAA data and review of literature," *The American Journal of Sports Medicine*, vol. 23, no. 6, pp. 694–701, 1995.

[7] S. Drawer and C. W. Fuller, "Propensity for osteoarthritis and lower limb joint pain in retired professional soccer players," *British Journal of Sports Medicine*, vol. 35, no. 6, pp. 402–408, 2001.

[8] H. Roos, "Are there long-term sequelae from soccer?" *Clinics in Sports Medicine*, vol. 17, no. 4, pp. 819–831, 1998.

[9] R. E. Outerbridge, "The etiology of chondromalacia patellae," *The Journal of Bone & Joint Surgery—British Volume*, vol. 43, pp. 752–757, 1961.

[10] H. J. Mankin, "The response of articular cartilage to mechanical injury," *The Journal of Bone & Joint Surgery—American Volume*, vol. 64, no. 3, pp. 460–466, 1982.

[11] N. A. Sgaglione, A. Miniaci, S. D. Gillogly, and T. R. Carter, "Update on advanced surgical techniques in the treatment of traumatic focal articular cartilage lesions in the knee," *Arthroscopy*, vol. 18, no. 2, pp. 9–32, 2002.

[12] A. G. McNickle, M. T. Provencher, and B. J. Cole, "Overview of existing cartilage repair technology," *Sports Medicine & Arthroscopy Review*, vol. 16, no. 4, pp. 196–201, 2008.

[13] K. Mithoefer, T. Mcadams, R. J. Williams, P. C. Kreuz, and B. R. Mandelbaum, "Clinical efficacy of the microfracture technique for articular cartilage repair in the knee: an evidence-based systematic analysis," *American Journal of Sports Medicine*, vol. 37, no. 10, pp. 2053–2063, 2009.

[14] J. W. Alford and B. J. Cole, "Cartilage restoration, part 2: techniques, outcomes, and future directions," *American Journal of Sports Medicine*, vol. 33, no. 3, pp. 443–460, 2005.

[15] E. L. Cain and W. G. Clancy, "Treatment algorithm for osteochondral injuries of the knee," *Clinics in Sports Medicine*, vol. 20, no. 2, pp. 321–342, 2001.

[16] H. Clarke, F. Cushner, and W. Scott, "Clinical algorithm for treatment of chondral injuries," in *Insall & Scott Surgery of the Knee*, W. N. Scott, Ed., pp. 433–437, Churchill Livingstone, Philadelphia, Pa, USA, 4th edition, 2005.

[17] A. J. Krych, H. W. Harnly, S. A. Rodeo, and R. J. Williams III, "Activity levels are higher after osteochondral autograft transfer mosaicplasty than after microfracture for articular cartilage defects of the knee: a retrospective comparative study," *The Journal of Bone & Joint Surgery—American Volume*, vol. 94, no. 11, pp. 971–978, 2012.

[18] L. Hangody and P. Füles, "Autologous osteochondral mosaicplasty for the treatment of full-thickness defects of weight-bearing joints: Ten years of experimental and clinical experience," *The Journal of Bone & Joint Surgery—American Volume*, vol. 85, no. 1, pp. 25–32, 2003.

[19] A. E. Gross, W. Kim, F. Las Heras, D. Backstein, O. Safir, and K. P. H. Pritzker, "Fresh osteochondral allografts for posttraumatic knee defects: long-term followup," *Clinical Orthopaedics and Related Research*, vol. 466, no. 8, pp. 1863–1870, 2008.

[20] R. F. LaPrade, J. Botker, M. Herzog, and J. Agel, "Refrigerated osteoarticular allografts to treat articular cartilage defects of the femoral condyles. A prospective outcomes study," *The Journal of Bone & Joint Surgery—American Volume*, vol. 91, no. 4, pp. 805–811, 2009.

[21] E. M. Samuelson and D. E. Brown, "Cost-effectiveness analysis of autologous chondrocyte implantation: a comparison of periosteal patch versus type I/III collagen membrane," *American Journal of Sports Medicine*, vol. 40, no. 6, pp. 1252–1258, 2012.

[22] M. Brittberg, A. Lindahl, A. Nilsson, C. Ohlsson, O. Isaksson, and L. Peterson, "Treatment of deep cartilage defects in the knee with autologous chondrocyte transplantation," *New England Journal of Medicine*, vol. 331, no. 14, pp. 889–895, 1994.

[23] Y. Tegner and J. Lysholm, "Rating systems in the evaluation of knee ligament injuries," *Clinical Orthopaedics and Related Research*, vol. 198, pp. 43–49, 1985.

[24] E. M. Roos, H. P. Roos, L. S. Lohmander, C. Ekdahl, and B. D. Beynnon, "Knee Injury and Osteoarthritis Outcome Score (KOOS)—development of a self-administered outcome measure," *Journal of Orthopaedic and Sports Physical Therapy*, vol. 28, no. 2, pp. 88–96, 1998.

[25] R. Kijowski, D. G. Blankenbaker, K. W. Davis, K. Shinki, L. D. Kaplan, and A. A. De Smet, "Comparison of 1.5- And 3.0-T MR imaging for evaluating the articular cartilage of the knee joint," *Radiology*, vol. 250, no. 3, pp. 839–848, 2009.

[26] S. Wong, L. Steinbach, J. Zhao, C. Stehling, C. B. Ma, and T. M. Link, "Comparative study of imaging at 3.0 T versus 1.5 T of the knee," *Skeletal Radiology*, vol. 38, no. 8, pp. 761–769, 2009.

[27] M. E. Reed, D. C. Villacis, G. F. Hatch III et al., "3.0-tesla MRI and arthroscopy for assessment of knee articular cartilage lesions," *Orthopedics*, vol. 36, no. 8, pp. e1060–e1064, 2013.

[28] M. L. Gray, D. Burstein, Y.-J. Kim, and A. Maroudas, "Magnetic resonance imaging of cartilage glycosaminoglycan: basic principles, imaging technique, and clinical applications," *Journal of Orthopaedic Research*, vol. 26, no. 3, pp. 281–291, 2008.

[29] P. Hindle, J. L. Hendry, J. F. Keating, and L. C. Biant, "Autologous osteochondral mosaicplasty or TruFit plugs for cartilage repair," *Knee Surgery, Sports Traumatology, Arthroscopy*, vol. 22, no. 6, pp. 1235–1240, 2014.

22

Clinical and Radiographic Evaluation of a Commercially Pure Cancellous-Structured Titanium Press Fit Total Hip Prosthetic Stem: Ten-Year Followup of the "Natural Hip" Femoral Stem

Thomas B. Pace,[1,2] James C. Karegeannes,[3] M. Jason Palmer,[1] Stephanie L. Tanner,[1] and Rebecca G. Snider[1]

[1] *Greenville Health System Department of Orthopaedics, 701 Grove Road, Greenville, SC 29605, USA*
[2] *University of South Carolina SOM, Greenville Health System, P.O. Box 27114, Greenville, SC 29616, USA*
[3] *Blue Ridge Bone and Joint, 129 McDowell Street, Asheville, NC 28801, USA*

Correspondence should be addressed to Thomas B. Pace; tpacemd@aol.com

Academic Editor: Neal L. Millar

This study evaluates the outcomes of 92 hip arthroplasties using a press fit, tapered, split tip, proximally porous ingrowth (CSTi) femoral stem (Zimmer Natural Hip) in consecutive hip arthroplasty patients followed for an average of ten years postoperatively (range 5–16 years). Patients were functionally and radiographically evaluated using Harris Hip Scores and plain radiographs assessing postarthroplasty groin or thigh pain and radiographic signs of stem subsidence, proximal femoral fixation, stress shielding, and related calcar resorption. At followup of 5–10 years, the incidence of groin pain and thigh pain was 9.1% and 3.6%, respectively. This incidence improved over time. Beyond 10 years of followup, groin pain was 2.7% and thigh pain zero. In 89% of cases, there was solid contact between the calcar and the undersurface of the stem collar. Five cases were revised for instability (5.4%). The Harris Hip Scores and the incidence of thigh or groin pain were very favorable compared to other reported press fit total hip arthroplasty stems and not significantly different across a broad age range. There were no cases of stem loosening of failure of bony ingrowth into the stem.

1. Introduction

Femoral component fixation in total hip arthroplasty by bone ingrowth evolved in response to loosening observed from cemented stems [1]. The goal of press fit femoral stem fixation is to obtain biologic fixation of the implant, and thereby a more durable implant to bone interlocking interface less likely to succumb to stress over time and osteoporotic geriatric femoral canal enlargement. Porous-coated acetabular components have performed well [2] and have become the standard implant for the majority of hip arthroplasty procedures in North America. Reports of early femoral stem designs raised concerns of proximal bone resorption, thigh pain from cylindrical cobalt chrome stems, and difficult revision surgery secondary to proximal femoral stress shielding associated with extensive ingrowth at the diaphyseal bone interface with the stem. A slightly roughened finish may not allow sufficient fixation for stem stability [3]. Noncircumferentially applied ingrowth surface allows particulate debris to enter the femoral canal leading to significant osteolysis of the femoral shaft [4]. Circumferentially applied ingrowth surface seals the canal from wear debris and decreases osteolysis within the canal [1, 5, 6]. Insufficient proximal ingrowth surface, even if applied circumferentially, also leads to early failure from inadequate fixation [7]. Proximal cortical atrophy may occur in response to stress shielding proximal to the region of bone ingrowth. Greater bone loss has been observed with implants that obtain fixation within the diaphysis [8, 9] compared with proximal fixation implants [10–12]. A medial collar further decreased the incidence of proximal medial cortex resorption [12]. Thigh pain, caused by the sharp elastic modulus transition from the rigid stem to the more flexible cortical bone [13], has been reported in up to 12–27 percent of patients after cementless arthroplasty

[6, 9, 14]. The rate of thigh pain has been reported as less than 10 percent in designs with a tapered [11, 15, 16] or slotted [17] distal stem.

The use of press fit total hip stems in various age groups has been reported to offer more benefits in younger patients [18] with increased incidence of thigh pain and or groin pain as well as aseptic loosening in patients over 75 years old.

The Natural Hip femoral stem (Zimmer, Warsaw, IN, USA) has been in clinical use since 1993. The midterm 4–8-year clinical results of this stem have reportedly been very successful [19]. This stem is a tapered, split tip, proximal ingrowth collared monolithic, titanium alloy component with an inset circumferential flush finish of commercially pure cancellous-structured titanium (CSTi) proximal to and under the collar. It has a 12-degree anteverted neck and tapered threaded 12/14 trunnion that accepts a modular head of either cobalt chrome or ceramic (see Figures 2, 3, and 4). The proximal metaphyseal region of the stem has a 4 mm anterior wedge shape built up to maximize proximal fit and fill for improved postsurgical rotational stability. The body is a straight stem tapered proximally and distally with a distal stem split in the coronal plane with 2 mm fins to lower the elastic modulus while allowing some distal canal rotational control. The spilt tip and fins are designed to expand to engage in osteoporotic Type C diaphyseal bone and press together in more dense Type A diaphyseal bone, thus allowing for sufficient fixation in both young and geriatric femurs. The distal two-thirds of the straight stem is grit blasted to provide a roughened metallic surface for bony "ongrowth" but not porous enough to allow bony ingrowth and thus potentially minimize the risk of proximal femur stress shielding, implant loosening, and subsequent clinical failure reported with some full stem ingrowth implant designs.

The goal of this retrospective case series is to evaluate both the intermediate clinical outcomes and the effectiveness of bony ingrowth stem fixation following implantation of the cementless Natural Hip stem in a consecutive THA series of older and younger osteoarthritic patients (age range 30–83) over a 5–16-year experience with a mean followup of 10 years.

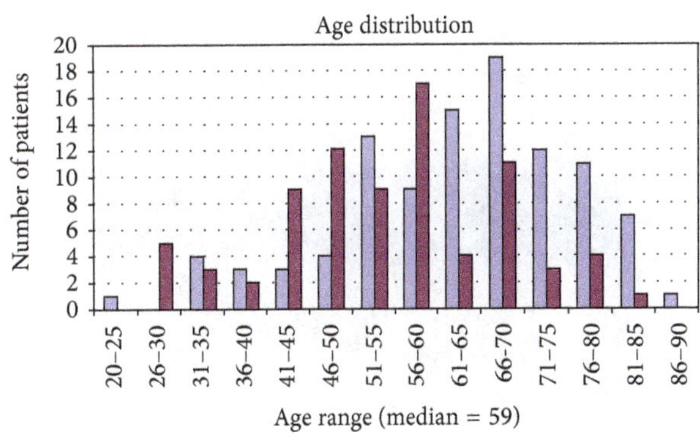

FIGURE 1

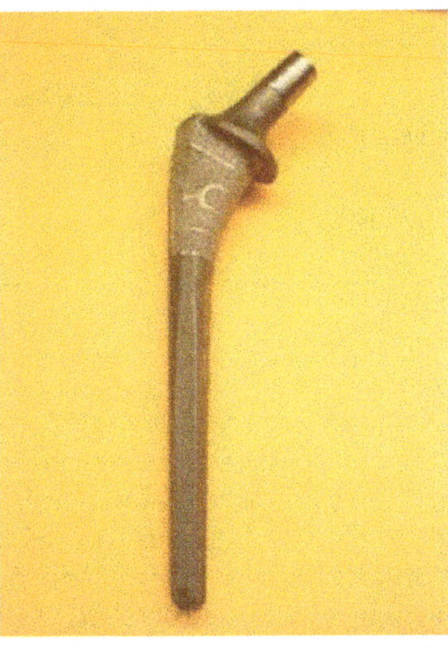

FIGURE 2: Natural Hip femoral stem.

2. Materials and Methods

Institutional Review Board approval was obtained for this study.

Serial office radiographs and clinical notes were retrospectively reviewed for 92 primary total hip and bipolar arthroplasties in 84 patients. All surgeries were performed from 1993 to 2000 using the Natural Hip uncemented femoral stem. Preoperative and postoperative clinical hip scores and radiographs were reviewed for all 84 patients.

The indication for hip arthroplasty was osteoarthritis in all patients. There were 48 female cases and 44 male cases with an average age at surgery of 61 years (24–86 years). Figure 1 shows patient's age distribution and percentages of males and females within each age range.

Surgery was performed by the senior author (TBP) using a posterolateral approach. The decision to use a cementless stem was based on intraoperative trial stem stability. Once the final broach was seated, torsional stability was assessed by applying a manual force to the broach handle. Lack of motion of the broach with enough torque force to rotate of the surgery extremity was interpreted as evidence for adequate bone quality and stem fixation to receive an uncemented stem.

The Sulzermedica (Zimmer) APR press fit acetabular component was used in 29 hips early in the series and the Sulzermedica (Zimmer) Intra-Op press fit cup was used in 63 hips later in the series. Of the total hip arthroplasties, cobalt chrome 28 mm heads were used in 41 hips, cobalt chrome 32 mm heads were used in 2 hips, and cobalt chrome 38 mm heads in 2 hips, Metasul (metal on metal) 28 mm heads were used in 12 hips, ceramic 28 mm heads in 34 hips, and one hip had a 32 mm ceramic head. Ceramic heads were used in younger patients, or those deemed by the senior author to be more physically active. Ten hips had a ceramic-zirconium 28 mm head. The duration of followup for each type of femoral head is described in Table 1.

Postoperative rehabilitation included weight bearing as tolerated with walker support for 3–6 weeks. Venous thrombosis event (VTE) prophylaxis was based on individualized

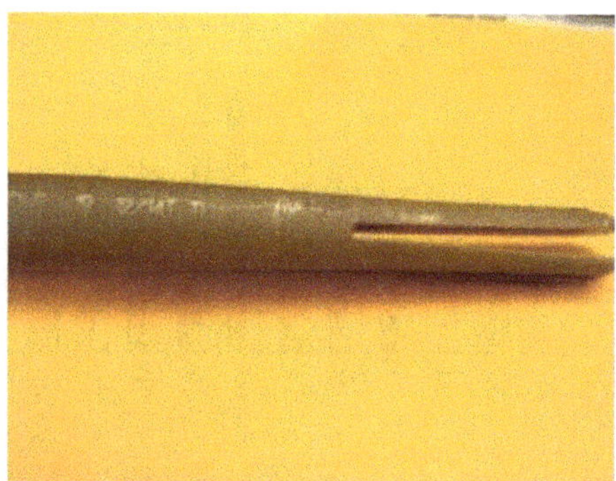

Figure 3: Natural Hip femoral stem, tapered split tip design.

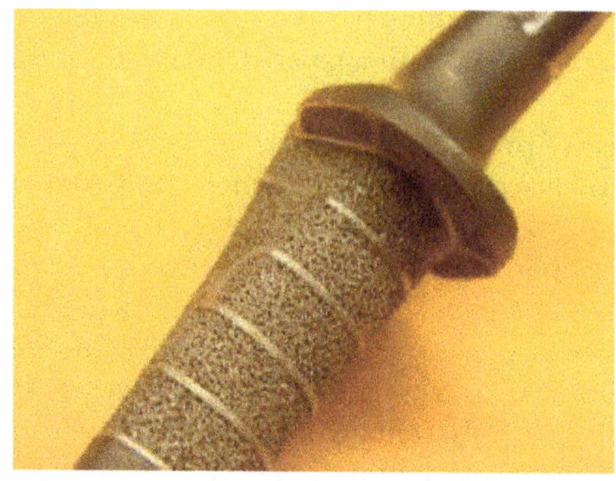

Figure 4: Natural Hip femoral stem circumferentially CSTi.

Table 1: Femoral head type and clinical follow-up time.

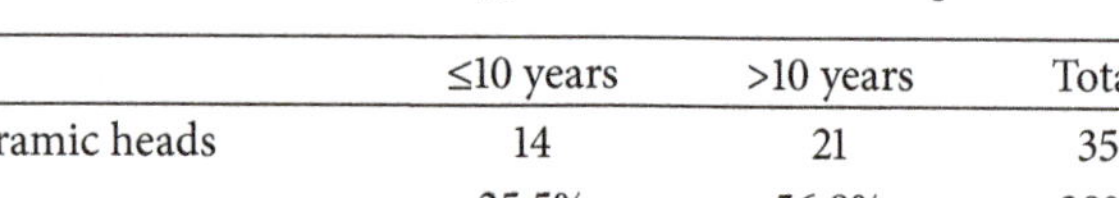

	≤10 years	>10 years	Total
Ceramic heads	14	21	35
	25.5%	56.8%	38%
Cobalt chrome heads	29	16	45
	53%	43%	48.9%
Metal on metal heads	12	0	12
	21.8%	0.0%	13%

patient risk assessment. For the standard at risk patient, this included oral warfarin 5 mg daily starting from the night of surgery until the prothrombin time was 15 seconds or until the INR (international normalized ratio) was 1.2 or greater, at which time the warfarin dosage was reduced to 2 mg daily. This was continued as has previously been reported for 4 weeks as a 2 mg per day mini fixed dose oral warfarin regimen [20]. For the patient without a higher VTE or bleeding risk assessment, once the hospital prothrombin time reached 15 seconds or INR levels reached 1.2–2.0, postdischarge monitoring was not done unless signs or symptoms of bleeding occurred [21]. For higher-risk VTE patients, higher-dose monitored oral warfarin was used (prothrombin time of 18–20 seconds or INR range 2.0–2.5). Early in the series, the hospital used a prothrombin time-based laboratory system (based on patients bleeding to clotting time in seconds verses a control) and later in the series the hospital converted to an INR-based bleeding time reporting system. All patients were counseled to avoid dislocation-prone lower extremity positioning of surgical leg internal rotation, adduction and maintain <90 hip flexion for 12 weeks following surgery.

Outcome data was collected at follow-up office visits by the senior author using the Harris Hip Scores (HHS) [22]. The score was recorded before surgery for all patients and at standard follow-up intervals after surgery of three, six, and twelve months, and then annually. The presence or absence of thigh or groin pain was determined from the Harris Hip Score functional assessment record.

Anteroposterior radiographs of the hip and pelvis and a Lowenstein lateral radiograph of the hip were obtained at each follow-up visit and compared with the immediate postoperative radiographs. Acetabular components were evaluated for radiolucent lines and osteolytic areas in the regions described by DeLee and Charnley [23]. The femoral components were evaluated for radiolucent lines and osteolytic areas described by Gruen et al. [24] and Johnston et al. [25]. Calcar round-off (defined as resorption of calcar bone back to the junction of collar and stem in zone VII) was also recorded. Erosion under the collar was defined as radiographic bone loss between 2 and 10 mm extending distally from the junction of the collar and stem. Calcar bone loss greater than 10 mm was considered structurally significant osteolysis. Stem subsidence was determined by measuring the distance from the proximal tip of the greater trochanter to the lateral shoulder of the prosthesis on successive radiographs [26]. This measurement was corrected for magnification using the known diameter of the prosthetic head to its measured diameter on the radiograph [27]. A change of 2 mm or more was considered evidence of subsidence. Heterotopic bone formation was evaluated at the second year following surgery and classified by the method of Brooker et al. [28].

The results were analyzed for the group as a whole based on longevity of followup (5–10 years and >10 years) and also evaluated based on patient's age at the time of arthroplasty (<55 years, 55–75 years, and >75 years).

3. Clinical Results

3.1. Harris Hip Scores (HHS). The average preoperative HHS score was 68 (range 58–87). At an average of 10-year followup (range 5–16 years), the HHS score average was 99 (range 70–100) (Table 2).

3.2. Groin/Thigh Pain. Six patients (6.5%) reported groin pain at final followup (average 9.2 years, range 6–11 years). Two patients (2.2%) reported thigh pain at final followup (average 8.4 years, range 7–10 years) (Table 2).

Complications including dislocations and revisions are shown in Table 3. Nine cases sustained a dislocation (9.8%). Four hips had isolated dislocations that remained stable after closed reduction and one was the only anterior dislocation in the series. Five hips (5.4%) had persistent instability that required cup revision surgery. Stability was restored in each of these cases using constrained liners and without any stem exchanges.

TABLE 2: Natural Hip clinical data compared by time of followup.

	5–10 years	>10 years	Total
Total cases	55	37	92
Average age	63	58	61
Range	31–83	30–82	30–83
Average Pre-op HHS	68	69	68
Range	58–87	58–87	58–87
Average HHS at last f/up	99	99	99
Range	93–100	70–100	70–100
Groin pain	5	1	6
	9.1%	2.7%	6.5%
Thigh pain	2	0	2
	3.6%	0%	2.2%

TABLE 3: Complications.

	5–10 years	>10 years	Total
Total cases	55	37	92
Infections	0	1	1
	0.0%	2.7%	1.1%
Dislocations	5	4	9
	9.1%	10.8%	9.8%
Revisions	3	2	5
	5.5%	5.4%	5.4%
Major bleeding	3	0	3
Symptomatic DVT	0	0	0
Symptomatic PE	0	0	0

3.3. *Infection.* Infection occurred in 1 case. The patient elected not to have additional surgery for personal/religious reasons and is currently being treated with suppressive therapy 12 years postoperatively with retained implants and oral antibiotic therapy successfully without cup or stem loosening.

3.4. *Major Bleeding.* Three cases had postsurgical wound hematomas that required surgical evacuation within 3 weeks of arthroplasty surgery. One resulted in the single infection report in this series. Each of these three cases was on chronic warfarin daily therapy prior to hip arthroplasty for stroke or heart valve related conditions and their postdischarge INR times were kept in the 2.0–2.5 range.

3.5. *Intraoperative Complications.* One (1%) intraoperative calcar fractures occurred while seating the press fit stem in a male patient 30 years of age. It was appreciated at the time of femoral stem insertion and treated with immediate femoral neck cerclage wiring at the time of primary hip arthroplasty. The patient was restricted to touch down weight bearing for 6 weeks and healed uneventfully. There were no postoperative periprosthetic fractures.

4. Radiographic Results

There were no cases of stem subsidence and one case of acetabular osteolysis. The incidence of proximal calcar resorption, osteolysis, and polyethylene wear as occurred over time is shown in Table 4.

TABLE 4: Natural Hip radiographic data points compared by time of followup.

	5–10 years	>10 years	Total
Total	55	37	92
Calcar contact	52	30	82
	94.5%	81.2%	89.2%
Calcar round-off	0	3	3
	0.0%	8%	3.3%
Calcar erosion	3	4	7
(>5 mm)	5.5%	10.8%	7.6%
Polywear			
1-2 mm	1	13	14
	1.8%	35.1%	15.2%
2-3 mm	0	4	4
	0.0%	10.8%	4.3%
3-4 mm	1	1	2
	2%	2.7%	2.2%
Osteolysis	0	1	1
	0.0%	2.7%	1.1%

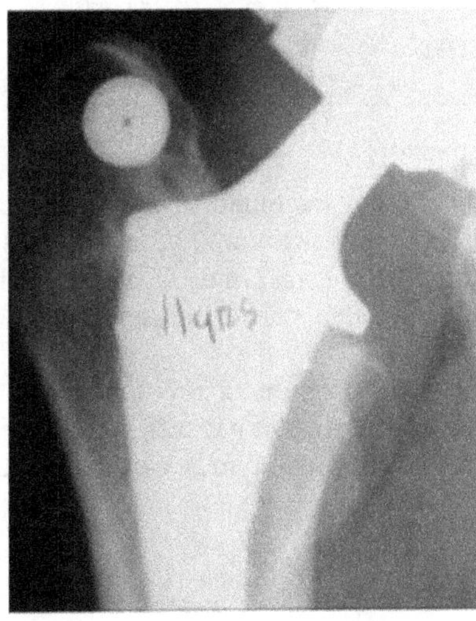

FIGURE 5: Radiograph of solid contact between the calcar and the cancellous-structured titanium under surface of the collar.

Eighty-two cases (89%) appeared to have solid contact between the calcar and the cancellous-structured titanium under surface of the collar. Of the 37 cases with beyond 10 years of followup, 30 (81%) had apparent calcar-collar bone contact (see Figure 5). Three of the hips (3.3%) had calcar bone "round-off" to the junction of the collar and stem (see Figure 6). Seven hips (7.6%) had 5–10 mm of focal subcollar calcar erosion of the Gruen zone VII (see Figure 7). Slowly progressive periprosthetic femoral radiolucent lines in Gruen zones I and VII were present in the one infected hip treated with suppressive antibiotic therapy. One case which also has 3-4 mm of polyethylene linear wear had focal osteolysis of the acetabular cup 16 years postoperatively.

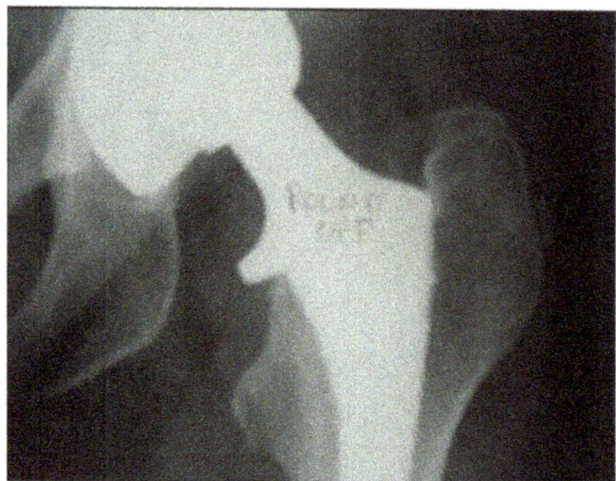

FIGURE 6: Radiograph showing calcar bone round-off to the junction of the collar and stem.

TABLE 5: Patient's age at time of surgery.

	<55 years $N = 27$	55–75 years $N = 56$	>75 years $N = 9$
Groin pain	3	5	1
Thigh pain	4	0	0
Avg. pre-op HHS (range)	68 (58–76)	68 (58–87)	68 (58–87)
Avg. pos-top HHS (range)	97.6 (95–100)	96 (95–100)	96 (76–100)

Heterotopic bone was found in 2 patients. The average followup for these patients was 10 years (range 8–12 years). One was Grade II, and 1 was Grade III as defined by Brooker et al. [28] and remained stable and asymptomatic at subsequent follow-up visits.

When the clinical results of this hip stem design were assessed relative to the age of patients at the time of arthroplasty, the pre-op and post-op follow-up HHS did not differ significantly (Table 5).

5. Discussion

This tapered, titanium, collared, split tip, proximally porous ingrowth, uncemented femoral stem design appears to address many of the historic concerns of cementless femoral stems in THA, namely, thigh pain in the early years, proximal femoral bone atrophy, and revision difficulty associated with diaphyseal press fit stem removal. The stem design worked equally well in both older and younger patients.

The presence of thigh pain in only two patients is consistent with literature reports of tapered, press fit, titanium stems. The lower modulus of titanium and slotted tip design that improve the transition from stem to host bone are thought to be the cause for the lower incidence of thigh pain.

One interesting feature of this stem design is the cancellous-structured titanium recessed ingrowth surface underneath the collar that contacts the calcar with full seating of the implant at the time of surgery. The finding that 89% of the patients in this series had apparent direct bone contact with the porous ingrowth surface under the collar suggests that a functional physiologic load is being applied

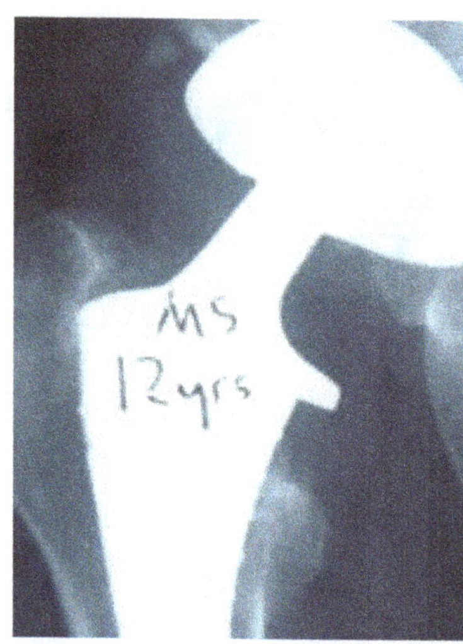

FIGURE 7: Radiograph of subcollar calcar erosion of Gruen zone VII.

through the collar and maintaining sufficient stress forces to avoid calcar bone regression. Furthermore, the finding that this pattern continued in 82% of the cases with beyond 10 years of followup suggests the physiological load sharing does not diminish over time. This coupled with the lack of any stem subsidence may indicate a favorable biomechanical load sharing construct of this stem design that minimizes proximal femur stress shielding. The 3% incidence of calcar round-off is significantly lower than other reports of up to 30% calcar round-off seen in other well functioning collarless press fit stem designs [29, 30].

The 10.8% incidence of nonstructural osteolysis referred to as erosion under the stem collar in the hips with 10 years or greater followup is lower than the rates reported with other bone ingrowth femoral stem designs [10, 12]. The limited osteolysis was felt to represent remote site osteolytic reaction secondary to polyethylene wear from the cup articulating surface. The fact that at 10 years 10.8% of the cases had subcalcar erosion suggests that the collar has some protective effect to seal of the medial calcar to polyethylene wear debris related osteolysis. The absence of femoral canal osteolysis and endosteal cavitation may indicate that the circumferential proximal bony ingrowth effectively seals the canal from wear debris as side from the focal subcalcar area.

One surgeon performed all arthroplasties utilizing the same stem insertion technique, which minimized intraoperative variables and is a potential strength of this study. The operating surgeon also performed all followups, including radiographic and Harris Hip Score assessment at the time of followup. This is a study weakness due to potential bias of the surgeon as some follow-up data is subjective. The stem function in this series is compared to the same stem results reported in another series [19] and functioned very similar to some cup impingement issues but otherwise low rates of failure related to stem loosening or thigh pain. What this paper contributes to the orthopaedic literature is the results of this press fit tapered stem not only in longitudinal followup but also across a wide spectrum of patient ages. While asymptomatic VTE was not reported here, the low incidence of symptomatic VTE is consistent with previous reports of good results utilizing a low or fixed 2 mg dose of oral warfarin program and consistent with current AAOS Clinical Guidelines for the Prevention of Symptomatic Pulmonary Embolism in Patients Undergoing Total Hip or Knee [29–31].

The overall dislocation rate of 9.8% and recurrent dislocation incidence of 5.4% are higher than those reported for primary hip arthroplasty. The significance of this is not clear from this study data. Possibilities include variations in acetabular cup positioning. All of the recurrent dislocations had 28 mm heads with some degree of linear polyethylene wear. Of the five dislocation cases that required revision surgery with subsequent stability, none of the cases exceeded 55 degrees of lateral inclination as measured on AP radiographs. The femoral neck geometry (12/14 taper) with 12 degrees of ante-version may predispose to impingement related instability. Hofmann reported midterm results of this femoral stem design with a 2.4% incidence of cup problems with two cases of polyethylene liner dislodgement [19]. This raises the question of a possible neck-cup-impingement-prone design issue. In the present series, the subsequent stability following closed reduction in the four hips with single instability episodes would suggest that isolated leg and body positioning was the primary factor leading to instability.

6. Conclusion

This hip stem design appears to function well with a variety of different femoral head types and was well tolerated across a broad age range of patients. This current 5–16-year report confirms the successful 4–8-year mid-term fixation results of the same stem design previously published. The clinical results of the stem fixation as reflected in HHS at the last clinical assessment showed equal results in all three age groups, all with excellent results. The clinical results did not deteriorate over time. The presence of the low profile collar appears to have some physiological effect on both loading the calcar and sealing the canal from debris related osteolysis. The findings from the current study show a rate of instability higher than expected and the reason for this is not clear. The minimal incidence of thigh and groin pain as well as the structural integrity of the proximal femoral bony ingrowth with limited calcar resorption suggests functional load sharing implant biomechanics with this tapered titanium split tip collared proximal (CSTi) press fit design at midterm followup.

Conflict of Interests

The authors declare that there is no conflict of interests regarding the publication of this paper.

Acknowledgments

The authors wish to thank Ms. Sandy Fowler and Mrs. Katharine A. Pace for their valuable contributions to the paper and data preparation.

References

[1] D. S. Hungerford and L. C. Jones, “The rationale for cementless total hip replacement,” *Orthopedic Clinics of North America*, vol. 24, no. 4, pp. 617–626, 1993.

[2] J. C. Clohisy and W. H. Harris, “The Harris-Galante porous-coated acetabular component with screw fixation. An average ten-year follow-up study,” *Journal of Bone and Joint Surgery A*, vol. 81, no. 1, pp. 66–73, 1999.

[3] W. J. Donnelly, A. Kobayashi, M. A. R. Freeman et al., “Radiological and survival comparison of four methods of fixation of a proximal femoral stem,” *Journal of Bone and Joint Surgery B*, vol. 79, no. 3, pp. 351–360, 1997.

[4] W. J. Maloney and S. T. Woolson, “Increasing incidence of femoral osteolysis in association with uncemented Harris-Galante total hip arthroplasty: a follow-up report,” *Journal of Arthroplasty*, vol. 11, no. 2, pp. 130–134, 1996.

[5] M. A. Mont and D. S. Hungerford, “Proximally coated ingrowth prostheses: a review,” *Clinical Orthopaedics and Related Research*, no. 344, pp. 139–149, 1997.

[6] J. S. Xenos, J. J. Callaghan, R. D. Heekin, W. J. Hopkinson, C. G. Savory, and M. S. Moore, “The porous-coated anatomic total hip prosthesis, inserted without cement. A prospective study with a minimum of ten years of follow-up,” *Journal of Bone and Joint Surgery A*, vol. 81, no. 1, pp. 74–82, 1999.

[7] C. Khalily and L. A. Whiteside, “Predictive value of early radiographic findings in cementless total hip arthroplasty femoral components: an 8- to 12-year follow-up,” *Journal of Arthroplasty*, vol. 13, no. 7, pp. 768–773, 1998.

[8] J. D. Bobyn, A. H. Glassman, H. Goto, J. J. Krygier, J. E. Miller, and C. E. Brooks, “The effect of stem stiffness on femoral bone resorption after canine porous-coated total hip arthroplasty,” *Clinical Orthopaedics and Related Research*, no. 261, pp. 196–213, 1990.

[9] J. L. Kronick, M. L. Barba, and W. G. Paprosky, “Extensively coated femoral components in young patients,” *Clinical Orthopaedics and Related Research*, no. 344, pp. 263–274, 1997.

[10] C. F. Burt, K. L. Garvin, E. T. Otterberg, and O. M. Jardon, “A femoral component inserted without cement in total hip arthroplasty: a study of the Tri-Lock component with an average ten-year duration of follow-up,” *Journal of Bone and Joint Surgery A*, vol. 80, no. 7, pp. 952–960, 1998.

[11] T. H. Mallory, W. C. Head, and A. V. Lombardi Jr., “Tapered design for the cementless total hip arthroplasty femoral component,” *Clinical Orthopaedics and Related Research*, no. 344, pp. 172–178, 1997.

[12] J. B. Meding, M. A. Ritter, E. M. Keating, P. M. Faris, and K. Edmondson, “A comparison of collared and collarless femoral components in primary cemented total hip arthroplasty: a randomized clinical trial,” *Journal of Arthroplasty*, vol. 14, no. 2, pp. 123–130, 1999.

[13] B. M. Dodge, R. Fitzrandolph, and D. N. Collins, “Noncemented porous-coated anatomic total hip arthroplasty,” *Clinical Orthopaedics and Related Research*, no. 269, pp. 16–24, 1991.

[14] R. B. Bourne, C. H. Rorabeck, M. E. Ghazal, and M. H. Lee, “Pain in the thigh following total hip replacement with a porous-coated anatomic prosthesis for osteoarthrosis. A five-year follow-up study,” *Journal of Bone and Joint Surgery A*, vol. 76, no. 10, pp. 1464–1470, 1994.

[15] S. M. Madey, J. J. Callaghan, J. P. Olejniczak, D. D. Goetz, and R. C. Johnston, “Charnley total hip arthroplasty with use of improved techniques of cementing. The results after a minimum

of fifteen years of follow-up," *Journal of Bone and Joint Surgery A*, vol. 79, no. 1, pp. 53–64, 1997.

[16] J. R. Mclaughlin and K. R. Lee, "Total hip arthroplasty with an uncemented femoral component. Excellent results at ten-year follow-up," *Journal of Bone and Joint Surgery B*, vol. 79, no. 6, pp. 900–907, 1997.

[17] H. U. Cameron, "The 3-6-year results of a modular noncemented low-bending stiffness hip implant: a preliminary study," *Journal of Arthroplasty*, vol. 8, no. 3, pp. 239–243, 1993.

[18] K. T. Mäkelä, A. Eskelinen, P. Pulkkinen, P. Paavolainen, and V. Remes, "Total hip arthroplasty for primary osteoarthritis in patients fifty-five years of age or older: an analysis of the Finnish Arthroplasty Registry," *Journal of Bone and Joint Surgery A*, vol. 90, no. 10, pp. 2160–2170, 2008.

[19] A. A. Hofmann, M. E. Feign, W. Klauser, C. C. VanGorp, and M. P. Camargo, "Cementless primary total hip arthroplasty with a tapered, proximally porous-coated titanium prosthesis: a 4- to 8-year retrospective review," *Journal of Arthroplasty*, vol. 15, no. 7, pp. 833–839, 2000.

[20] M. J. Vives, W. J. Hozack, P. F. Sharkey, L. Moriarty, B. Sokoloff, and R. H. Rothman, "Fixed minidose versus-adjusted low-dose warfarin after total joint arthroplasty: a randomized prospective study," *Journal of Arthroplasty*, vol. 16, no. 8, pp. 1030–1037, 2001.

[21] J. R. Lieberman, J. Wollaeger, F. Dorey et al., "The efficacy of prophylaxis with low-dose warfarin for prevention of pulmonary embolism following total hip arthroplasty," *Journal of Bone and Joint Surgery A*, vol. 79, no. 3, pp. 319–325, 1997.

[22] W. H. Harris, "Traumatic arthritis of the hip after dislocation and acetabular fractures: treatment by mold arthroplasty. An end-result study using a new method of result evaluation," *Journal of Bone and Joint Surgery A*, vol. 51, no. 4, pp. 737–755, 1969.

[23] J. G. DeLee and J. Charnley, "Radiological demarcation of cemented sockets in total hip replacement," *Clinical Orthopaedics and Related Research*, vol. 121, pp. 20–32, 1976.

[24] T. A. Gruen, G. M. McNeice, and H. C. Amstutz, "'Modes of failure' of cemented stem-type femoral components. A radiographic analysis of loosening," *Clinical Orthopaedics and Related Research*, no. 141, pp. 17–27, 1979.

[25] R. C. Johnston, R. H. Fitzgerald Jr., W. H. Harris, R. Poss, M. E. Muller, and C. B. Sledge, "Clinical and radiographic evaluation of total hip replacement. A standard system of terminology for reporting results," *Journal of Bone and Joint Surgery A*, vol. 72, no. 2, pp. 161–168, 1990.

[26] C. A. Engh, P. Massin, and K. E. Suthers, "Roentgenographic assessment of the biologic fixation of porous-surfaced femoral components," *Clinical Orthopaedics and Related Research*, no. 257, pp. 107–128, 1990.

[27] M. J. Griffith, M. K. Seidenstein, D. Williams, and J. Charnley, "Socket wear in Charnley low friction arthroplasty of the hip," *Clinical Orthopaedics and Related Research*, vol. 137, pp. 37–47, 1978.

[28] A. F. Brooker, J. W. Bowerman, R. A. Robinson, and L. H. Riley Jr., "Ectopic ossification following total hip replacement. Incidence and a method of classification," *Journal of Bone and Joint Surgery A*, vol. 55, no. 8, pp. 1629–1632, 1973.

[29] J. R. McLaughlin and K. R. Lee, "Total hip arthroplasty with an uncemented tapered femoral component," *Journal of Bone and Joint Surgery A*, vol. 90, no. 6, pp. 1290–1296, 2008.

[30] J. B. Meding, E. M. Keating, M. A. Ritter, P. M. Faris, and M. E. Berend, "Minimum ten-year follow-up of a straight-stemmed, plasma-sprayed, titanium-alloy, uncemented femoral component in primary total hip arthroplasty," *Journal of Bone and Joint Surgery A*, vol. 86, no. 1, pp. 92–97, 2004.

[31] N. A. Johanson, P. F. Lachiewicz, J. R. Lieberman et al., "AAOS clinical practice guideline summary prevention of symptomatic pulmonary embolism in patients undergoing total hip or knee arthroplasty," *Journal of the American Academy of Orthopaedic Surgeons*, vol. 17, pp. 183–196, 2009.

23

Open Reduction and Internal Fixation of Displaced Supracondylar Fracture of Late Presentation in Children

Ram K. Shah,[1] Raju Rijal,[2] Rosan P. Shah Kalawar,[2] Sujit R. Shrestha,[1] and Niraj Kumar Shah[3]

[1]*Nepal Medical College, Jorpati, Kathmandu, Nepal*
[2]*B.P. Koirala Institute of Health Sciences, Dharan, Nepal*
[3]*Department of General Surgery, PGIMER, Chandigarh, India*

Correspondence should be addressed to Ram K. Shah; rkshah786@gmail.com

Academic Editor: Werner Kolb

Background. In late presentation of cases there is dilemma whether to wait for osteotomy later or do open reduction on arrival. The purpose of this prospective multicentric study is to evaluate the functional outcome of open reduction and internal fixation (ORIF) with crossed Kirschner wires fixation and early joint motion in the late presentation of supracondylar fractures in children. *Methods.* A total of 21 children, with an average delay of 20.3 days, with displaced type III Gartland supracondylar fracture, were treated by ORIF with crossed Kirschner wires fixation and early joint motion. Average follow-up was 12 months. *Results.* Flynn's criteria were used to evaluate the outcome. All of them had more functional range of motion of the injured elbow than the published reports. *Conclusions.* Most of the surgeons in the developing world prefer ORIF for optimal results. Thus it appears to be justifiable to go for ORIF with K-wires even in the late presentation of supracondylar fractures. The overall results are encouraging. However, the small number of cases and lack of control group are the limitations of this study. The study is ongoing and so the full report with more cases will be presented later.

1. Introduction

Supracondylar fractures are one of the most common elbow fractures seen in paediatric orthopaedic clinics worldwide [1]. These fractures comprise 55% to 75% of elbow fractures and approximately 3% of all fractures in children [2, 3]. Between 10% and 20% of cases report late for treatment in developing countries [4]. Late presentation is defined as roughly more than 2 days after injury [5] and objectively is defined as when a callus is visible in X-rays, but a fracture line is still visible.

A delay in presentation for treatment at a proper hospital may result from poor transportation, ignorance, and/or inability of the child's parents. Sometimes, lack of skilled personnel or suitable resources can delay or deny suitable treatment in a hospital in poor countries. In developing countries, the percentage of late presentation is much higher because of poor health care delivery systems and patients reaching the tertiary care centre late from a long distance [6].

Malunion resulting in cubitus varus is common in 10%–30% of cases regardless of the method of treatment. This deformity does not improve with remodelling [5].

The treatment modalities implicated in late presenting cases are as follows:

(i) Continuous traction of the arm to gradually reduce the fracture, which avoids the risk of vascular complications and iatrogenic ulnar nerve injury but has the disadvantage of prolonged hospital stay [7].

(ii) Early wedge osteotomy 1–4 months after injury but before adolescence [8].

(iii) Open reduction and internal fixation [9, 10].

Table 1: Flynn's criteria for grading [14].

Result	Rating	Cosmetic factor (carrying angle loss) (degrees)	Functional factor (motion loss) (degrees)
Satisfactory	Excellent	0–5	0–5
	Good	5–10	5–10
Unsatisfactory	Fair	10–15	10–15
	Poor	Over 15	Over 15

There is not much literature regarding specific treatment guidelines for late presentation of supracondylar fracture in children, so the treatment method remains controversial.

2. Materials and Methods

This is a prospective and multicentric study in Nepal with follow-up at 2, 4, 12, and 24 weeks and finally at 1 year. Average follow-up was 1 year. Between August 2012 and January 2014, a total of 21 patients sought treatment with a delay between 15 and 30 days (average 20.3 days) after the injury. The reason for the delay was inadequate treatment in 18 patients and ignorance in 3 patients. A total of 110 cases of displaced type III Gartland supracondylar fracture were treated at these centres within the study period in the years from 2012 to 2014. Out of 110 cases only 21 (19.1%) cases were included in the study.

Patients who had a callus but a visible fracture line on their radiograph were included in the study. Those with open fracture, intra-articular fracture, stable supracondylar fracture (Gartland type I), or fracture with a callus without a visible fracture line were excluded from the study.

Detailed examination of the neurological and vascular status of the limb was performed. Anteroposterior and lateral radiograph of the elbow were obtained from the injured and normal elbows, and the Baumann angle was measured.

Open reduction using a posterior approach with midline triceps split was performed. All visible calluses were removed to clean and recreate the fracture. Then, the anatomic reduction of fracture fragments was stabilized with crossed K-wires and checked under an image intensifier for reduction and stability. In one patient, more than one K-wire was inserted for laterally better stability. K-wires were buried under the skin, which reduces the chance of infection and lowers the risk of early removal of an infected K-wire and subsequent displacement of fracture fragments [11].

Skin sutures were removed at 2 weeks, and the back slab was removed for early mobilization of the elbow when it is pain-free. The buried K-wires were removed at 12 weeks after fracture consolidation.

All patients were discharged 48 hours after the surgery. At 12 weeks, the range of motion and carrying angle were measured with a goniometer and graded according to Flynn's criteria (Table 1). The Baumann angle was measured for radiological assessment [12]. The patients were also evaluated for functional range of motion of the injured elbow, which is established as 75–120 degrees of flexion with an arc of motion of 45 degrees necessary for feeding and toilet purposes [13].

3. Results

All fractures united. All the cases were followed up for one year. Two patients were lost to follow-up after 6 weeks and so they were excluded from the study.

The average age of the patients was 7.4 years (range: 5–10 years) with 9 males and 12 females with left elbow being the predominant injury side, 12 out of 21. All injuries were Gartland type III injuries and closed fractures.

The average delay time of presentation to us was 20.3 days (range: 15–30 days).

The average range of motion loss of the injured elbow compared to the normal elbow was 42.1 degrees (range: 5–70 degrees) and the average carrying angle loss was 16.4 degrees (range: 0–30 degrees). The mean Baumann angle of the injured elbow was 78.1 degrees (range: 70–85 degrees) compared to 72.8 degrees (range: 70–80 degrees) for the normal elbow. Cubitus varus was seen in 12 patients (57.1%), 3 patients had carrying angle gain (14.3%), three had carrying angle loss but the elbow was in the valgus position (14.3%), and 3 patients had no varus deformity (14.3%).

Patients were graded according to Flynn's criteria, which take into account range of motion loss (functional factor) and carrying angle loss (cosmetic factor) [14]. The overall rating is made on the basis of greater clinical loss of functional or cosmetic factors. Three patients (14.3%) had an excellent rating and a satisfactory result, and 18 patients (85.7%) had poor ratings and unsatisfactory results (Table 2).

All patients had painless and useful range of motion at the last follow-up. The flexion of the elbow ranged from 110 to 145 degrees (average of 127.1 degrees). The extension ranged from 0 degrees to limitation of full extension by 40 degrees (average of 22.8 degrees lag). All of our patients had a more functional range of motion of the injured elbow than established by Vasen et al. [13] (Table 3).

Three patients had iatrogenic ulnar nerve palsy due to technical error, which spontaneously recovered after the medial buried K-wire was removed, as it had impinged the ulnar nerve, which was observed when the K-wires were removed. Beyond this, no other intraoperative complications or postoperative complications were observed in the study. There was no radiographic evidence of heterotopic ossification in our study.

Eighteen parents were satisfied regarding the useful range of movement and appearance of the elbow, while 3 parents were unsatisfied regarding the appearance of the elbow (Figure 1).

4. Discussion

The prognosis of displaced supracondylar humeral fracture with late presentation in children is unfavourable if the child presents one day after injury [15] (Table 4).

According to Flynn's criteria [14], 14.3% (3 cases) of patients had satisfactory results and 85.7% (18 cases) had

TABLE 2: Overall grading of patients according to Flynn's criteria [14].

Grading	Cosmetic factor (carrying angle loss)	Functional factor (motion loss)	Overall number (%)
Satisfactory			
Excellent	0°–5°	0°–5°	
Good	5°–10°	0°–5°	3 (14.3%)
Fair	10°–15°	10°–15°	
Unsatisfactory			
Poor	Over 15°	Over 15°	18 (85.7%)

TABLE 3: Functional range of motion obtained.

Number of cases	Flexion (degrees)	Extension (degrees)	Arc of motion (degrees)	Useful arc of motion (%) (compared with Vasen et al. [13])*
3	125	35 lag	90	200
3	140	15 lag	95	277.8
3	115	45 lag	70	155.5
3	145	5 lag	140	311.1
3	130	0	130	288.9
3	105	20 lag	85	188.9
3	130	40 lag	90	200

*Functional elbow range of motion established as 75–120° flexion with arc of motion of 45°.

unsatisfactory results. The incidence of cubitus varus was 57.1% (12 patients). However, all our patients obtained more than double the functional range of motion established by Vasen et al. [13] for activities of daily living (Table 3).

Lal and Bhan [8] obtained 35% incidence (20 patients) of cubitus varus among patients who had open reduction 11–17 days after the injury, but 70% of them (14 patients) had an arc of motion of less than 90 degrees. Compared with this study, our results had a higher incidence of cubitus varus (57.1%), but the arc of motion achieved was more. Only 2 patients (28.6%) had an arc of motion of less than 90 degrees compared to 14 patients (70%) in their study. Ali et al. [11] reported 12% poor results after open reduction because of limited movement. Reitman et al. [10] reported cubitus varus in 13 of 52 patients (25%) after open reduction and K-wire fixation. Mahaisavariya [7] included children presenting up to 3 weeks after injury. Lal and Bhan [8] included children up to 4 months after the injury in their series but for early wedge osteotomy rather than open reduction and internal fixation.

To the best of our knowledge, there has not been any study beyond 3 weeks of delay, so we took up the task to operate on injured elbows and evaluate the functional and cosmetic outcome in those children with callus formation but a visible fracture line on a radiograph, which included children with delays up to 30 days after injury.

Some authors [16] prefer to let the fracture malunite and later perform a corrective osteotomy to avoid myositis ossificans and stiffness. Theoretically, the fracture should be left alone until solid union occurs and the patient regains full range of motion of the elbow to full extension, and then corrective osteotomy is scheduled [8]. However, in our part of the world, the parents of the children want treatment upon presentation and do not accept corrective osteotomy at a later date. Moreover, the patients are not compliant and are lost to follow-up when such advice is given. Considering these circumstances, we feel that it is justified to offer them treatment by open reduction and internal fixation of displaced fractures with crossed K-wires.

The Flynn et al. [14] grading system is more severe than that of Aronson and Prager [17], and loss of range of motion greater than 15 degrees compared to the normal elbow is graded as an unsatisfactory result. However, clinically, the patient has a useful range of motion for activities of daily living.

In all of our patients anatomical reduction was achieved. However, the resulting deformity at the elbow made it difficult to predict the outcome. Displaced supracondylar fractures of the humerus almost always unite, but malunion resulting in cubitus varus is common. Its reported incidence ranges from 10 to 57% regardless of the method of treatment [18, 19]. The deformity does not improve with time, as seen in our study [20].

In our study the range of motion of the injured elbow improved with time. There was improvement in the range of motion at the 6-month follow-up relative to the 3-month follow-up. The initial decrease in range of motion could be due to the posterior approach, which provides adequate exposure but results in scarring of posterior soft tissue and increased elbow stiffness [21]. However, movement of the elbow nearly always recovers after healing of a supracondylar fracture in children [12].

Open reduction and internal fixation are a better treatment option in displaced supracondylar fractures of the humerus in patients presenting even late after injury in our

Table 4

	Study	Year	Journal	Number	Presentation	Mean delay	Hospital stay	Treatment	Mean follow-up	Complications	Functional outcome
1	Lal and Bhan [8]	1991	Int. Orthop. 1991; 15: 189–191.	20	11–17 days					35% varus	
2	Leet et al. [23]	1994–1999	J Pead. Ortho. 2002; 22: 203–207	158	2.7 hrs–6.6 days	21 hrs	26 min–6 days	CRIF/ORIF with crossed K-wires	16.7 wks	1.26% varus <1% pin-tract infection	
3	Devnani [5]	Jan. 1990–Dec. 2001	Cl Ortho. 2005; 431: 36–41	28	2–21 days	5.6 days	14 days	CRIF/ORIF with crossed K-wires	24 mths	18%. >10 deg. varus	good 71%, fair 4%, poor 25%
4	Mahaisavariya [7]	1994 through 2004	Techniques in Orthopaedics 2006; 21 (2): 150–157	9	1–4 mths	3.2 mths		Simple wedge osteotomy and fixation by 2 K-wires combined with TBW loop	13.3 mths (5–48)		
5	Tiwari et al. [22]	Feb. 2002–June 2003	J. of Ortho. Surg. 2007; 15 (2): 177–82	40	2–12 days	4 days	41 hrs	CRIF/ORIF with crossed K-wires	18 mths	5% >15 deg. varus 10% nerve palsy (5% R, 2.5% M, U each) 5% Trochlear necrosis 7.5% stiffness ROM loss > 15 deg.	88%, Flynn's criteria
6	Eren et al. [6]	Jan. 1992 to Feb. 2005	J. Child Orthop. (2008) 2: 21–27	31	2–19 days	6 days	2 days	ORIF with crossed K-wires	4 yrs (2–11 yrs)	22.5% cubitus varus 6.5% pin-tract infections	
7	Dua et al. [24]	July 2003–June 2007	Chinese J. of Traumatology, 2011; 14 (1): 14–19	40	12 hrs–3 days	17.55 hrs	12 hrs	CRIF with crossed K-wires	15 mths (12–24)	5% mild myositis	95% excellent Flynn's criteria

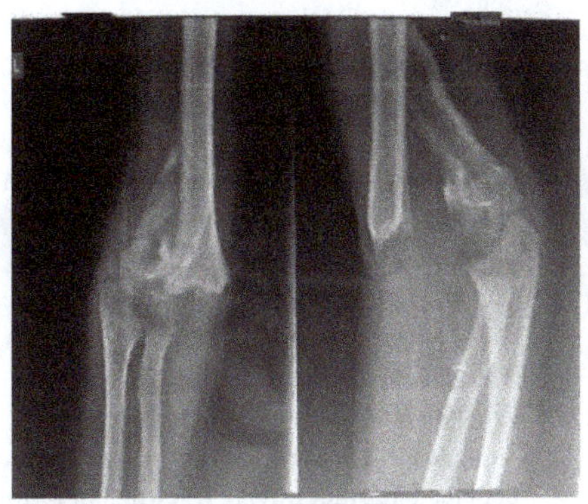

(a) 4-week-old fracture with callus formation

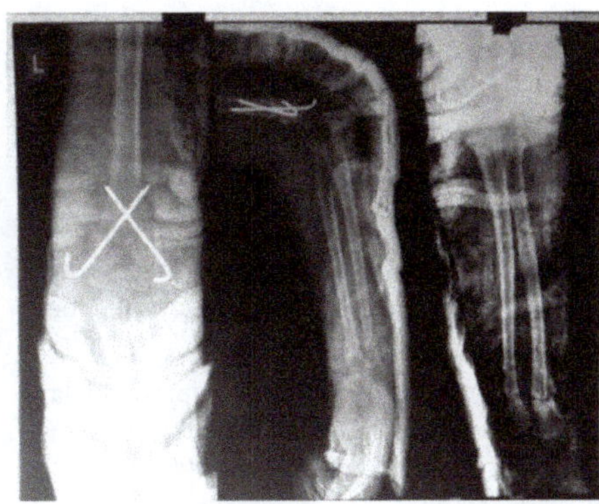

(b) Open reduction, removal of callus, and internal fixation with crossed K-wires

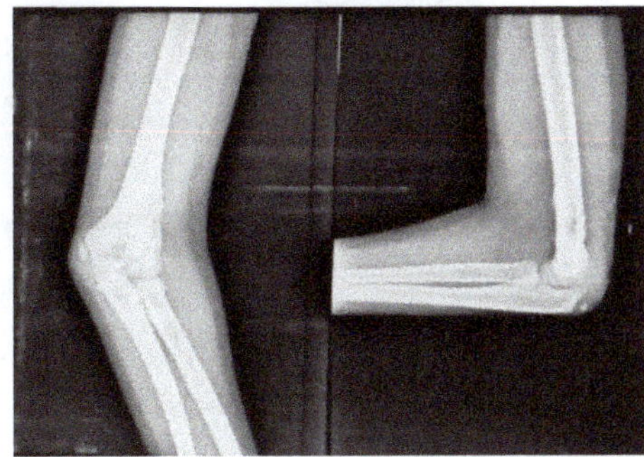

(c) Final healing of fracture after 6 months

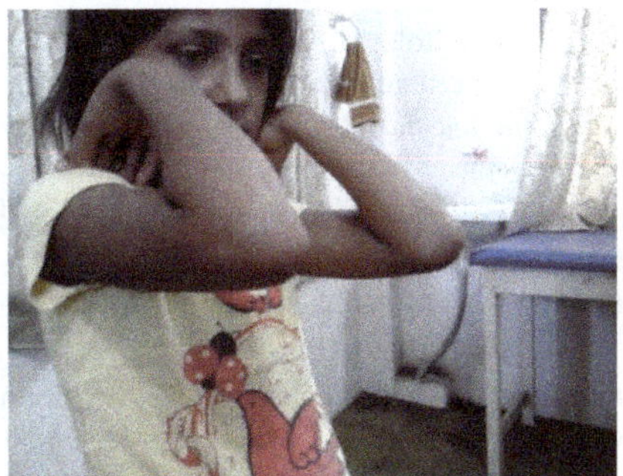

(d) Functional result after 6 Months

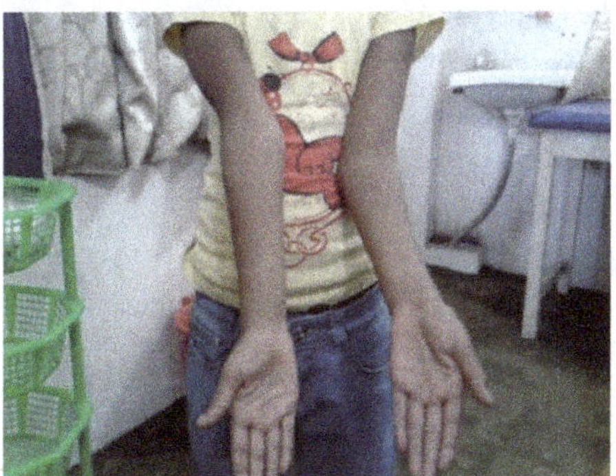

(e) Functional result after 6 Months

FIGURE 1: Clinical result of a case.

set-up. This approach minimises the risk of complications and the need for continuous traction or corrective osteotomy [22].

Disclosure

This is a Level 1 prospective study as all patients were enrolled within the same duration with more than 80% follow-up for the investigation of the effect of the treatment on the outcome.

Conflict of Interests

The authors declare that there is no conflict of interests regarding the publication of this paper.

References

[1] J. C. Cheng and W. Y. Shen, "Limb fracture pattern in different pediatric age groups: a study of 3350 children," *Journal of Orthopaedic Trauma*, vol. 7, no. 1, pp. 15–22, 1993.

[2] J. C. Y. Cheng, T. P. Lam, and N. Maffulli, "Epidemiological features of supracondylar fractures of the humerus in Chinese children," *Journal of Pediatric Orthopaedics Part B*, vol. 10, no. 1, pp. 63–67, 2001.

[3] K. E. Wilkins, "Supracondylar fractures of the distal humerus," in *Rockwood and Wilkins' Fractures in Children*, J. M. Flynn, D. L. Skaggs, and P. M. Waters, Eds., pp. 487–557, Lippincott Williams & Wilkins, Philadelphia, Pa, USA, 7th edition, 2010.

[4] A. Devnani, "Late presentation of supracondylar fractures of humerus in children," in *Neglected Musculoskeletal Disorders*,

A. K. Jain and S. Kumar, Eds., pp. 335–342, Jaypee Brothers Medical, 1st edition, 2011.

[5] A. S. Devnani, "Late presentation of supracondylar fracture of the humerus in children," *Clinical Orthopaedics and Related Research*, vol. 431, pp. 36–41, 2005.

[6] A. Eren, M. Güven, B. Erol, and M. Čakar, "Delayed surgical treatment of supracondylar humerus fractures in children using a medial approach," *Journal of Children's Orthopaedics*, vol. 2, no. 1, pp. 21–27, 2008.

[7] B. Mahaisavariya, "Late treatment of displaced supracondylar fractures of the humerus using early wedge osteotomy," *Techniques in Orthopaedics*, vol. 21, no. 2, pp. 150–157, 2006.

[8] G. M. Lal and S. Bhan, "Delayed open reduction for supracondylar fractures of the humerus," *International Orthopaedics*, vol. 15, no. 3, pp. 189–191, 1991.

[9] A. J. Weiland, S. Meyers, V. T. Tolo, H. L. Berg, and J. Mueller, "Surgical treatment of displaced supracondylar fracture of the humerus in children," *The Journal of Bone & Joint Surgery—American Volume*, vol. 60, pp. 657–661, 1978.

[10] R. D. Reitman, P. Waters, and M. Millis, "Open reduction and internal fixation for supracondylar humerus fractures in children," *Journal of Pediatric Orthopaedics*, vol. 21, no. 2, pp. 157–161, 2001.

[11] A. Ali, A. Q. Mohammad, and A. Zain, "Pin tract infection rates between percutaneous and buried K wire in supracondylar fracture of humerus in children," *Pakistan*, vol. 26, no. 2, pp. 146–150, 2010.

[12] P. Worlock, "Supracondylar fractures of the humerus. Assessment of cubitus varus by the Baumann angle," *The Journal of Bone & Joint Surgery—British Volume*, vol. 68, no. 5, pp. 755–757, 1986.

[13] A. P. Vasen, S. H. Lacey, M. W. Keith, and J. W. Shaffer, "Functional range of motion of the elbow," *The Journal of Hand Surgery*, vol. 20, no. 2, pp. 288–292, 1995.

[14] J. C. Flynn, J. G. Matthews, and R. L. Benoit, "Blind pinning of displaced supracondylar fracture of the humerus in children, sixteen years experience with long term follow up," *The Journal of Bone and Joint Surgery. American Volume*, vol. 56, no. 2, pp. 263–272, 1974.

[15] J. A. Wilson, "Injuries of the elbow," in *Watson-Jones Fractures and Joint Injuries*, vol. 2, pp. 583–649, Churcill Livingstone, Edinburgh, UK, 6th edition, 2000.

[16] W. J. Mitchell and J. P. Adams, "Supracondylar fractures of the humerus in children," *Journal of the American Medical Association*, vol. 175, pp. 235–252, 1961.

[17] D. D. Aronson and B. I. Prager, "Supracondylar fractures of the humerus in children: a modified technique for closed pinning," *Clinical Orthopaedics and Related Research*, vol. 219, pp. 174–184, 1987.

[18] R. T. Davis, J. T. Gorczyca, and K. Pugh, "Supracondylar humerus fractures in children: comparison of operative treatment methods," *Clinical Orthopaedics and Related Research*, vol. 376, pp. 49–55, 2000.

[19] A. S. Devnani, "Lateral closing wedge supracondylar osteotomy of humerus for post-traumatic cubitus varus in children," *Injury*, vol. 28, no. 9-10, pp. 643–647, 1997.

[20] M. Carcassonne, M. Bergoin, and H. Hornung, "Results of operative treatment of severe supracondylar fractures of the elbow in children," *Journal of Pediatric Surgery*, vol. 7, no. 6, pp. 676–679, 1972.

[21] T. Gosens and K. J. Bongers, "Neurovascular complications and functional outcome in displaced supracondylar fractures of the humerus in children," *Injury*, vol. 34, no. 4, pp. 267–273, 2003.

[22] A. Tiwari, R. K. Kanojia, and S. K. Kapoor, "Surgical management for late presentation of supracondylar humeral fracture in children," *Journal of Orthopaedic Surgery*, vol. 15, no. 2, pp. 177–182, 2007.

[23] A. I. Leet, F. Juan, and E. Edward, "Delayed treatment of type 3 supracondylar fractures of the humerus," *Journal of Pediatric Orthopaedics*, vol. 22, pp. 203–207, 2002.

[24] A. Dua, K. K. Eachempati, R. Malhotra, L. Sharma, and M. Gidaganti, "Closed reduction and percutaneous pinning of displaced supracondylar fractures of humerus in children with delayed presentation," *Chinese Journal of Traumatology*, vol. 14, no. 1, pp. 14–19, 2011.

Risk Factors for Recurrent Shoulder Dislocation Arthroscopically Managed with Absorbable Knotless Anchors

Raffaele Russo,[1] Fabio Cautiero,[1] and Giuseppe Della Rotonda[2]

[1] *Orthopaedic and Traumatology Department, Ospedale dei Pellegrini, 80134 Napoli, Italy*
[2] *Royal Berkshire Hospital, London Road, Reading RG1 5AN, UK*

Correspondence should be addressed to Fabio Cautiero; fabiocau@inwind.it

Academic Editor: Doron Norman

Purpose. To evaluate the clinical outcome and risk factors for recurrent dislocation after arthroscopic stabilization with absorbable knotless anchor. *Methods.* We treated 197 patients affected by anterior shoulder instability, either traumatic or atraumatic with the same arthroscopic suture technique. We recorded age at surgery and number and type of dislocations (traumatic/atraumatic). Of the 197 patients, 127 (65.4%) were examined with a mean follow-up of 5.6 years (range: 25–108 months). Eighty-one shoulders were evaluated with the Rowe score and 48 with the Simple Shoulder Test (SST). *Results.* The mean Rowe score was 90.8, while the mean SST score was 10.9. Recurrence occurred in 10 cases (7.7%) but only in 4 cases was atraumatic, which reduces the real recurrence rate to 3.1%. Patients with recurrence were significantly younger at surgery than patients who did not relapse ($P = 0.040$). Moreover, neither the number ($P = 0.798$) nor the type of shoulder instability ($P = 0.751$), or the amount of glenoid bone loss ($P = 0.184$) significantly affected the probability of recurrence. *Conclusions.* In a patient population with involuntary monodirectional anterior shoulder instability, use of absorbable knotless anchor was reliable and resulted in a good outcome. In this series the statistical significant risk factors for recurrent dislocation were age of patient.

1. Introduction

Unidirectional shoulder instability is a very frequent condition that generally responds well to arthroscopic surgery. However, arthroscopic procedures can fail due to such factors as patient age [1], number of previous dislocations and rehabilitation program [2], chondral and bone defects [3], sports activity [4], insufficient soft-tissue tensioning [5], failure of surgical devices [6], and bone quality [7].

Very little is known about risk factors associated with recurrence of shoulder instability after arthroscopic treatment. There appears to be no statistically significant differences in outcome using absorbable versus non absorbable sutures [8]. However, severe osteoarthritis has been associated with metal anchors [9]. Other complications have been reported in patients treated with bioknotless anchors. Athwal et al. [10] reported four failures that led to destructive glenoid osteolysis, anchor pull-out, and subsequent severe damage of the articular surface. Barber [11] described 2 failures: one due to rapid degradation of the suture anchor; the other because the upper part of the anchor and a portion of the eyelet became loose bodies as the anchor absorbed. Freehill et al. [12] reported synovitis, implant debris, and full-thickness chondral damage in 10 of 52 patients. Meyer and Gerber [6] described 2 cases of instability recurrence after arthroscopic Bankart repair. During reoperation, all sutures were correctly knotted around the labrum but were intact and torn out of the anchor eyelets. There was no sign of anchor displacement (3 anchors in each patient). The authors described these cases as "unambiguous structural suture anchor failure."

The purpose of our study was to identify the risk factors of recurrent dislocation and complications in anterior shoulder instability treated with arthroscopic absorbable knotless anchors in a large series of patients with anterior unidirectional shoulder instability.

2. Materials and Methods

From September 2001 to December 2007, 197 patients affected by unidirectional shoulder instability were operated on by the senior surgeon (RR) of our hospital; 127 patients (100 men and 27 women) were available for the minimum follow-up of 24 months. Both shoulders were affected in 2/127 patients for a total of 129 shoulders followed-up. The average age at surgery was 27.8 years (range 16–48 years). After surgery, all patients were monitored by the same surgical team. In addition, the 129 shoulders were also independently assessed at a minimum follow-up of 24 months by two surgeons working outside the surgical team.

Patients were selected based on the following inclusion criteria: (1) clinical history of recurrent anterior shoulder instability, whether traumatic or not; (2) Bankart lesion, also associated with superior labral anterior posterior (SLAP) lesions and rotator cuff lesions; (3) absence of severe bone defects at the anteroinferior glenoid edge (less than 20% of the unaffected contralateral side, as preoperatively assessed). Patients were excluded if one of the following conditions was present: (1) multidirectional, posterior, and voluntary instability; (2) previous surgical stabilization; (3) incomplete passive range of motion; (4) first dislocation; (5) large Hill-Sachs lesions.

Fifty-one (39.5%) cases were related to sports activities, and 16 of these patients (12.4%) practiced high-risk contact sports. All patients had a history of anterior traumatic or atraumatic dislocation, and preoperative examination revealed a positive apprehension and relocation test without passive limitation of range of motion. Sulcus sign for shoulder laxity and rotator cuff tests were performed in all cases. Sixty-five patients (50.4%) underwent a preoperative radiographic evaluation according to Bernageau and Patte [13]. Magnetic resonance imaging was performed in 90 patients (69.8%). Arthro-MRI was performed in 26 patients including athletes (20.1%) and arthro-CT scan in 10 cases (7.8%). In one patient affected by bilateral anterior shoulder instability we used one CT scan to evaluate both shoulders.

We use an instrumental imaging like MRI, arthro-MRI, or arthro-CT scan to evaluate lesion of the glenoideal labrum and glenohumeral ligaments.

From 2001 to 2004, we used the nonobjective method described by Burkhart and de Beer [14] to evaluate the glenoid bone. From 2005, we evaluated bone loss using the "PICO" CT scan technique [15] and treated arthroscopically those patients with a maximum bone loss of 15%. All patients were treated with the arthroscopic technique described by Thal [16] using bioknotless anchors (De Puy Mitek, Raynham, MA). During this procedure, it is important to make a good capsular south-north shift and a capsular bumper on the glenoid rim. In hyperlaxity cases, rather than closing the rotator interval we use an appropriate number of anchors to fix the ligaments on the glenoid. From 2001, we also treated associated superior labral anterior to posterior (SLAP) lesions with absorbable knotless anchors using the surgical technique subsequently described by Yian et al. [17].

As shown in Table 1, during surgery, we found a Bankart lesion in all 129 patients, and, in 21 of them, the lesion was associated with a SLAP lesion. In 4 patients the Bankart lesion was associated with a partial rotator cuff lesion that was treated with debridement. Seven patients had a Bony-Bankart lesion and 14 an anterior labral periosteal sleeve avulsion (ALPSA) lesion.

Table 1: Type of lesion detected at surgery.

Type of lesion	Number
Bankart	129
Bankart with SLAP	21
Bankart with rotator cuff lesion	4
Bony-Bankart	7
ALPSA	14

The shoulder was immobilized for 4 weeks in a sling in adduction-internal rotation. After this period, patients were allowed to remove the brace intermittently and start rehabilitation with the Lyon protocol in water [18]. When the shoulder reached the complete passive range of motion, active movement was begun with strengthening exercises according to the Hawkins et al.'s Protocol [19]. Regular sports practice was allowed 8 months after surgery.

In our protocol a postoperative MRI is not expected.

3. Statistical Analysis

Statistical analysis was designed to assess whether there was a correlation between risk factors and recurrent shoulder instability treated with absorbable knotless anchors. We performed a separate statistical analysis for the Rowe and the SST groups. The level of stability at 24 months of follow-up was the dependent variable (Rowe stability score, SST results). Age (≤20 years, >20 years), number of dislocations (<5 or ≥5) and type (traumatic or not traumatic) of shoulder dislocation (traumatic or not traumatic), difficulty in shoulder movements (Rowe movement score ≤15, >15), and functions (Rowe function score <30, ≥30) were the independent variables when the Rowe group was evaluated. Age (≤20 years, >20 years), number of shoulder dislocations (<5 or ≥5), and type of shoulder dislocation (whether traumatic or not) were the independent variables considered for the subjects evaluated by means of the SST questionnaire. The bivariate association of the dependent variable with the independent variables was analyzed using the Chi-square test or the Fisher exact test (when the expected frequencies were less than 5). The effect of the independent variables on the postoperative shoulder stability was investigated using a multiple logistic regression model.

We also analyzed the distribution of relapses according to age at intervention, shoulder dislocations number, and type (whether traumatic or not). Because of the small number of relapses, we used a nonparametric approach, namely, the Wilcoxon rank test for quantitative variables and the Fisher exact test for the qualitative variables. We used survival analysis to evaluate the relapse-free probability. The Kaplan-Maier method was applied considering age at intervention, number, and type of shoulder dislocation as factors that could affect the probability of relapse. The log-rank test was used to compare strata. A level of probability equal to 0.05 was

TABLE 2: Main features of patients evaluated by the Rowe score according to the level of shoulder stability.

	Level of stability		
	Score 30 $n = 19$	Score 50 $n = 62$	P
Age [n (%)]			
≤20 years	4 (21.0)	16 (25.8)	0.770*
>20 years	15 (79.0)	46 (74.2)	*Fisher exact test
No. of shoulder dislocations N. (%)			
<5	9 (47.4)	29 (46.8)	0.964
≥5	10 (52.6)	33 (53.2)	Chi-square test
Traumatic dislocation N. (%)			
No	7 (36.8)	19 (30.6)	0.613
Yes	12 (63.2)	43 (69.4)	Chi-square test
Difficulty in movement N. (%)			
≤15 score	7 (36.8)	4 (6.5)	0.003
≥20 score	12 (63.2)	58 (93.5)	Chi-square test
Difficulty in function N.nd (%)			
<30 score	11 (57.9)	18 (29.0)	0.03
=30 score	8 (42.1)	44 (71.0)	Chi-square test

chosen to assess statistical significance; all the analyses were performed using the SAS program versus 9.1.

4. Results

At minimum follow-up of 24 months, 79 patients (total number of shoulders 81; 2 cases were bilateral) were assessed. The main features of patients according to the level of shoulder stability evaluated by the Rowe score are shown in Table 2. Sixty-two of the 81 shoulders (76.5%) had a stability score of 50 and 18 a stability score of 30. The latter patients had significantly greater difficulty in movement (Rowe movement score ≤15, $P = 0.003$) and in function (Rowe function score <30, $P = 0.03$) than those with a stability score of 50. The level of shoulder stability was not significantly associated with the patients' age, or with the number or type of shoulder dislocations. Only one patient in the Rowe group relapsed; consequently, this variable was not included in the analysis.

We performed a multiple logistic regression analysis to evaluate the effect of age, number and type of dislocations, difficulty in movement, and function on the level of shoulder stability in patients with a low Rowe stability score (Table 3). Among the factors considered in the analysis, difficulty of movement was statistically significant. In fact, the probability of having a low level of shoulder stability was 6.41 times higher in patients with a Rowe movement score ≤15 than in patients with a Rowe movement score ≥20. The 95% CI of the odds ratio was particularly large due to the small number of patients who had both a Rowe movement score ≤15 and a Rowe stability score of 30 (7 of a total of 11 subjects with a Rowe movement score ≤15).

TABLE 3: Effect of age, number and type of dislocations, movement,and function on shoulder instability (Rowe stability score = 30).

	Odds ratio	95% CI LL	95% CI UL	P
Age: ≤20 versus >20	1.13	0.29	4.38	0.857
N. dislocations: ≤5 versus <5	0.86	0.27	2.72	0.798
Traumatic dislocation: yes versus no	0.83	0.25	2.77	0.751
Movement score: ≤15 versus ≥20	5.95	1.21	29.41	0.029
Function score: <30 versus 30	1.86	0.51	6.76	0.350

95% CI: confidence interval; LL: lower level; UL: upper level.

TABLE 4: Main features of patients evaluated by the SST questionnaire according to shoulder stability.

	Stability		
	No $n = 18$	Yes $n = 30$	P
Age [n (%)]			
≤20 years	6 (33.3)	2 (6.7)	0.040
>20 years	12 (66.7)	28 (93.3)	Chi-square test
No. of shoulder dislocations [n (%)]			
<5	7 (38.9)	16 (53.3)	0.332
≥5	11 (61.1)	14 (46.7)	Chi-square test
Traumatic dislocation [n (%)]			
No	6 (33.3)	15 (50.0)	0.260
Yes	12 (66.7)	15 (50.0)	Chi-square test
Recurrence [n (%)]			
No	9 (50.0)	30 (100.0)	<0.001*
Yes	9 (50.0)	0 (0.0)	*Fisher exact test

In the SST group, constituted by 48 patients (Table 4), an unstable shoulder was significantly more frequent in patients aged ≤20 years ($P = 0.040$). A number of dislocations ≥5 and traumatic dislocations were more frequent in patients with an unstable shoulder than in patients with a stable shoulder, but the difference was not statistically significant. No relapse occurred in patients with a stable shoulder; 50% of patients with unstable shoulder relapsed ($P < 0.001$).

The distribution of relapses according to the type of shoulder dislocation, the year of surgery, the age at surgery, and the number of dislocations is shown in Table 5. Patients who relapsed were significantly younger at surgery than patients who did not relapse. Up to the end of 2004, we treated

Table 5: Features of the 10 cases of dislocation recurrence.

Case number	Age at surgery	Type of lesion	Time from surgery	Type of instability	Cause of recurrence
1	22	Bankart + ALPSA	3 years	Traumatic	Traumatic
2	25	Bankart + ALPSA	2 years	Not traumatic	Traumatic
3	34	Bankart	1 year	Traumatic	Traumatic
4	22	Bankart + ALPSA	1 year	Traumatic	Traumatic
5	23	Bankart + SLAP	3 months	Traumatic	Traumatic
6	19	Bankart + ALPSA	1 year	Traumatic	Not traumatic
7	18	Bankart	1 year	Traumatic	Traumatic
8	20	Bankart + ALPSA	1 year	Traumatic	Not traumatic
9	21	Bankart	1 year	Traumatic	Not traumatic
10	20	Bankart + ALPSA	18 months	Traumatic	Not traumatic

Table 6: Distribution of recurrence dislocation in relation to type and number of dislocations and age at surgery.

	Relapse		
	No $n = 119$	Yes $n = 10$	P
Traumatic dislocations [n (%)]			
No	46 (38.7)	1 (10.0)	0.092
Yes	73 (61.3)	9 (90.0)	Fisher exact test
Year of intervention [n (%)]			
<2005	64 (53.8)	4 (40.0)	0.184
≥2005	55 (46.2)	6 (60.0)	Fisher exact test
Number of dislocations			
[Median (25th–75th percentile)]	4 (2–6)	4 (3–5)	0.922*
Age			*Wilcoxon rank test
Years [median (25th–75th percentile)]	24.1 (21.6–27.2)	21.6 (19.1–22.4)	0.016* *Wilcoxon rank test

cases with a glenoid bone loss less than 25% and thereafter cases with a glenoid bone loss lower than 15%. The incidence of recurrence did not differ statistically between these two groups (data not shown).

Table 6 shows the patient's age, lesion at surgery, type of instability, and cause of redislocation in our cohort. The probability of remaining relapse-free was significantly higher in subjects who were 20 years old at surgery. Neither the number nor the type of shoulder dislocations significantly affected the probability of relapsing. The dislocation recurrence rate was 7.7% (10 cases). Recurrence was due to a trauma in 60% of cases and was spontaneous in the remaining 40%.

In the 80 cases treated for nontraumatic instability, the apprehension test in external rotation at 90° of abduction was positive in 5/80 patients (6.2%); pain was present in 2 patients (2.5%), while apprehension and pain were present in 3 (3.7%). In all cases treated for traumatic instability (n = 117), the apprehension test was positive in 15 patients (13%) while 38 patients (33%) reported apprehension and pain.

Fifty-one (39.5%) patients were involved in sports and 16 of them (12.4%) practiced high-risk contact sports. Thirty-eight (74.5%) of these patients resumed their sport at preinjury level and 10 (19.6%) at a lower level, whereas 3 (5.8%) could not resume sport either because of pain during sports practice (n = 2) or due to relapse.

We did not observe any case of synovitis or anchor mobilization. There was only one case of chondral damage (0.07%), which could have been related to the use of articular infusion of local anesthetic.

5. Discussion

Arthroscopic treatment has evolved to become the main surgical option in the management of anterior shoulder instability given the comparable outcome of open and arthroscopic techniques: 10% of failure [20]. However, the use of absorbable versus not absorbable and of knotted versus knotless anchors is still controversial because of the lack of data about the frequency and complications associated with arthroscopic techniques [21]. To our knowledge, there are no reports of large series of patients treated with knotless absorbable anchors. Thal et al. [22] evaluated 73 consecutive patients, with 5 cases (6.9%) of failure of knotless anchors in patients aged 22 years or younger; however follow-up was short. Oh et al. [23] reported that 5 cases out of 37 (13.5%) treated with absorbable suture anchors perceived mild pain during the apprehension test without a sense of instability and one case (2.7%) with a sense of instability during normal daily activity.

Age at surgery, number of dislocations, type of dislocation, hyperlaxity glenoid bone loss, and Hill Sachs lesions have been reported to be risk factors for recurrence [1, 3–7]. In our study of 129 shoulders with unidirectional anterior instability for a minimum 2-year follow-up, we found that age of 20 years or lower was a significant risk factor ($P = 0.011$) for recurrence in patients managed with the arthroscopic Bankart repair technique using absorbable knotless anchors. Patients who were significantly younger at surgery did not relapse (see Table 4). The incidence of recurrence was higher in patients who had more than 5 dislocations or whose previous dislocation was traumatic, but the difference was not statistically significant.

Many of our patients (76.5%) had a high level of stability and good recovery of motion without stiffness. There was only case (0.07%) of chondral damage. We did not observe any cases of synovitis or anchor mobilization. Fifty-one of our patients (39.5%) had practiced sports before surgery: 16 of them (29.4%) practiced contact or collision sports and 36 (70.6%) noncollision sports. Thal et al. reported failure in 42/72 patients (7.1%) who practiced contact or collision sports and in 30 who did not (6.7%) [22]. Konrad et al. [24] reported that 29/35 patients (83%) with traumatic, unidirectional anterior shoulder instability treated with arthroscopic transglenoid fixation were able to return to their preoperative level of sports activity. In a prospective randomized study on absorbable versus nonabsorbable sutures for arthroscopic treatment of anterior shoulder instability in athletes, Monteiro et al. [8] reported 50 patients randomly assigned to two groups: one treated with absorbable and the other one with nonabsorbable sutures. They obtained excellent results in 22 patients (90.5%) of the former group and in 21 patients (87.5%) of the latter group. In our experience, 38/51 cases (74.5%) returned to sports at preinjury level, 10 (19.6%) at a lower level, while 3 (5.8%) could not resume sports activity due to relapse. In our series, the recurrent dislocation rate was 7.7%, but it should be stressed that recurrence was traumatic in 6 cases and spontaneous in 4 cases, so the true recurrence rate was 3.1%.

6. Conclusions

The risk factors for recurrent shoulder dislocation arthroscopically managed with absorbable knotless anchors in our series were age, number, and type of dislocation. The use of bioabsorbable materials did not increase the risk of synovitis, anchor mobilization, stiffness, or chondral damage. Correct execution of the arthroscopic technique and careful patient selection based on the patient's age, type of dislocation, and glenoideal bone loss are the key to a successful clinical outcome and a recurrence-free outcome.

Conflict of Interests

The authors declare that there is no conflict of interests.

Acknowledgment

The authors thank Jean Ann Gilder (Scientific Communication Srl.) for revising and editing the text.

References

[1] F. Postacchini, S. Gumina, and G. Cinotti, "Anterior shoulder dislocation in adolescents," *Journal of Shoulder and Elbow Surgery*, vol. 9, no. 6, pp. 470–474, 2000.

[2] S. H. Kim, K. I. Ha, M. W. Jung, M. S. Lim, Y. M. Kim, and J. H. Park, "Accelerated rehabilitation after arthroscopic Bankart repair for selected cases: a prospective randomized clinical study," *Arthroscopy*, vol. 19, no. 7, pp. 722–731, 2003.

[3] T. J. Gill, R. F. Warren, C. A. Rockwood Jr., E. V. Craig, R. H. Cofield, and R. J. Hawkins, "Complications of shoulder surgery," *Instructional Course Lectures*, vol. 48, pp. 359–374, 1999.

[4] H. H. Handoll, M. A. Almaiyah, and A. Rangan, "Surgical versus non-surgical treatment for acute anterior shoulder dislocation," *Cochrane Database of Systematic Reviews*, no. 1, Article ID CD004325, 2004.

[5] H. E. Segmüller, M. G. Hayes, and A. D. Saies, "Arthroscopic repair of glenolabral injuries with an absorbable fixation device," *Journal of Shoulder and Elbow Surgery*, vol. 6, no. 4, pp. 383–392, 1997.

[6] D. C. Meyer and C. Gerber, "Failure of anterior shoulder instability repair caused by eyelet cutout of absorbable suture anchors," *Arthroscopy*, vol. 20, no. 5, pp. 521–523, 2004.

[7] C. R. Good and J. D. MacGillivray, "Traumatic shoulder dislocation in the adolescent athlete: advances in surgical treatment," *Current Opinion in Pediatrics*, vol. 17, no. 1, pp. 25–29, 2005.

[8] G. C. Monteiro, B. Ejnisman, C. V. Andreoli, A. C. Pochini, and M. Cohen, "Absorbable versus nonabsorbable sutures for the arthroscopic treatment of anterior shoulder instability in athletes: a prospective randomized study," *Arthroscopy*, vol. 24, no. 6, pp. 697–703, 2008.

[9] M. Ozbaydar, B. Elhassan, and J. J. P. Warner, "The use of anchors in shoulder surgery: a shift from metallic to bioabsorbable anchors," *Arthroscopy*, vol. 23, no. 10, pp. 1124–1126, 2007.

[10] G. S. Athwal, S. M. Shridharani, and S. W. O'Driscoll, "Osteolysis and arthropathy of the shoulder after use of bioabsorbable knotless suture anchors: a report of four cases," *Journal of Bone and Joint Surgery A*, vol. 88, no. 8, pp. 1840–1845, 2006.

[11] F. A. Barber, "Biodegradable shoulder anchors have unique modes of failure," *Arthroscopy*, vol. 23, no. 3, pp. 316–320, 2007.

[12] M. Q. Freehill, D. J. Harms, S. M. Huber, D. Atlihan, and D. D. Buss, "Poly-L-lactic acid tack synovitis after arthroscopic stabilization of the shoulder," *The American Journal of Sports Medicine*, vol. 31, no. 5, pp. 643–647, 2003.

[13] J. Bernageau and D. Patte, "The radiographic diagnosis of posterior dislocation of the shoulder," *Revue de Chirurgie Orthopedique et Reparatrice de l'Appareil Moteur*, vol. 65, no. 2, pp. 101–107, 1979.

[14] S. S. Burkhart and J. F. de Beer, "Traumatic glenohumeral bone defects and their relationship to failure of arthroscopic Bankart repairs: Significance of the inverted-pear glenoid and the humeral engaging Hill-Sachs lesion," *Arthroscopy*, vol. 16, no. 7, pp. 677–694, 2000.

[15] P. Baudi, P. Righi, D. Bolognesi et al., "How to identify and calculate glenoid bone deficit," *La Chirurgia degli Organi di Movimento*, vol. 90, no. 2, pp. 145–152, 2005.

[16] R. Thal, "A Knotless suture anchor: technique for use in arthroscopic Bakart repair," *Arthroscopy*, vol. 17, no. 2, pp. 213–218, 2001.

[17] E. Yian, C. Wang, P. J. Millett, and J. J. P. Warner, "Arthroscopic repair of SLAP lesions with a bioknotless suture anchor," *Arthroscopy*, vol. 20, no. 5, pp. 547–551, 2004.

[18] J.-P. Liotard, T. B. Edwards, A. Padey, G. Walch, and A. Boulahia, "Hydrotherapy rehabilitation after shoulder surgery," *Techniques in Shoulder & Elbow Surgery*, vol. 4, no. 2, pp. 44–49, 2003.

[19] R. J. Hawkins, R. Litchfield, J. Atkins, G. Hagerman, and C. J. Dillman, "Rehabilitation of the shoulder," *Annales Chirurgiae et Gynaecologiae*, vol. 85, no. 2, pp. 173–184, 1996.

[20] P. Bacilla, L. D. Field, and F. H. Savoie III, "Arthroscopic Bankart repair in a high demand patient population," *Arthroscopy*, vol. 13, no. 1, pp. 51–60, 1997.

[21] G. M. Gartsman, T. S. Roddey, and S. M. Hammerman, "Arthroscopic treatment of anterior-inferior glenohumeral instability. Two to five-year follow-up," *Journal of Bone and Joint Surgery*, vol. 82, no. 7, pp. 991–1003, 2000.

[22] R. Thal, M. Nofziger, M. Bridges, and J. J. Kim, "Arthroscopic Bankart repair using knotless or BioKnotless suture anchors: 2- to 7-year results," *Arthroscopy*, vol. 23, no. 4, pp. 367–375, 2007.

[23] J. H. Oh, H. K. Lee, J. Y. Kim, S. H. Kim, and H. S. Gong, "Clinical and radiologic outcomes of arthroscopic glenoid labrum repair with the bioknotless suture anchor," *The American Journal of Sports Medicine*, vol. 37, no. 12, pp. 2340–2348, 2009.

[24] G. G. Konrad, V. Rössler, P. C. Kreuz, and N. P. Südkamp, "Sports activity and proprioceptive ability after arthroscopic capsulolabral repair of post-traumatic shoulder instability," *Zeitschrift für Orthopädie und Unfallchirurgie*, vol. 147, no. 4, pp. 452–456, 2009.

25

Reducing Shoulder by Vertical Traction: A One-Man Method for Shoulder Reduction

Hayat Ahmad Khan,[1] Younis Kamal,[1] Mohammad Ashraf Khan,[1] Munir Farooq,[1] Naseemul Gani,[1] Nazia Hassan,[2] Adil Bashir Shah,[1] and Mohammad Shahid Bhat[1]

[1] *Department of Orthopaedics, B & J Hospital, GMC Srinagar, Kashmir 190005, India*
[2] *GMC Srinagar, Kashmir, India*

Correspondence should be addressed to Hayat Ahmad Khan; drhayatkhan@gmail.com

Academic Editor: Shyu-Jye Wang

Fifty percent of joint dislocations reported to the emergency department are of shoulder joint. Various techniques are used to reduce the shoulder and Spaso technique is the least known to the orthopaedic residents which is a simple one-man vertical traction method of shoulder reduction. We evaluated the effectiveness of vertical traction method for anterior shoulder dislocation by orthopaedic residents. Sixty consecutive patients of anterior glenohumeral dislocation attending the emergency department of our hospital were taken up for the study. The reduction was done using Spaso technique. Right shoulder was dislocated in 40 patients and 31 patients had recurrent shoulder dislocation. In 55 patients, shoulder was reduced without the use of any anaesthesia. In patients where no anaesthesia was used, the time of traction ranged from 45 seconds to 5 minutes, while under anaesthesia the time of traction ranged from 1 to 4 minutes. Twenty-one patients had associated greater tuberosity fracture which did not affect the method of reduction and all of them were reducible. No complication was reported, and all the patients were satisfied with the method. In conclusion vertical traction method is a good technique for reducing anterior shoulder dislocation with an easy learning curve among the residents and no complication has been reported so far.

1. Introduction

Of all the joint dislocations encountered in the accident and emergency departments, shoulder joint takes half of the share [1]. Krøner et al. (1989) reported the annual incidence of 17 per 100000 [2]. More and more people now indulge in recreational and sports activity which may be the cause for increased incidence of glenohumeral dislocation. Majority of shoulders are dislocated anteriorly (90–98%) with trauma being the main cause [3, 4]. Whatever the cause is, the joint needs to be reduced ideally. The method has to be quick, effective, and least painful to the patient without causing any iatrogenic injury. Many reduction techniques for shoulder joint have been documented with each having its advantages and disadvantage [5–7]. The relatively new technique of anterior shoulder joint reduction is the Spaso technique which is the one-man vertical traction method of reduction [8]. We conducted a prospective study to report our experience of using this technique to reduce shoulder. This is first study being conducted in India or even Asia to the best of our knowledge. It is also first of its kind given that only orthopaedic residents are involved in the study.

2. Aims and Objectives

Aim of this study was to evaluate the effectiveness of vertical traction method for anterior shoulder dislocation by orthopaedic residents.

3. Material and Methods

Sixty consecutive patients of anterior glenohumeral dislocation attending the Emergency Department of Bone and Joint Hospital were taken up for the study after the clinical and radiological diagnosis was made. The reduction was attempted by one of the authors. Demographic data including

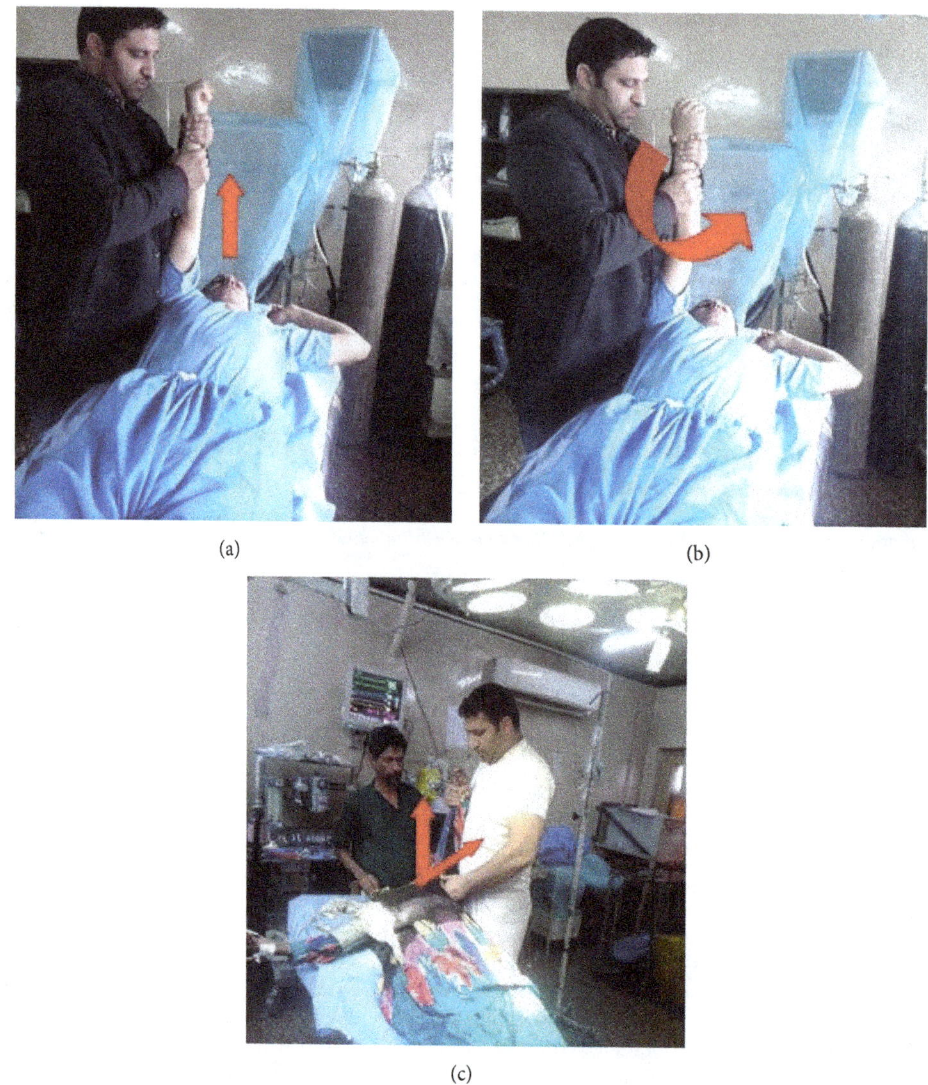

FIGURE 1: Method of shoulder reduction. Figure showing the method of shoulder reduction. (a) Vertical traction, (b) external rotation, and (c) palpation of humeral head being done. Red arrow shows the direction of force.

age, site, associated fracture of greater tuberosity, history of previous dislocation, any joint laxity, and number of manipulation attempts were noted on the patients case sheet. Mode of trauma and time since dislocation were noted. All patients gave consent for the procedure and the study was performed in accordance with the ethical standards and was approved by ethical committee.

The technique used was similar to that used by Spaso himself.

3.1. Technique. Patients were asked to lie down supine on the bed. Procedure was explained to the patients so that apprehension was over. Since the original article has not mentioned about the anaesthesia used, we followed up all cases without anaesthesia and reserved anaesthesia for patients where it was necessary. As advised by Spaso the affected limb was held at wrist and slowly elevated (forward flexion) and vertical traction was applied. While maintaining vertical traction, the shoulder was slightly externally rotated. A clunk was heard or felt when reduction was done (Figures 1, 2, and 3).

The patient tends to lift up the shoulder off the bed or stop the surgeon with opposite hand in case of discomfort. We stopped the further movement of the limb while maintaining the traction. Most of the times pain subsided allowing further traction. If reduction did not come, the head was palpated with the other hand and gently pushed. If still reduction was unsuccessful, anaesthesia was given and above procedure is repeated under anaesthesia.

After reduction, shoulder immobiliser was applied and patients were followed up in outpatient department.

3.2. Review of Other Reduction Methods

3.2.1. Hippocrates Method. With the patient lying supine, the physician's foot is placed in the patient's axilla against the chest wall while leaning backward. The affected arm is

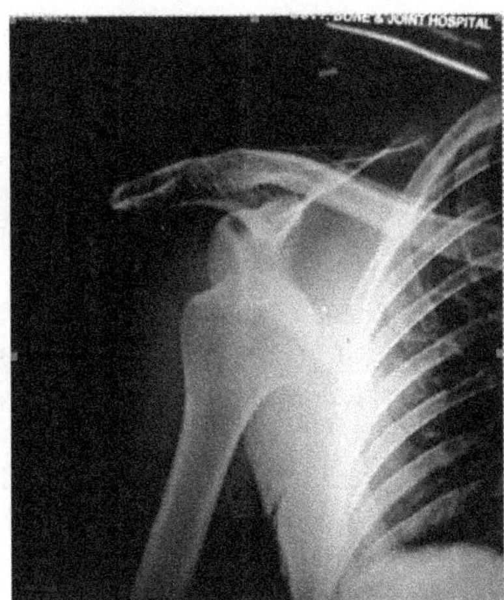

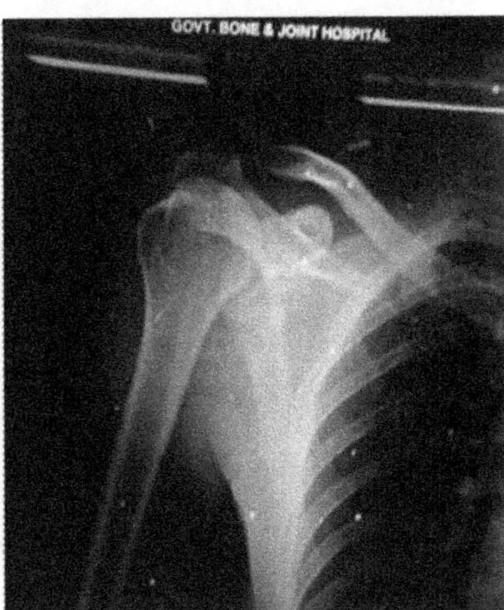

FIGURE 2: X-rays showing dislocated and reduced shoulder joint.

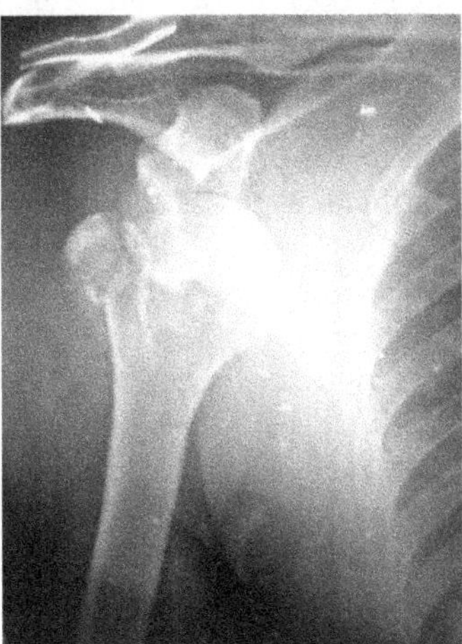

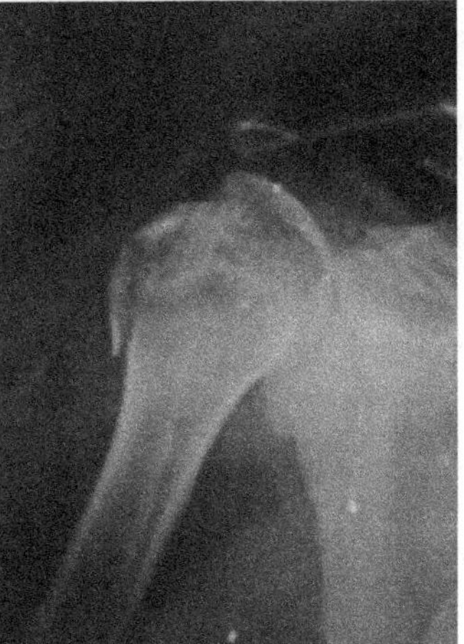

FIGURE 3: X-rays showing dislocated and reduced shoulder with fractured greater tuberosity.

abducted and gentle traction is applied steadily for about a minute. The foot acts as a counterforce and as a lever to push the humeral head laterally while the physician pulls the head toward the patient's foot along the surface of the glenoid.

3.2.2. Milch Technique. The patient lies supine or head elevated 30°. The physician stands on the affected side and places the ipsilateral hand upon the patients shoulder so that the fingers support the top of the shoulder, while the thumb is applied to the under surface of the dislocated humeral head to hold it in place. The elbow of the affected arm is put into 90° flexion. The physician gently *abducts* the arm into the overhead position with opposite hand and *externally rotates it.* The humeral head in the axilla is then pushed over the glenoid rim with direct pressure of the thumb.

Axial traction may be applied with countertraction via the hand or a foot upon the top of the shoulder (this was not in Milch's original description).

3.2.3. Kocher. It uses external rotation to roll the humeral head over the anterior glenoid rim. In this method the arm is flexed at elbow and pressed against the body. It is then rotated outwards till resistance is felt. The upper arm is then lifted in sagittal plane and turned inwards. Kocher did not use traction in his original description.

3.2.4. External Rotation Method. In this method the patient can be supine, sitting, or 45° recumbent. The affected arm is adducted against the torso. The elbow is flexed to 90°. The upper arm is externally rotated slowly and gently, using the forearm as a lever by grasping the wrist with one hand and the elbow with the other hand.

3.2.5. Scapular Manipulation Methods. In this method the patient is kept prone. The shoulder is kept in 90° of forward flexion and external rotation. The forearm is suspended from the stretcher with the wrist secured and the elbow flexed. Forward traction is maintained with about 5–7 Kg of hanging weight to the wrist or with manual traction for 5–10 minutes. With the patient relaxed, the physician pushes medially on the tip of the scapula with both thumbs and

Table 1

Number of patients Total 60	Male $N = 38$ (63.3%)	Females $N = 22$ (36.7%)
Side	Right $n = 40$ (64%)	Left $n = 20$ (33%)
Age group	Range [20 years to 75 years]	
Success rate 100%	$N = 55$ (91.67%) Without anaesthesia	$N = 5$ (8.33%) Under anaesthesia

lifts it occasionally while externally rotating the superior and medial aspects of the scapula.

4. Results

Among the cohort of 60, we had 38 males and 22 females. Right shoulder was dislocated in 40. And 31 patients had recurrent shoulder dislocation. Age group was between 20 and 75. Time of reporting to hospital ranged from 30 min to 2 weeks.

In 55 patients, shoulder was reduced without the use of any anaesthesia. Among the cases, ten were referred from the peripheral health centres and few attempts to reduce the shoulder were already made. Five patients were first tried without anaesthesia but the shoulder could not be reduced. Under anaesthesia all the shoulders were reduced by the same technique.

In patients where no anaesthesia was used, the time of traction ranged from 45 seconds to 5 minutes while under anaesthesia the time of traction ranged from 1 minute to 4 minutes. Twenty-one patients had associated greater tuberosity fracture and only two needed fixation.

Thirty-one patients had recurrent dislocation. Twenty-eight shoulders were previously reduced by other methods and all of them regarded this technique as better than the previous one. The demography of the patients is given in Table 1.

Table 2 summarizes the various techniques given by various authors and the percentage in which the premedication was used. Studies with more than 50 cases have been included. Also the authors in all the studies are male authors as in our case; we presume the female doctors who work in emergency centres can learn the technique as this has an easy learning curve.

5. Discussion

The method of reducing the shoulder joint is as old as the history of medical science. Different methods are given in the literature and most of the orthopaedicians have the opinion that one should use a method of reduction with which he is well versed. The review done by Ashton and Hassan [20] suggested that the individual preference for the method of reduction is not supported by evidence. In 2006 Kuhn presented the study showing that little data exists to predict best method of reduction or the type of anaesthesia [21].

Various methods used for shoulder reduction are still being practiced and various operators give good results. Traditional traction countertraction, Kocher's, Stimson's, scapular manipulation and Milch maneuver [10, 16, 22–24]. The number of methods available itself signifies that none of them is an ideal method and different methods need to be compared under a randomised control to know the effectiveness.

The complications associated with traction countertraction methods include axillary nerve injury, fractures of humeral head or shaft, and even capsular damage.

Also the countertraction causes muscle spasm which makes reduction more difficult or even impossible and may be the cause for need of general anaesthesia. In vertical traction method, all the forces are acting in the same direction and there is no force of opposition. The Spaso technique relies on sound biomechanical principles in that in the overhead position, all of the shoulder muscles course directly upwards inserting into the humerus thereby assisting reduction to the anatomical position [8, 11]. This contrasts with the methods performed with the arm at the side, where each of the shoulder muscles is running in a different direction usually requiring the use of more force or more sedation and hence the risk of fracture is increased.

Spaso method is the least known method among the techniques. The reason may be that the original study was published in the nonindexed journal and most of the orthopaedicians had no access to that. However Yuen et al. [25] have promoted the technique and published paper using the same technique. They further emphasised that further studies need to be conducted for knowing the effectiveness of technique. We took the initiative because this technique needed only single operator and no such study has been conducted at an orthopaedic centre which is overburdened by the road traffic accidents, infective cases, and multiple trauma patients.

We see almost 100 to 120 shoulder dislocation patients per year besides other orthopaedic trauma. Being a tertiary care institute and catering for a population of five millions, it is always a busy trauma centre. Also the analgesics like pethidine and morphine are not available for the masses in the developing countries like ours. This study was different from that conducted by Yuen et al. as no pethidine, valium, or morphine was used.

We were able to reduce all our patients with this technique although five patients needed anaesthesia. Presence of greater tuberosity fracture did not affect the method of reduction and all of them were reducible. Two patients were operated on for fixation of greater tuberosity. Of the five patients who needed anaesthesia, all had dislocations for the first time and two had greater tuberosity fracture.

No complication was reported in any of the patients and all patients were satisfied with the method. Few patients complained of pain after procedure which subsided after few hours. No patient had severe pain during or after the procedure.

6. Conclusion

Vertical traction method is a good technique for reducing anterior shoulder dislocation with an easy learning curve

TABLE 2: Table showing various studies conducted so far by various authors using different techniques. Only studies having fifty ($n \geq 50$) or more cases have been included.

Study type	Reduction method	Year	Author	No. of patients	Success rate	Complications	Without premedication
Case series	Snow bird looped technique	1995	Westin et al. [4]	118	114 (97%)	0%	93%
Case series	Autoreduction	1997	Ceroni et al. [9]	100	60 (60%)	0%	70%
Case series	Milch	1981	Russell et al. [10]	76	68 (89%)	0%	69%
Case series	Milch	1982	Janecki and Shahcheragh [6]	50	50 (100%)	0%	34%
RCT	Milch	1986	Beattie et al. [11]	56	39 (70%)	0%	NA
Case series	Milch	1992	Johnson et al. [12]	142	122 (86%)	0%	73%
Case series	Modified Milch	1989	Canales Cortés et al. [13]	128	107 (84%)	NA	33%
Case series	Modified Milch	1992	Garnavos [14]	75	71 (95%)	0%	100%
RCT	Kocher	1986	Beattie et al. [11]	55	40 (73%)	2%	NA
Case series	External rotation	1977	Leidelmeyer [15]	50	50 (100%)	0%	0%
Case series	External rotation	1979	Mirick et al. [16]	85	68 (80%)	0%	NA
Case series	External rotation	1986	Danzl et al. [17]	100	78 (78%)	1%	0%
Case series	Scapular manipulation	1982	Anderson et al. [18]	51	47 (92)	0%	34%
Case series	Scapular manipulation-seated	1993	McNamara [19]	61	48 (79%)	0%	64%
Present study	Spaso technique	2013-2014	Khan et al.	60	100%	0%	91.67%

among the residents and no complication has been reported so far.

Competing Interests

The authors declare that they have no competing interests.

Authors' Contributions

All authors contributed equally to this work.

Acknowledgments

The authors thank M. C. Yuen for providing them with the necessary material and help whenever required.

References

[1] R. Blake and J. Hoffman, "Emergency department evaluation and treatment of the shoulder and humerus," *Emergency Medicine Clinics of North America*, vol. 17, no. 4, pp. 859–876, 1999.

[2] K. Krøner, T. Lind, and J. Jensen, "The epidemiology of shoulder dislocations," *Archives of Orthopaedic and Trauma Surgery*, vol. 108, no. 5, pp. 288–290, 1989.

[3] J. A. Hill, "Epidemiologic perspective on shoulder injuries," *Clinics in Sports Medicine*, vol. 2, no. 2, pp. 241–247, 1993.

[4] C. D. Westin, E. A. Gill, M. E. Noyes, and M. Hubbard, "Anterior shoulder dislocation: a simple and rapid method for reduction," *American Journal of Sports Medicine*, vol. 23, no. 3, pp. 369–371, 1995.

[5] K. K. Eachempati, A. Dua, R. Malhotra, S. Bhan, and J. R. Bera, "The external rotation method for reduction of acute anterior dislocations and fracture-dislocations of the shoulder," *Journal of Bone and Joint Surgery A*, vol. 86, no. 11, pp. 2431–2434, 2004.

[6] C. J. Janecki and G. H. Shahcheragh, "The forward elevation maneuver for reduction of anterior dislocations of the shoulder," *Clinical Orthopaedics and Related Research*, vol. 164, pp. 177–180, 1982.

[7] H. R. Manes, "A new method of shoulder reduction in the elderly," *Clinical Orthopaedics and Related Research*, vol. 147, pp. 200–202, 1980.

[8] S. Miljesic and A.-M. Kelly, "Reduction of anterior dislocation of the shoulder: the Spaso technique," *Emergency Medicine*, vol. 10, no. 2, pp. 173–175, 1998.

[9] D. Ceroni, H. Sadri, and A. Leuenberger, "Anteroinferior shoulder dislocation: an auto-reduction method without analgesia," *Journal of Orthopaedic Trauma*, vol. 11, no. 6, pp. 399–404, 1997.

[10] J. A. Russell, E. M. Holmes III, D. J. Keller, and J. H. Vargas III, "Reduction of acute anterior shoulder dislocations using the milch technique: a study of ski injuries," *Journal of Trauma: Injury, Infection and Critical Care*, vol. 21, no. 9, pp. 802–804, 1981.

[11] T. F. Beattie, D. J. Steedman, A. McGowan, and C. E. Robertson, "A comparison of the Milch and Kocher techniques for acute anterior dislocation of the shoulder," *Injury*, vol. 17, no. 5, pp. 349-352, 1986.

[12] G. Johnson, W. Hulse, and A. McGowan, "The Milch Technique for reduction of anterior shoulder dislocations in an accident and emergency department," *Archives of Emergency Medicine*, vol. 9, no. 1, pp. 40–43, 1992.

[13] V. Canales Cortés, L. García-Dihinx Checa, and J. Rodriguez Vela, "Reduction of acute anterior dislocations of the shoulder without anaesthesia in the position of maximum muscular relaxation," *International Orthopaedics*, vol. 13, no. 4, pp. 259–262, 1989.

[14] C. Garnavos, "Technical note: modifications and improvements of the milch technique for the reduction of anterior dislocation of the shoulder without premedication," *Journal of Trauma*, vol. 32, no. 6, pp. 801–803, 1992.

[15] R. Leidelmeyer, "Reduced! A shoulder, subtly and painlessly," *The Journal of Emergency Medicine*, vol. 9, pp. 223–234, 1977.

[16] M. J. Mirick, J. E. Clinton, and E. Ruiz, "External rotation method of shoulder dislocation reduction," *Journal of the American College of Emergency Physicians*, vol. 8, no. 12, pp. 528–531, 1979.

[17] D. F. Danzl, S. J. Vicario, G. L. Gleis, J. R. Yates, and D. L. Parks, "Closed reduction of anterior subcoracoid shoulder dislocation. Evaluation of an external rotation method," *Orthopaedic Review*, vol. 15, no. 5, pp. 311–315, 1986.

[18] D. Anderson, R. Zvirbulis, and J. Ciullo, "Scapular manipulation for reduction of anterior shoulder dislocations," *Clinical Orthopaedics and Related Research*, vol. 164, pp. 181–183, 1982.

[19] R. M. McNamara, "Reduction of anterior shoulder dislocations by scapular manipulation," *Annals of Emergency Medicine*, vol. 22, no. 7, pp. 1140–1144, 1993.

[20] H. R. Ashton and Z. Hassan, "Best evidence topic report. Kocher's or Milch's technique for reduction of anterior shoulder dislocations," *Emergency Medicine Journal*, vol. 23, no. 7, pp. 570–571, 2006.

[21] J. E. Kuhn, "Treating the initial anterior shoulder dislocation—an evidence-based medicine approach," *Sports Medicine and Arthroscopy Review*, vol. 14, no. 4, pp. 192–198, 2006.

[22] H. Milch, "Treatment of dislocation of the shoulder," *Surgery*, vol. 3, pp. 732–738, 1938.

[23] L. A. Stimson, "An easy method of reducing dislocations of the shoulder and hip," *Med Record*, vol. 57, pp. 356–357, 1900.

[24] M. Daya, "Shoulder," in *Rosen's Emergency Medicine. Concepts and Clinical Practice*, J. A. Marx, R. S. Hockberger, and R. M. Walls, Eds., pp. 576–606, Mosby, St. Louis, Mo, USA, 5th edition, 2002.

[25] M.-C. Yuen, P.-G. Yap, Y.-T. Chan, and W.-K. Tung, "An easy method to reduce anterior shoulder dislocation: the Spaso technique," *Emergency Medicine Journal*, vol. 18, no. 5, pp. 370–372, 2001.

26

Clinical and Radiological Outcome of the Newest Generation of Ceramic-on-Ceramic Hip Arthroplasty in Young Patients

Avishai Reuven,[1] Grigorios N. Manoudis,[1] Ahmed Aoude,[2] Olga L. Huk,[1] David Zukor,[1] and John Antoniou[1]

[1] *Department of Orthopaedics, McGill University, Jewish General Hospital, 3755 Cote-St.-Catherine Road, Room E-003, Montreal, QC, Canada H3T 1E2*

[2] *Medical School, University of Montreal, P.O. Box 6128, Station Centre-Ville, Montreal, QC, Canada H3C 3J7*

Correspondence should be addressed to Grigorios N. Manoudis; gregmanou@yahoo.com

Academic Editor: Mel S. Lee

Ceramic-on-ceramic articulations have become an attractive option for total hip arthroplasty in young patients. In this study, we retrospectively evaluated the short- to midterm clinical and radiographic results in 51 consecutive patients (61 hips) using the newest generation of ceramic implants. Results obtained in our study showed positive clinical and radiological outcomes. Both HHS and UCLA activity scores doubled after surgery and tended to increase over time. There was one infection requiring a two-stage revision and a case of squeaking that began 2 years postoperatively after a mechanical fall. The overall survival rate of the implants was 98.4% at six years with revision for any reason as the end point. Based on these results, fourth generation ceramics offer a viable option for young and active patients.

1. Introduction

One of the most challenging problems that orthopaedic surgeons are facing today is the increasing number of young and active patients requiring long lasting and reliable primary total hip arthroplasty (THA) [1]. It is well known that bearing surface wear and particle-driven osteolysis remain the major factors threatening the longevity and limiting the performance of the implant [2, 3]. Ceramic-on-ceramic (CC) hip articulations made form alumina have become an attractive option for young and active patients who require THA. This is partially due to the excellent wear characteristics and outstanding tribological properties of alumina over metal-on-polyethylene (MP) bearings [4, 5]. In addition, the inert nature of alumina gives the CC surfaces a great advantage over metal-on-metal (MM) surfaces [6].

Alumina CC bearings have a long history of use [7]. Initial attempts of ceramic-on-ceramic THA had high failure rates that were mainly related to bad design and flaws in the material [8, 9]. Further advancements in alumina manufacturing technology such as hot isostatic pressing led to the fabrication of a highly purified alumina (BIOLOX forte; CeramTec AG, Plochingen, Germany) with increased material density, decreased grain structure, and less impurities [10, 11]. All these material improvements yielded a noticeable decrease in the rate of implant components fracture and chipping [12, 13]. Despite the advancements made in the quality of alumina ceramic, substantial concerns remain regarding CC bearings including stripe wear, limited sizing option, squeaking, and ceramic implant fracture. Limitations of pure alumina characteristics required the development of an advanced ceramic material.

Ceramic composites were the next step in the development of CC bearings. The newest generation of BIOLOX delta ceramic bearings was introduced in 2000 by CeramTec AG (Plochingen, Germany). BIOLOX delta is an alumina-matrix composite (AMC) consisting of 81.6% aluminium oxide, 17% yttria-stabilized tetragonal zirconia particles, and traces (1.4%) of chromium dioxide and strontium crystals engineered to increase material density and reduce grain size (less than 0.8 μm compared with the grain size of alumina 1–5 μm) [14–16]. With these improvements, the risk for crack propagation and component fracture was minimized. Laboratory mechanical and hip simulator wear tests have shown that these manufacturing advances have indeed resulted in a high-strength material with increased fracture toughness and lower wear rates over pure alumina [15, 17].

These enhanced mechanical properties should decrease the ceramic fracture rate, allowing the manufacturing of thinner acetabular liner inserts and therefore the use of larger femoral head options. This increased head size should improve joint stability and reduce dislocation rates [18, 19]. One study also suggests that material properties of the AMC may lead to a different wear response and may decrease or eliminate squeaking [17]. These favorable material characteristics make AMC a very promising material and particularly desirable for long lasting bearing surfaces. However, AMC has a relatively short clinical history and further monitoring is necessary.

The aim of this study was to retrospectively evaluate the short- to midterm clinical and radiographic outcome after primary total hip replacements using the fourth generation ceramic BIOLOX delta implants.

2. Material and Methods

Prior to the onset of the study, institutional review board approval was obtained. We conducted a retrospective evaluation of all patients who received a cementless CC BIOLOX delta THA between December 2004 and December 2009. Our exclusion criteria were a previous total hip replacement, previous hemiarthroplasty, or fusion on the ipsilateral side. In all, we evaluated 60 hips in 50 patients. Among these patients, 10 underwent staged bilateral THAs. There were 10 males (11 hips) and 40 females (49 hips) (Table 1). The mean age at the time of the surgery was 41.8 years (range 21–56 years). All patients underwent primary hip arthroplasty for both noninflammatory and inflammatory degenerative joint diseases. Preoperative diagnoses were osteoarthritis (40%), developmental dysplasia of the hip (22%), rheumatoid arthritis (13%), avascular necrosis (7%), juvenile rheumatoid arthritis (5%), and other causes (11%). Three arthroplasty surgeons performed all procedures through a direct lateral (77%) or posterior approach (23%). Bilateral cases were conducted on separate dates with a mean interval of 10.3 months (3–42 months) between the two procedures.

Twenty-five hips (42%) received 28 mm ceramic heads and 35 hips (58%) received 36 mm ceramic heads, depending on patient anatomy and implant stability. Head size was determined by the inner diameter of the ceramic liner for the corresponding cup size. All patients received one of four cementless Pinnacle acetabular cups (Pinnacle 100, Pinnacle 300, Pinnacle Bantam, Pinnacle Multihole II; DePuy Warsaw, IN) and one of five cementless femoral stems (Summit, Prodigy, Trilock, Corail, or S-ROM; DePuy, Warsaw, IN) (Table 1). Acetabular fixation with screws was used based on the patient's bone quality.

All patients were evaluated clinically and radiographically at 6 weeks, 3 months, and one year postoperatively, followed by subsequent annual examinations. Minimum followup for this study was 2 years, and average followup was 4.6 years (range 2–6.8 years). Preoperative and postoperative Harris hip score (HHS) [20] was recorded. HHS score of 90 points or more was defined as an excellent outcome; 80 to 89 points, a good outcome; 70 to 79 points, a fair outcome; and less than 70 points, a poor outcome. Activity score was assessed preoperatively and postoperatively using the University of California, Los Angeles (UCLA) activity level rating scale from 1 to 10 [21]. Presence of hip squeaking and all postoperative complications were documented. In each visit, serial anteroposterior (AP) radiographs of the pelvis and AP and lateral radiographs of the operated side were obtained. Radiographic analysis was performed using Einzel-Bild-Roentgen-Analyse (EBRA) by two of the authors (AR and AA).

Survival analysis was performed with use of the Kaplan-Meier method [22]. The patient demographics were calculated with arithmetic mean and all errors are reported as standard deviation. A nonparametric Mann-Whitney U test was conducted to determine the significance between preoperative and the last postoperative HHS and UCLA activity scores. All other comparisons between different time

TABLE 1: Demographic data.

Characteristic	Finding
Number of hips	60
Number of patients	50
Age (range)*	41.8 (21–56)
Gender	10 males/40 females
Side of surgery	31 right/29 left
Etiology	
Osteoarthritis	24 (40%)
Congenital dislocation	13 (22%)
Rheumatoid arthritis	8 (13%)
Avascular necrosis	4 (7%)
Juvenile rheumatoid arthritis	3 (5%)
Developmental dysplasia	1 (2%)
Multiple causes	7 (11%)
Femoral head	
BIOLOX delta 28 mm	25 hips (42%)
BIOLOX delta 36 mm	35 hips (58%)
Femoral stem	
S-ROM	41 (69%)
Prodigy	11 (18%)
Summit	3 (5%)
Corail	3 (5%)
Trilock	2 (3%)
Acetabular cup	
Pinnacle 100	37 (62%)
Pinnacle 300	19 (31%)
Pinnacle Bantam	3 (5%)
Pinnacle Multihole II	1 (2%)

*This value is reported as the mean in years.

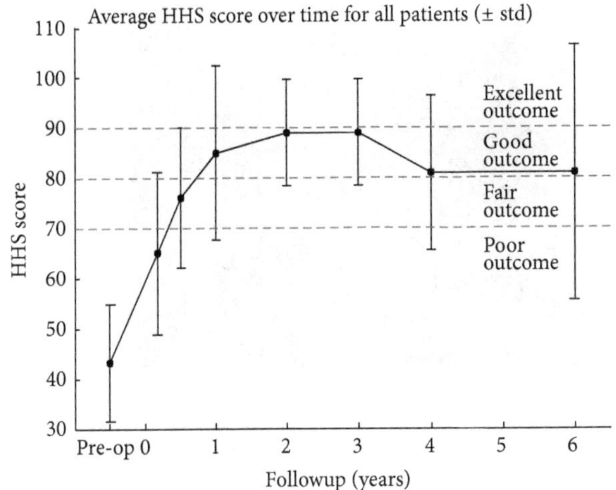

FIGURE 1: Average and standard deviation (SD) values of HHS scores for all patients over time.

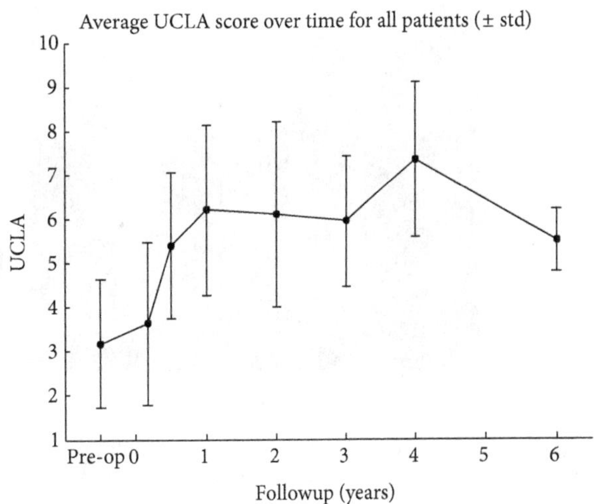

FIGURE 2: Average and standard deviation (SD) values of UCLA activity scores for all patients over time.

points of followup groups were performed using a nonparametric Kruskal-Wallis test followed by a Dunn's multiple comparisons. GraphPad Prism software (GraphPad Software, La Jolla, CA, USA) was used for all data analyses. A P value of less than 0.05 was considered to be statistically significant.

3. Results

All 50 patients had complete clinical and radiographic data at 2 years of followup.

The mean HHS and UCLA scores at last followup significantly improved ($P = 0.00087$) from their preoperative values. The mean HHS score for all patients at their last followup was 88 points (range, 40–99). The mean UCLA activity score was 6 (range, 2–10). Table 3 shows the number of hips showing excellent (HHS > 90), good (90 > HHS > 80), fair (80 > HHS > 70), or poor (HHS < 70) outcomes based on HHS score for all patients as well as those who received 36 mm and 28 mm femoral heads. In all cases, excellent outcomes were observed in 67% of hips, while poor results were only observed in minority of 5% of hips. There were no outcome differences between the two head diameters.

We also looked at the evolution of HHS and UCLA activity score over time. Both scores significantly increased until 4 years postoperatively reaching a plateau thereafter (Figures 1 and 2).

At the time of the final followup, there was no radiographic evidence of component loosening and no evidence of implant subsidence, liner fracture or dislocation. All components were stable and osseous-integrated. The mean acetabular inclination and anteversion were 46 degrees (range, 28 to 58 degrees) and 7 degrees (range, 2 to 22 degrees), respectively (Table 2).

There was a case of deep infection requiring a two-stage revision. One female patient presented with audible repetitive "squeaking" noise that began after a fall 2 years postoperatively. She had a 36 mm head and she was able to

TABLE 2: Clinical and radiographic results at the last followup.

	Preoperative	Final followup
Clinical parameters*		
Harris hip score	45	88 (40–90)
UCLA activity score	3	6 (2–10)
Radiographic parameters*		
Acetabular anteversion	n/a	7° (2°–22°)
Acetabular inclination	n/a	46° (28°–56°)

*The values are reported as the mean.
n/a = not applicable.

TABLE 3: The number of hips showing the clinical outcome based on HHS score.

Total	Excellent	Good	Fair	Poor	
60	40 (67%)	9 (15%)	8 (13%)	3 (5%)	All THAs
25	18 (72%)	4 (16%)	3 (12%)	0 (0%)	28 mm THRs
35	22 (63%)	5 (14%)	5 (14%)	3 (9%)	36 mm THRs

reproduce the squeaking in the office with walking. The cup was found to be in a nonoptimal position, measuring 58° of inclination and 19° of anteversion (Figures 3(a) and 3(b)). The patient was completely pain-free and she refused a revision surgery. The third patient presenting with poor result was a female patient with juvenile rheumatoid arthritis and reduced mobility.

The Kaplan-Meier survival with revision for any reason as the end point was 98.4% at 6 years. In summary, no patients showed osteolysis, one patient had audible squeaking, and only one patient required revision surgery for infection. Both HHS and UCLA activity scores significantly improved after surgery and tended to increase over time. Of all procedures, 72% of 28 mm heads and 63% of 36 mm heads had excellent HHS outcomes. No statistically significant difference was noted between 28 mm and 36 mm heads in both HHS

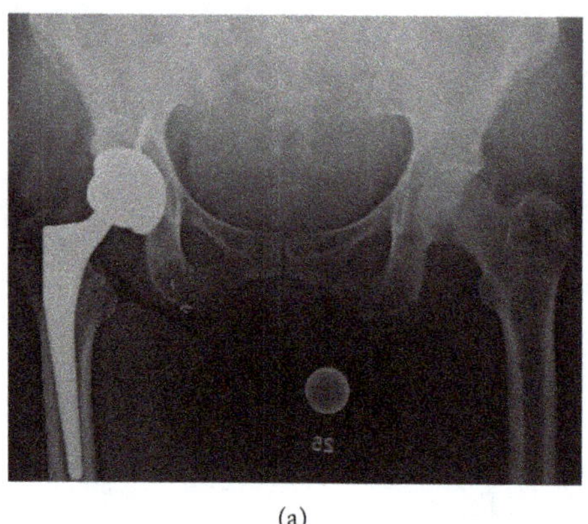

(a)

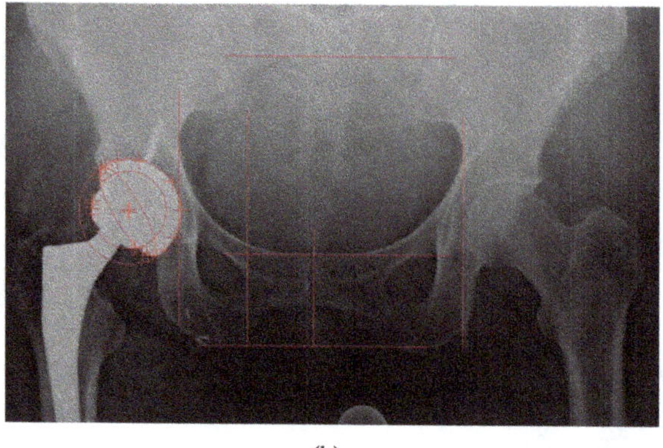

(b)

Figure 3: (a) AP radiograph of the patient presenting with audible hip squeaking. (b) Analysis with the EBRA software revealed cup inclination of 58 degrees and anteversion of 19 degrees.

($P = 0.277$) and UCLA activity score ($P = 0.1029$) at the last followup or at any time point of followup.

4. Discussion

Wear debris-induced osteolysis and subsequent implant loosening are major factors limiting the survivorship and performance of THA. This problem may be overcome with the use of CC bearings known to produce the lowest volumetric wear rate and reduced incidence of periprosthetic osteolysis [23, 24]. Despite their elevated hardness and toughness, the CC surfaces are not immune to wear or surface damage and concerns arising about ceramic implants are chipping and component fracture, stripe wear, and the poorly understood phenomenon of squeaking [12]. Moreover, the lack of large modular options continues to exist [10, 13, 19]. The BIOLOX delta AMC was developed to address some of the drawbacks of currently available alumina designs. Its increased fracture toughness combined with the wider range of head sizes make this implant an attractive selection. In this study our aim was to evaluate the short- and midterm outcome of this new material.

One of the major disadvantages of the alumina ceramic bearing is the risk of fracture. Although sporadic, these component fractures can be catastrophic and continue to be a clinical concern for both surgeon and patient [12]. The CC fracture failure is principally related to the crack propagation and is favoured by stress concentration zones caused by microstructural flaws either at the surface or within the material [25]. Incremental advances in the manufacturing process, design, and quality control of alumina components have addressed these issues improving significantly the structural characteristics and fracture toughness of pure alumina [26].

Currently, component fractures with modern CC bearings are rare (0.004%) [26, 27]. Both D'Antonio et al. [23] and Lusty et al. [5] showed no ceramic bearing fractures in 213 and 301 primary alumina-on-alumina THAs, respectively, at an average of five years. The estimated risk of fracture of these implants is from 0.03% to 0.05% for femoral heads and from 0.017% to 0.013% for the alumina ceramic acetabular insert and is more likely to occur within the first three years following implantation [27]. Furthermore, fractures of 28 mm heads occur more frequent than 32 mm and 36 mm heads [28]. Because of the BIOLOX delta's increased fracture toughness and burst strength, the expectation is that fracture would occur with far less frequency than the estimated fracture rate of alumina ceramic heads (0.02%) [27, 29]. In our study, there was no incidence of head or liner fracture. Moreover, there was no difference between 28 mm and 32 mm heads in terms of clinical and radiological outcome.

In their prospective randomized study, D'Antonio et al. showed that liners that were not fully seated were prone to peripheral chipping during impaction [30]. They observed a peripheral chip in 1.2% of cases; however, none of these resulted in a fracture or in revision surgery. A subsequent design encased the ceramic acetabular component in a titanium sleeve, which eliminates the risk of insertional chips [28, 30].

Recognition of squeaking in ceramic articulations as a clinical problem has increased recently [16, 17, 31] with its incidence ranging from 0.48% to 7% [11, 18, 32]. Squeaking has been shown to be due to ceramic or metal wear, component factors, implant design, impingement, implant positioning [11, 18], and patient characteristics [27]. Squeaking often occurs in younger, heavier, and taller patients [33]. Edge loading appears to be the predominant causative factor for squeaking [33]. Ki et al. showed that increased BMI and certain cup designs were more prone to squeaking [34]. Swanson et al. reviewed 233 patients comparing 4 implant combinations representing 4 manufacturers and found that Trident acetabular cups paired with Stryker Accolade femoral stems showed a dramatically higher incidence of squeaking. They concluded that prosthetic design plays a key role in squeaking occurrence [35]. Another significant cause of squeaking is cup design that results in premature femoral neck-acetabular component rim impingement such as the presence of modular ceramic liner designs that are placed within a titanium encasement with extended rims [29, 34]. Most studies report that squeaking is rare with no clinical consequences [17], but in some studies, squeaking has led to revision [32, 36]. Yang et al. also suggested that squeaking can be reduced due to material properties, such as the wear response of BIOLOX delta [17]. In our study squeaking was noted in only one patient with increased inclination of the acetabular component.

Our study has certain limitations. The number of patients is relatively small, three surgeons were involved using two different approaches, and four acetabular cups matched with five femoral stems were implanted. We also recognize that our study is of relatively short duration with a minimum followup of two years and a mean followup of just over four years. To the best of our knowledge, this is the first study reporting the survival and functional outcome of solely fourth generation ceramic delta implants.

5. Conclusion

Alumina-based ceramic composite materials, with its superior mechanical properties and excellent wear behavior, have been successfully implanted and have offered outstanding performance in the last 11 years. This retrospective study demonstrates that BIOLOX delta bearings provided good to excellent overall functioning outcomes with no implant related complications or osteolysis. An increase in head size did not lead to significantly different HHS and UCLA activity score results. However, the duration of followup is relatively short. Therefore, we cannot conclude whether this new ceramic material will outperform other bearing couplings over time. Long-term follow-up studies are needed to determine the stability and reliability of fourth generation ceramic articulation in THA. However, based on the results we observed and those already present in the literature, fourth generation ceramic bearing couplings appear to be very promising and should be considered for young and active patients.

Conflict of Interests

The authors declare that there is no conflict of interests regarding the publication of this paper.

Acknowledgment

This research was done in the Jewish General Hospital, Department of Orthopaedic Surgery.

References

[1] S. Kurtz, K. Ong, E. Lau, F. Mowat, and M. Halpern, "Projections of primary and revision hip and knee arthroplasty in the United States from 2005 to 2030," *Journal of Bone and Joint Surgery A*, vol. 89, no. 4, pp. 780–785, 2007.

[2] W. H. Harris, "Wear and periprosthetic osteolysis the problem," *Clinical Orthopaedics and Related Research*, no. 393, pp. 66–70, 2001.

[3] J. H. Dumbleton, M. T. Manley, and A. A. Edidin, "A literature review of the association between wear rate and osteolysis in total hip arthroplasty," *Journal of Arthroplasty*, vol. 17, no. 5, pp. 649–661, 2002.

[4] J. Y. Jeong, Y.-M. Kim, S. Y. Kang, K.-H. Koo, S. S. Won, and J. K. Hee, "Alumina-on-alumina total hip arthroplasty: a five-year minimum follow-up study," *Journal of Bone and Joint Surgery A*, vol. 87, no. 3, pp. 530–535, 2005.

[5] P. J. Lusty, C. C. Tai, R. P. Sew-Hoy, W. L. Walter, W. K. Walter, and B. A. Zicat, "Third-generation alumina-on-alumina ceramic bearings in cementless total hip arthroplasty," *Journal of Bone and Joint Surgery A*, vol. 89, no. 12, pp. 2676–2683, 2007.

[6] P. S. Christel, "Biocompatibility of surgical-grade dense polycrystalline alumina," *Clinical Orthopaedics and Related Research*, no. 282, pp. 10–18, 1992.

[7] P. Boutin, "Total hip arthroplasty using a ceramic prosthesis. Pierre Boutin (1924–1989)," *Clinical Orthopaedics and Related Research*, vol. 379, pp. 3–11, 2000.

[8] R. S. Nizard, L. Sedel, P. Christel, A. Meunier, M. Soudry, and J. Witvoet, "Ten-year survivorship of cemented ceramic-ceramic total hip prosthesis," *Clinical Orthopaedics and Related Research*, no. 282, pp. 53–63, 1992.

[9] L. Sedel, R. S. Nizard, L. Kerboull, and J. Witvoet, "Alumina-alumina hip replacement in patients younger than 50 years old," *Clinical Orthopaedics and Related Research*, no. 298, pp. 175–183, 1994.

[10] R. J. Heros and G. Willmann, "Ceramics in total hip arthroplasty: history, mechanical properties, clinical results, and current manufacturing state of the art," *Seminars in Arthroplasty*, vol. 9, pp. 114–122, 1998.

[11] Y.-Z. Cai and S.-G. Yan, "Development of ceramic-on-ceramic implants for total hip arthroplasty," *Orthopaedic Surgery*, vol. 2, no. 3, pp. 175–181, 2010.

[12] G. Willmann, "Cerami femoral head retrieval data," *Clinical Orthopaedics and Related Research*, no. 379, pp. 22–28, 2000.

[13] K. Kawanabe, K. Tanaka, J. Tamura et al., "Effect of alumina femoral head on clinical results in cemented total hip arthroplasty: old versus current alumina," *Journal of Orthopaedic Science*, vol. 10, no. 4, pp. 378–384, 2005.

[14] M. Kuntz, N. Schneider, and R. Heros, "Controlled zirconia phase transformation in biolox delta—a feature of safety," *Ceramics in Orthopeadics*, pp. 79–83, 2006.

[15] J. Y. Jeong, Y.-M. Kim, S. Y. Kang, K.-H. Koo, S. S. Won, and J. K. Hee, "Alumina-on-alumina total hip arthroplasty: a five-year minimum follow-up study," *Journal of Bone and Joint Surgery A*, vol. 87, no. 3, pp. 530–535, 2005.

[16] S. A. Sexton, W. L. Walter, M. P. Jackson, R. De Steiger, and T. Stanford, "Ceramic-on-ceramic bearing surface and risk of revision due to dislocation after primary total hip replacement," *Journal of Bone and Joint Surgery B*, vol. 91, no. 11, pp. 1448–1453, 2009.

[17] C. C. Yang, R. H. Kim, and D. A. Dennis, "The squeaking hip: a cause for concern-disagrees," *Orthopedics*, vol. 30, no. 9, pp. 739–742, 2007.

[18] K. Mai, M. E. Hardwick, R. H. Walker, S. N. Copp, K. A. Ezzet, and C. W. Colwell Jr., "Early dislocation rate in ceramic-on-ceramic total hip arthroplasty," *HSS Journal*, vol. 4, no. 1, pp. 10–13, 2008.

[19] D. J. Berry, M. Von Knoch, C. D. Schleck, and W. S. Harmsen, "Effect of femoral head diameter and operative approach on risk of dislocation after primary total hip arthroplasty," *Journal of Bone and Joint Surgery A*, vol. 87, no. 11, pp. 2456–2463, 2005.

[20] W. H. Harris, "Traumatic arthritis of the hip after dislocation and acetabular fractures: treatment by mold arthroplasty. An end-result study using a new method of result evaluation," *Journal of Bone and Joint Surgery A*, vol. 51, no. 4, pp. 737–755, 1969.

[21] S. Lerouge, O. Huk, L. H. Yahia, and L. Sedel, "Characterization of in vivo wear debris from ceramic-ceramic total hip arthroplasties," *Journal of Biomedical Materials Research A*, vol. 32, no. 4, pp. 627–633, 1996.

[22] E. L. Kaplan and P. Meier, "Nonparametric estimation from incomplete observations," *Journal of the American Statistical Association*, vol. 53, no. 282, pp. 457–481, 1958.

[23] J. D'Antonio, W. Capello, M. Manley, M. Naughton, and K. Sutton, "Alumina ceramic bearings for total hip arthroplasty: five-year results of a prospective randomized study," *Clinical Orthopaedics and Related Research*, no. 436, pp. 164–171, 2005.

[24] R. L. Barrack, C. Burak, and H. B. Skinner, "Concerns about ceramics in THA," *Clinical Orthopaedics and Related Research*, no. 429, pp. 73–79, 2004.

[25] D. Hannouche, C. Nich, P. Bizot, A. Meunier, R. Nizard, and L. Sedel, "Fractures of ceramic bearings: history and present status," *Clinical Orthopaedics and Related Research*, no. 417, pp. 19–26, 2003.

[26] J. A. D'Antonio and K. Sutton, "Ceramic materials as bearing surfaces for total hip arthroplasty," *Journal of the American Academy of Orthopaedic Surgeons*, vol. 17, no. 2, pp. 63–68, 2009.

[27] M. Hamadouche, P. Boutin, J. Daussange, M. E. Bolander, and L. Sedel, "Alumina-on-alumina total hip arthroplasty: a minimum 18.5-year follow-up study," *Journal of Bone and Joint Surgery A*, vol. 84, no. 1, pp. 69–77, 2002.

[28] J. A. D'Antonio, W. N. Capello, M. T. Manley, M. Naughton, and K. Sutton, "A titanium-encased alumina ceramic bearing for total hip arthroplasty: 3- to 5-year results," *Clinical Orthopaedics and Related Research*, no. 441, pp. 151–158, 2005.

[29] Y.-C. Ha, S.-Y. Kim, H. J. Kim, J. J. Yoo, and K.-H. Koo, "Ceramic liner fracture after cementless alumina-on-alumina total hip arthroplasty," *Clinical Orthopaedics and Related Research*, no. 458, pp. 106–110, 2007.

[30] J. A. D'Antonio, W. N. Capello, B. Bierbaum, M. Manley, and M. Naughton, "Ceramic-on-ceramic bearings for total hip arthroplasty: 5-9 year follow-up," *Seminars in Arthroplasty*, vol. 17, no. 3-4, pp. 146–152, 2006.

[31] C. A. Jarrett, A. S. Ranawat, M. Bruzzone, Y. C. Blum, J. A. Rodriguez, and C. S. Ranawat, "The squeaking hip: a phenomenon of ceramic-on-ceramic total hip arthroplasty," *Journal of Bone and Joint Surgery A*, vol. 91, no. 6, pp. 1344–1349, 2009.

[32] C. Restrepo, J. Parvizi, J. Purtill, P. Sharkey, W. Hozack, and R. Rothman, "The noisy ceramic hip: is component malposition the problem?" in *Proceedings of the 16th Annual Meeting of the American Association of Hip and Knee Surgeons*, American Association of Hip and Knee Surgeons, Rosemont, Ill, USA, 2006.

[33] S. J. C. Stanat and J. D. Capozzi, "Squeaking in third- and fourth-generation ceramic-on-ceramic total hip arthroplasty: meta-analysis and systematic review," *Journal of Arthroplasty*, vol. 27, no. 3, pp. 445–453, 2012.

[34] S.-C. Ki, B.-H. Kim, J.-H. Ryu, D.-H. Yoon, and Y.-Y. Chung, "Squeaking sound in total hip arthroplasty using ceramic-on-ceramic bearing surfaces," *Journal of Orthopaedic Science*, vol. 16, no. 1, pp. 21–25, 2011.

[35] T. V. Swanson, D. J. Peterson, R. Seethala, R. L. Bliss, and C. A. Spellmon, "Influence of prosthetic design on squeaking after ceramic-on-ceramic total hip arthroplasty," *The Journal of arthroplasty*, vol. 25, no. 6, pp. 36–42, 2010.

[36] W. L. Walter, G. C. O'Toole, W. K. Walter, A. Ellis, and B. A. Zicat, "Squeaking in ceramic-on-ceramic hips: the importance of acetabular component orientation," *Journal of Arthroplasty*, vol. 22, no. 4, pp. 496–503, 2007.

27

McHale Operation in Patients with Neglected Hip Dislocations: The Importance of Locking Plates

Mark Eidelman,[1] Alexander Katzman,[1] Michael Zaidman,[1] and Yaniv Keren[2]

[1] *Pediatric Orthopedic Surgery Unit, Rambam Health Care Campus, P.O. Box 9602, 31096 Haifa, Israel*
[2] *Department of Orthopedic Surgery, Rambam Health Care Campus, P.O. Box 9602, 31096 Haifa, Israel*

Correspondence should be addressed to Yaniv Keren; y_keren@rambam.health.gov.il

Academic Editor: Padhraig O'Loughlin

Neglected hip dislocation in patients with cerebral palsy is a challenge for the pediatric orthopedic surgeon. Many patients experience pain, limitation of hip motion, and sitting and hygiene problems. Arthrodesis, proximal femoral head resection, and subtrochanteric valgus osteotomy are effective salvage procedures for patients with painful hip dislocation and restricted hip motion when reconstruction of the hip is not possible. Osteopenia is one of the problems that can complicate the postoperative course in these patients. Postoperative cast immobilization may further worsen the osteopenia and can predispose to fractures of the femur after cast removal. Standard plating of the proximal osteotomy may not always provide adequate stability of the fixation. In order to prevent postoperative osteoporotic fractures we use locking plates, without casting. Since 2003 until 2011, we operated on 9 patients (14 hips) with painful neglected hip dislocations. The first three patients (five hips) were operated on using standard nonlocking plates. All other patients (nine hips) were operated on using locking plates. During the followup, the hardware failed in one of these cases. All patients treated with locking plates had not been casted postoperatively, and none had loss of fixation or fractures during the followup.

1. Introduction

Neglected hip dislocation in patients with cerebral palsy is not an unusual problem in patients with severe neurological involvement [1–4]. Usually these patients are nonambulators categorized as gross motor function classification system (GMFCS) of five. Nearly 90 percent of GMFCS IV patients develop some degree of hip displacement [1]. The ideal treatment for hip displacement (dislocation or subluxation) is hip reconstruction combining soft tissue release, varus derotational osteotomy of the femur, and pelvic osteotomy [5–8]. When the femoral head is severely deformed and the acetabulum is too shallow for hip reduction, salvage procedures might be indicated. These patients usually experience hip pain, and their condition does not allow appropriate sitting or adequate nursing and hygiene (Figure 1). Described salvage procedures for nonreconstructible hips include proximal femoral head resection [4, 9, 10], valgus osteotomy [11–13], hip arthrodesis [14, 15], and total hip arthroplasty [16]. In 1990, McHale et al. described their technique of subtrochanteric valgus osteotomy in 5 patients with spastic quadriplegia [11]. All patients were nonambulators and all achieved reasonable results after the procedure. This procedure became popular in cases in which hip reconstruction is not feasible. The technique involves using standard nonlocking plates and spica casting postoperatively to further secure the fixation. Known complications after the McHale procedure are persistent pain, femur fracture, and hardware failure [17].

Patients with severe cerebral palsy frequently suffer from osteopenia, disuse osteoporosis, and bone fragility [18, 19]. In fact, cerebral palsy is the most prevalent childhood condition associated with osteoporosis [20]. Furthermore, bone volumetric density decreases with increasing GMFCS level [21]. This condition may lead to hardware loosening and failure.

In addition, application of a spica cast following surgery in cerebral palsy patients may be associated with osteopenic disuse fractures, mostly distal femur and proximal tibia [5, 7, 22, 23].

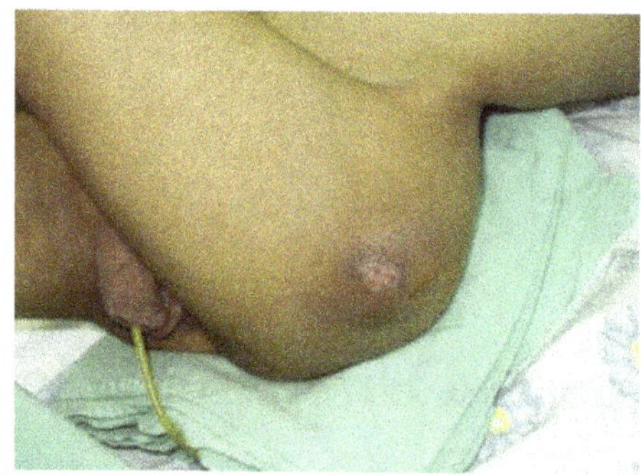

FIGURE 1: Neglected hip dislocation complicated by hip contracture, nursing difficulties, and subsequent pressure sores.

In modern fracture surgery, locking plates gained increasing popularity due to increased rigidity and fracture site stability. These benefits can be precious when treating severe osteoporotic bones, as seen in nonambulatory cerebral palsy patients. Moreover, using these plates might eliminate the need for further securing the fixation with casts and may lead to decreased morbidity following surgery. These plates have been described as alternatives to traditional nonlocking plates in cerebral palsy patients undergoing proximal femoral varus osteotomy [24]. These plates provided stable fixation and are advantageous in osteoporotic bone.

In this study we describe a modification of the original McHale procedure. Instead of using standard plates, we use locking plates, which in turn allow us not to use spica casts postoperatively.

2. Patients and Methods

During 9 years (2003–2011) we operated on 9 patients (14 hips), with neglected hip dislocations (Table 1). All patients had cerebral palsy with spastic diplegia. All patients were GMFCS level 5. Mean age at the time of operation was 18.3 years (range 14–23). All patients suffered from limitation of abduction on the site of the dislocated hip, pain during sitting, and hygiene problems. Five patients were never operated on before, two underwent adductor release, and two others underwent soft tissue release and varus derotation osteotomy.

2.1. Operative Technique. A bump should be placed underneath the sacrum in order to improve access to the affected hip joint. Anterolateral Watson-Jones approach gives excellent exposure to the hip joint and proximal femur (Figure 2(a)). Resection of the femoral head (Figure 2(b)) is performed while the ligamentum teres is preserved for further attachment to the iliopsoas tendon. Subtrochanteric open wedge valgus osteotomy is performed distal to the lesser trochanter taking into account that 3 holes of the LCP plate should be proximal to the created osteotomy. After attachment of the ligamentum teres to the iliopsoas tendon, as originally described by McHale, a 4.5 mm LCP plate (locking compression plate, Synthes) is prebent and contoured to accommodate to the shape of the femur after the osteotomy. The plate is then fixed to the femur using locking screws. An abduction pillow is used for the first 3 weeks after the operation. Gentle passive range of motion and sitting in a wheelchair is allowed immediately following surgery.

3. Results

Mean follow-up period was 74.8 weeks. The first 3 patients were operated on using standard nonlocking broad DCP plates (dynamic compression plate, Synthes). No spica cast was applied following surgery. One patient with bilateral procedure (Figure 3(a)) had lost plate fixation on the right side two weeks postoperatively. The patient was reoperated on using a LCP plate, and a spica cast was applied postoperatively for 3 weeks (Figure 3(b)). After removal of the spica cast pain and swelling were noted over the distal thigh and radiographs revealed a supracondylar femoral fracture (Figure 3(c)). Since then, we changed our protocol and the last six patients were operated on using 4.5 mm LCP plates (Figures 4(a) and 4(b)). Spica cast was not applied postoperatively. All nine patients achieved the preoperative goal: prolonged sitting, unrestricted abduction with easier change of diapers, and perineal care. In the LCP group, none had loss of fixation or post operative fractures.

4. Discussion

Hip displacement is common in nonambulatory cerebral palsy patients with severe neuromuscular involvement. According to Soo et al. [1], the incidence of hip displacement ranges from 0% in patients with gross motor function classification system level 1 (GMFCS) to 90% in patients with GMFCS level 5. Restriction of abduction, pain, pressure sores, and difficulty with sitting and perineal hygiene are well described [2, 3, 12, 25]. However, some advocate that the incidence of pain in patients with hip dislocation is low and neither hip displacement nor osteoarthritis is associated with hip pain. Noonan et al. suggested that surgical treatment should be based on the presence of pain and contracture and not on radiographic appearance of dislocation [26].

The treatment of hip subluxation and dislocation might be challenging. Early careful monitoring may prevent dislocation [27]. However, neglected hip displacement is still common in severely disabled patients with cerebral palsy. Surgical treatment for neglected hip dislocations includes constructive or salvage procedures, from total hip arthroplasty [16], to hip reconstruction [6, 7], subtrochanteric valgus osteotomy without resection of the femoral head [13], resection of the femoral head [9, 28, 29], resection of the femoral head with articulated hip distraction [30], and subtrochanteric valgus osteotomy with femoral head resection [11, 12]. Arthrodesis [14] is another option for nonreconstructible hips.

In 1978 Castle and Schneider [9] described proximal femoral resection and interposition arthroplasty in 12 patients and 14 hips (Castle procedure). The proximal femoral head was resected below the lesser trochanter, and a capsular flap across the acetabulum was constructed. The quadriceps muscle was sutured around the resected end of the femur. Postoperatively all patients were placed in Russell's traction

TABLE 1

N	Age/sex	Diagnosis/GMFCS	Previous hip surgeries	Fixation side	Postoperative spica cast	Followup (weeks)	Complications
1	14/F	Spastic diplegia Bilateral hip dislocation GMFCS 4	STR and VDRO	Nonlocking plate Unilateral	No	108	No
2	16/F	Spastic diplegia GMFCS 5	STR	Nonlocking plating Bilateral Reoperation on the Rt side using locking plate	Initially no 3 weeks of spica following reoperation	103	Loss of fixation on the right femur Reoperation and supracondylar fracture after cast removal
3	19/M	Spastic diplegia GMFCS 5	No	Nonlocking plating Bilateral	For 4 weeks	95	No
4	17	Spastic diplegia GMFCS 5	STR and VDRO	Bilateral LCP	No	87	No
5	23	Spastic diplegia GMFCS 5	No	Unilateral LCP	No	81	No
6	19	Spastic diplegia GMFCS 5	No	Bilateral LCP	No	69	No
7	21	Spastic diplegia GMFCS 5	No	Unilateral LCP	No	56	No
8	19	Spastic diplegia GMFCS 5	STR	Unilateral LCP	No	49	Skin irritation that resolved after plate removal
9	17	Spastic diplegia GMFCS 5	No	Bilateral LCP	No	26	No

STR: soft tissue release.
VDRO: varus derotational osteotomy.
GMFCS: gross motor function classification system.
F: female.
M: male.

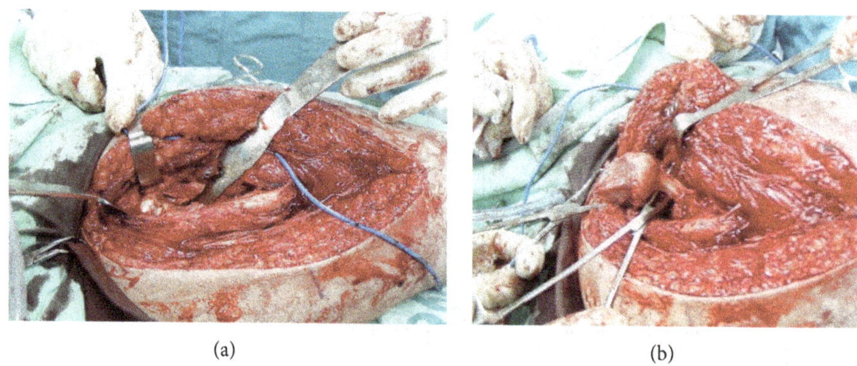

(a) (b)

FIGURE 2: (a) Watson-Jones approach; note wide exposure of the femoral head and proximal shaft. (b) Resection of the femoral head with preservation of ligamentum teres.

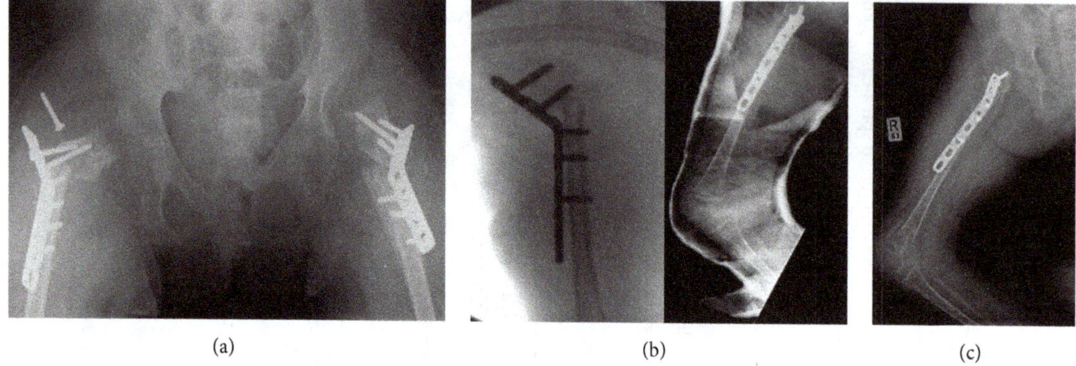

(a) (b) (c)

FIGURE 3: (a) Bilateral procedure with fixation failure on the right side two weeks postoperatively. (b) Reoperation using a LCP plate and a spica cast. (c) Supracondylar femoral fracture after removal of spica cast.

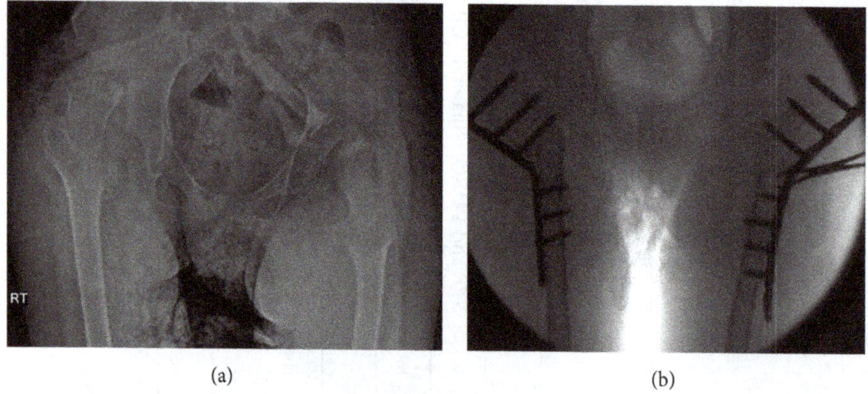

(a) (b)

FIGURE 4: (a) Preoperative radiograph of bilateral hip displacement. Dislocation on the right hip and subluxation on the left hip. (b) Postoperative radiograph of bilateral modified McHale operation, using locking compression plates, and no spica cast.

until healing of soft tissues. These measures were taken in order to prevent recurrence of pain and deformity and proximal migration with gradual adduction deformity. Knaus and Terjesen [28] and Widmann et al. [29] described a similar procedure utilizing interposition of the iliopsoas and gluteal muscles to the hip capsule with improvement of pain, sitting ability, and perineal care.

McHale et al. presented their technique in 1990 in order to lessen the problems associated with the previously described procedures, especially proximal migration of the femur. In their method, placement of the lesser trochanter in the acetabulum prevents proximal migration. Removing the femoral head prevents the pressure generated from the prominence of the femoral head. Furthermore, this technique moves the abductor force laterally. This in turn directs the remaining femur strongly into the acetabulum. According to Leet et al., in the McHale operation, compared to proximal head resection and traction, the length of stay in the hospital is shorter, the postoperative superior migration of the femoral head is less pronounced, and the surgical and medical complications are lower [12].

To our view, the main drawbacks of the McHale procedure are the use of nonlocking plates in osteoporotic bones and the need for spica casting postoperatively. Using modern locking plates provides better stability and eliminates the need for spica casting, with its potential for femur fractures after cast removal.

5. Conclusion

The McHale procedure is widely used due to its effectiveness in achieving the goals of pain relief, increased range of motion, and improved seating ability. This technique was proved to be safe with few complications compared to other salvage procedures. Still, loosening and post spica casting fracture are, to our view, the major drawbacks of the procedure, due to decreased bone mass in these patients. We suggest a modification of using locking plates with no casting postoperatively. To our experience, this change in the technique is reliable and useful and provides the benefits of the original McHale procedure, with lessened morbidity. Therefore we believe that locking plate stabilization of subtrochanteric valgus osteotomy provides the most stable fixation without the need for post operative casting.

Conflict of Interests

The authors declare no conflict of interests regarding the publication of this paper.

References

[1] B. Soo, J. J. Howard, R. N. Boyd et al., "Hip displacement in cerebral palsy," *The Journal of Bone & Joint Surgery*, vol. 88, no. 1, pp. 121–129, 2006.

[2] R. L. Samilson, P. Tsou, G. Aamoth, and W. M. Green, "Dislocation and subluxation of the hip in cerebral palsy. Pathogenesis, natural history and management," *The Journal of Bone & Joint Surgery*, vol. 54, no. 4, pp. 863–873, 1972.

[3] J. E. Lonstein and K. Beck, "Hip dislocation and subluxation in cerebral palsy," *Journal of Pediatric Orthopaedics*, vol. 6, no. 5, pp. 521–526, 1986.

[4] R. B. Abu-Rajab and G. C. Bennet, "Proximal femoral resection-interposition arthroplasty in cerebral palsy," *Journal of Pediatric Orthopaedics B*, vol. 16, no. 3, pp. 181–184, 2007.

[5] S. J. Mubarak, F. G. Valencia, and D. R. Wenger, "One-stage correction of the spastic dislocated hip. Use of pericapsular acetabuloplasty to improve coverage," *The Journal of Bone & Joint Surgery*, vol. 74, no. 9, pp. 1347–1357, 1992.

[6] F. Miller, H. Girardi, G. Lipton, R. Ponzio, M. Klaumann, and K. W. Dabney, "Reconstruction of the dysplastic spastic hip with peri-ilial pelvic and femoral osteotomy followed by immediate mobilization," *Journal of Pediatric Orthopaedics*, vol. 17, no. 5, pp. 592–602, 1997.

[7] R. Brunner and J. U. Baumann, "Long-term effects of intertrochanteric varus-derotation osteotomy on femur and acetabulum in spastic cerebral palsy: an 11-to 18-year follow-up study," *Journal of Pediatric Orthopaedics*, vol. 17, no. 5, pp. 585–591, 1997.

[8] M. Inan, P. G. Gabos, M. Domzalski, F. Miller, and K. W. Dabney, "Incomplete transiliac osteotomy in skeletally mature adolescents with cerebral palsy," *Clinical Orthopaedics and Related Research*, no. 462, pp. 169–174, 2007.

[9] M. E. Castle and C. Schneider, "Proximal femoral resection-interposition arthroplasty," *The Journal of Bone & Joint Surgery*, vol. 60, no. 8, pp. 1051–1054, 1978.

[10] S. Ackerly, C. Vitztum, B. Rockley, and B. Olney, "Proximal femoral resection for subluxation or dislocation of the hip in spastic quadriplegia," *Developmental Medicine and Child Neurology*, vol. 45, no. 7, pp. 436–440, 2003.

[11] K. A. McHale, M. Bagg, and S. S. Nason, "Treatment of the chronically dislocated hip in adolescents with cerebral palsy with femoral head resection and subtrochanteric valgus osteotomy," *Journal of Pediatric Orthopaedics*, vol. 10, no. 4, pp. 504–509, 1990.

[12] A. I. Leet, K. Chhor, F. Launay, J. Kier-York, and P. D. Sponseller, "Femoral head resection for painful hip subluxation in cerebral palsy: is valgus osteotomy in conjunction with femoral head resection preferable to proximal femoral head resection and traction?" *Journal of Pediatric Orthopaedics*, vol. 25, no. 1, pp. 70–73, 2005.

[13] K. A. Hogan, M. Blake, and R. H. Gross, "Subtrochanteric valgus osteotomy for chronically dislocated, painful spastic hips," *The Journal of Bone & Joint Surgery*, vol. 88, no. 12, pp. 2624–2631, 2006.

[14] L. Root, J. R. Goss, and J. Mendes, "The treatment of the painful hip in cerebral palsy by total hip replacement or hip arthrodesis," *The Journal of Bone & Joint Surgery*, vol. 68, no. 4, pp. 590–598, 1986.

[15] P. M. M. B. Fucs, C. Svartman, R. M. C. Assumpção, H. H. Yamada, and D. R. Rancan, "Is arthrodesis the end in spastic hip disease?" *Journal of Pediatric Rehabilitation Medicine*, vol. 4, no. 3, pp. 163–169, 2011.

[16] B. S. Raphael, J. S. Dines, M. Akerman, and L. Root, "Long-term followup of total hip arthroplasty in patients with cerebral palsy," *Clinical Orthopaedics and Related Research*, vol. 468, no. 7, pp. 1845–1854, 2010.

[17] A. van Riet and P. Moens, "The McHale procedure in the treatment of the painful chronically dislocated hip in adolescents and adults with cerebral palsy," *Acta Orthopaedica Belgica*, vol. 75, no. 2, pp. 181–188, 2009.

[18] E. Aronson and S. B. Stevenson, "Bone health in children with cerebral palsy and epilepsy," *Journal of Pediatric Health Care*, vol. 26, no. 3, pp. 193–199, 2012.

[19] S. D. Apkon and H. H. Kecskemethy, "Bone health in children with cerebral palsy," *Journal of Pediatric Rehabilitation Medicine*, vol. 1, no. 2, pp. 115–121, 2008.

[20] C. M. Houlihan and R. D. Stevenson, "Bone density in cerebral palsy," *Physical Medicine and Rehabilitation Clinics of North America*, vol. 20, no. 3, pp. 493–508, 2009.

[21] T. Al Wren, D. C. Lee, R. M. Kay, F. J. Dorey, and V. Gilsanz, "Bone density and size in ambulatory children with cerebral palsy," *Developmental Medicine & Child Neurology*, vol. 53, no. 2, pp. 137–141, 2011.

[22] P. F. Sturm, B. A. Alman, and B. L. Christie, "Femur fractures in institutionalized patients after hip spica immobilization," *Journal of Pediatric Orthopaedics*, vol. 13, no. 2, pp. 246–248, 1993.

[23] L. Root, F. J. LaPlaza, S. N. Brourman, and D. H. Angel, "The severely unstable hip in cerebral palsy. Treatment with

open reduction, pelvic osteotomy, and femoral osteotomy with shortening," *The Journal of Bone & Joint Surgery*, vol. 77, no. 5, pp. 703–712, 1995.

[24] E. Rutz and R. Brunner, "The pediatric LCP hip plate for fixation of proximal femoral osteotomy in cerebral palsy and severe osteoporosis," *Journal of Pediatric Orthopaedics*, vol. 30, no. 7, pp. 726–731, 2010.

[25] J. W. Pritchet, "The untreated unstable hip in severe cerebral palsy," *Clinical Orthopaedics and Related Research*, vol. 173, pp. 169–172, 1983.

[26] K. J. Noonan, J. Jones, J. Pierson, N. J. Honkamp, and G. Leverson, "Hip function in adults with severe cerebral palsy," *The Journal of Bone & Joint Surgery*, vol. 86, no. 12, pp. 2607–2613, 2004.

[27] G. Hägglund, S. Andersson, H. Düppe, H. Lauge-Pedersen, E. Nordmark, and L. Westbom, "Prevention of dislocation of the hip in children with cerebral palsy. The first ten years of a population-based prevention programme," *The Journal of Bone & Joint Surgery*, vol. 87, no. 1, pp. 95–101, 2005.

[28] A. Knaus and T. Terjesen, "Proximal femoral resection arthroplasty for patients with cerebral palsy and dislocated hips," *Acta Orthopaedica*, vol. 80, no. 1, pp. 32–36, 2009.

[29] R. F. Widmann, T. T. Do, S. M. Doyle, S. W. Burke, and L. Root, "Resection arthroplasty of the hip for patients with cerebral palsy: an outcome study," *Journal of Pediatric Orthopaedics*, vol. 19, no. 6, pp. 805–810, 1999.

[30] M. Lampropulos, M. H. Puigdevall, D. Zapozko, and H. R. Malvárez, "Proximal femoral resection and articulated hip distraction with an external fixator for the treatment of painful spastic hip dislocations in pediatric patients with spastic quadriplegia," *Journal of Pediatric Orthopaedics B*, vol. 17, no. 1, pp. 27–31, 2008.

28

Enhanced Recovery Protocol Reduces Transfusion Requirements and Hospital Stay in Patients Undergoing an Elective Arthroplasty Procedure

Kirsten Juliette de Burlet,[1] James Widnall,[1] Cefin Barton,[1] Veera Gudimetla,[2] and Stephen Duckett[1]

[1]*Department of Orthopaedic Surgery, Leighton Hospital, Crewe CW1 4QJ, UK*
[2]*Department of Anaesthetics, Leighton Hospital, Crewe CW1 4QJ, UK*

Correspondence should be addressed to Kirsten Juliette de Burlet; kjdeburlet@gmail.com

Academic Editor: Padhraig O'Loughlin

Background. Enhanced recovery (ER) for elective total hip or total knee replacement has become common practice. The aim of this study is to evaluate the impact of ER on transfusion rates and incidence of venous thromboembolism (VTE). *Methods.* A comprehensive review was undertaken of all patients who underwent primary hip or knee arthroplasty surgery electively between January 2011 and December 2013 at our institution. ER was implemented in August 2012, thus creating two cohorts: the traditional protocol (TP) group and the ER group. Outcome measurements of length of stay, postoperative transfusion, thromboembolic complications, and number of readmissions were assessed. *Main Findings.* 1262 patients were included. The TP group contained a total of 632 patients and the ER group contained 630 patients. Postoperative transfusion rate in the ER group was reduced with 45% ($P \leq 0.05$). There was no statistical difference in postoperative VTE complications. The length of stay was reduced from 5.5 days to 4.8 days ($P < 0.05$). *Conclusions.* There was no difference in the number of readmissions. ER has contributed to a significant decrease in transfusions after elective arthroplasty surgery, with no increase in the incidence of thromboembolic events. Furthermore, it has significantly reduced inpatient length of stay.

1. Introduction

Several studies advocating enhanced recovery (ER) or fast-track protocol for elective total hip or total knee replacement have been published and it is becoming the common practice for arthroplasty surgery in most hospitals in the United Kingdom. ER protocols are commonly developed and tailored to given units routine practice, but common themes include preoperative patient education, perioperative administration of tranexamic acid and defined standards for anaesthesia and postoperative analgesia, fluid management, and early mobilisation. This multidisciplinary approach has been proven to be beneficial for the patient with a significant reduction of early postoperative complications and a reduction in length of stay (LOS) [1–5].

Intravenous administration of tranexamic acid prior to surgery has been proven to reduce perioperative blood loss and postoperative transfusion rate [6, 7]. There have been historic concerns regarding increased risk of thromboembolism with its use but several recent studies appear to contradict this view [8].

Reducing LOS with a given ER protocol has obvious potential cost benefits and there is increasing evidence that it does not lead to an increase in the number of readmissions [1–3]. Furthermore, a combined multidisciplinary approach and comprehensive preoperative patient education have resulted in higher patient satisfaction scores [1, 9–11].

Our aim was to evaluate the ER protocol in our hospital. Our main outcome measures were transfusion rate, number of VTE complications, and overall LOS.

Table 1: Traditional protocol versus enhanced recovery protocol.

	Traditional protocol	Enhanced recovery protocol
Preoperative	(i) Generic patient education	(i) Patient education and emphasis on active patient participation—"joint school" (ii) Energy drink 2 hrs before surgery (iii) Premedication: omeprazole 20 mg PO and gabapentin 300 mg PO
Perioperative	(i) General or spinal anaesthesia according to anaesthetist's preferences	(i) Spinal anaesthesia: 3 mL of 0.5% levobupivacaine (ii) Antibiotics: 1.2 g co-amoxiclav (iii) Tranexamic acid 1 g IV (iv) Medication: Paracetamol 1g IV, Ondansetron 4 mg IV, Dexamethasone 6.6 mg IV (v) Local infiltration: 100 mL of 0.2% ropivacaine with 1 in 100000 adrenaline and 50 mLs of plain 0.2% ropivacaine for skin and subcutaneous tissues
Postoperative	(i) Enoxaparin 48 hrs after surgery (ii) Analgesia and fluid management according to consultants preferences (iii) Involving femoral/sciatic nerve blocks and PCAs for all patients (iv) Physiotherapy without a specific postoperative protocol—mobilised when nerve blocks wear off at variable duration	(i) Enoxaparin started the same day (ii) Multimodal analgesia management by acute pain team and ward staff using oxycodone regime. No PCA/nerve blocks (iii) Fluid monitoring (iv) Early mobilisation with physiotherapy—the same day or early next day

2. Materials and Methods

The ER protocol was officially implemented in our institution in August 2012. Initially a pilot protocol was implemented in May 2012 based on the existing protocol from the Robert Jones and Agnes Hunt Orthopaedic Hospital in Oswestry, United Kingdom. The pilot protocol was audited and after minor adjustments the current protocol (shown in Table 1) was implemented. Prior to implementation, there was a formal educational process for all staff involved including physiotherapist, nursing staff, and occupational therapists. For this study we retrospectively included all patients who underwent an elective total hip or total knee replacement between January 2011 and December 2013. Any revision arthroplasty procedures were excluded. Thus, two cohorts were created in accordance with their date of operation: the traditional protocol (TP) group and the ER group. We retrospectively collected all the data from operation notes, discharge letters, laboratory, and radiology reports. Ninety-day complication and readmission rates were included.

The preoperative management, perioperative management, and postoperative management of the TP and the ER protocol are shown in Table 1. Patients were initially assessed in the orthopaedic outpatient department, where they were counselled about what to expect during their inpatient journey. They also received a patient information leaflet. Post-operative analgesia included OxyContin 10–20 mg PO every 12 hours for the first three days, Gabapentin 300 mg at night for five days, Naproxen every 12 hours (if not contraindicated, eGFR < 60 mLs/min/m^2), omeprazole 20 mg PO for 5 days (continued when NSAID was continued), and Paracetamol 1 g four times a day IV which was changed to oral after 24 hrs.

All patients received antibiotic prophylaxis within 60 minutes prior to incision. Co-amoxiclav (Augmentin®) 1.2 g was administered intravenously according to our hospital policy. Patients who were allergic to penicillin received Teicoplanin (Targocid®) 600 mg IV instead.

The surgical implants used did not change during the study period. All procedures were performed by 5 experienced arthroplasty consultants. No wound drains were used.

Patients were discharged home when the following criteria were met: postoperative pain was well controlled; the individual was able to move independently using appropriate walking aids, voiding urine normally and opening their bowels at least once after surgery. These criteria did not change during our study period. There was a follow-up phone call from the orthopaedic ward 48 hours after discharge to ensure that the patients continued to recover as expected and to give individuals opportunity to express any concerns.

Postoperative blood transfusion was considered when a haemoglobin (Hb) drop of more than 40 g/L was seen or when the postoperative Hb was lower than 80 g/L for patients with no cardiovascular history and 90 g/L for patients with a significant cardiovascular history. Oral supplementary iron tablets were prescribed when a patient had a moderate Hb drop of <30 g/L or a postoperative Hb of 90–110 g/L.

Comparison between the two cohorts was performed with Student's t-test and Chi-square test, and Mann-Whitney U tests were used to analyse differences. Data analyses were performed using SPSS® software (SPSS 20, Chicago,

TABLE 2: Patient characteristics.

	Traditional protocol (n = 638)	Enhanced protocol (n = 629)	P value
Age (mean [SD])	69.6 [9.1]	69.5 [10.2]	0.072
Gender			
Female (%)	352 (55.2%)	343 (54.5%)	0.819
Procedure (%)			
THR	323 (50.6%)	324 (51.5%)	0.753
TKR	315 (49.4%)	305 (48.5%)	
Length of stay (mean/median (range))	5.5/4.0 (2–92)	4.8/4.0 (1–41)*	<0.001
Readmission	21 (3.3%)	17 (2.7%)	0.539

Note: length of stay is in days. There is no significant difference in age, gender, operation, and readmission. There is a significant difference for length of stay, $P = 0.001$, using Mann-Whitney's test.
*Value is significant.

Illinois, USA). A P value of <0.05 was considered statistically significant.

3. Results

A total of 1267 patients were included, 638 in the traditional protocol (TP) group and 629 in the enhanced recovery (ER) group. There were no significant differences in age or gender between the two groups and the distributions of THR and TKR were equal between the groups (Table 2). The length of stay (LOS) was significantly shorter in the ER group (P = 0.001). There were 21 (3.3%) readmissions in the traditional protocol group and 17 (2.7%) in the ER group; this was not statistically significant.

In total 76 patients received a blood transfusion during the study period (Table 3). In the TP group, the number of transfusions was 49 (7.7%) and in the ER group it was 27 (4.3%); this was a statistically significant difference ($P \le 0.001$). Patients undergoing a THR during the study period were more likely to receive a blood transfusion (n = 49 (7.6%)) compared to patients who underwent a TKR (n = 27 (4.4%)) (P = 0.011). There was a drop in the number of patients who underwent a blood transfusion between the TR group and the ER group for both procedures. In the TR group 33 (10.2%) patients who had a THR needed a blood transfusion; this number was 16 (4.9%) for the ER group. This was also found to be statistically significant difference (P = 0.008). For the TKR patients, 19 (6.0%) received a blood transfusion in the TP group and 8 (2.6%) received a blood transfusion in the ER group (P = 0.029). The odds ratio for receiving a blood transfusion in the ER group was 0.45 (95% CI: 0.27 to 0.74).

There was no difference in the mean preoperative, postoperative, or discharge haemoglobin level for the patients who underwent a blood transfusion. The number of units transfused was equal between the TP group and the ER group.

Table 4 shows the mean LOS in days per different category. For patients undergoing a THR or TKR the mean

TABLE 3: Transfusion.

	Traditional protocol (n = 52)	Enhanced protocol (n = 24)	P value
Procedure (n (%))			
THR	33 (63.5%)	16 (66.7%)	0.008
TKR	19 (36.5%)	8 (33.3%)	0.029
Hemoglobin (g/L)			
Preop.	118.3 [13.0]	125.7 [12.7]	0.957
Postop.	78.3 [8.3]	89.9 [14.1]	0.021
Discharge	100.0 [7.4]	106.0 [11.5]	0.125
Units (mean)	2.14 [0.6]	2.15 [0.6]	0.772
Anticoagulant (n)			
Aspirin/clopidogrel	4 (8.2%)	4 (14.8%)	0.366
Warfarin	10 (20.4%)	6 (22.2%)	0.952

Note: this table only shows data of the patients who received a blood transfusion in our cohort. Less patients were transfused in the ER group ($P \le 0.001$). There was no statistical difference between the other values in this table (Chi-square test).

TABLE 4: Length of stay.

	Traditional protocol (n = 638)	Enhanced recovery (n = 629)	P value
Operation (mean [SD])			
THR	5.8 [7.0]	4.7 [3.3]	<0.001
TKR	5.2 [4.0]	4.9 [3.5]	0.012
Blood transfusion			
No	5.1 [5.1]	4.5 [3.0]	<0.001
Yes	10.3 [9.2]	10.8 [6.3]	0.416
Age (yr)			
30–50	4.1 [1.4]	3.7 [4.7]	0.002
50–60	4.2 [2.4]	4.0 [2.1]	0.457
60–70	4.5 [3.6]	3.9 [1.9]	0.001
70–80	6.3 [7.1]	5.2 [4.0]	<0.001
80–91	8.4 [7.6]	7.0 [3.9]	0.372
Gender			
Male	5.4 [6.3]	4.6 [3.9]	<0.001
Female	5.7 [5.2]	4.9 [2.9]	0.002

Note: length of stay is a mean value in days. All outcomes are significantly different (Mann-Whitney's test).

LOS dropped significantly ($P \le 0.001$ and 0.012, resp.). However, the most significant drop was seen for the patients undergoing a THR. Patients undergoing a blood transfusion stayed in hospital longer compared to patients who did not undergo a blood transfusion ($P \le 0.001$). A correlation between increasing age and a longer LOS was demonstrated. Female patients undergoing a THR or a TKR were more likely to stay in hospital longer (P = 0.001). Seventy-one (5.6%) patients were discharged to an *intermediate care facility*; no difference was found in this number between the ER group and TP group.

Table 5: Complications.

	Traditional protocol ($n = 638$)	Enhanced protocol ($n = 629$)
Thromboembolic complications		
PE	2 (0.3%)	2 (0.3%)
DVT	7 (1.1%)	5 (0.8%)
Other cardiovascular complications	2 (0.3%)	3 (0.5%)
Cerebrovascular complications	3 (0.5%)	1 (0.2%)
Other complications		
Pneumonia	13 (2.0%)	8 (1.3%)
Haematoma	2 (0.3%)	1 (0.2%)
Wound infection	8 (1.3%)	7 (1.1%)
Gastric ulcer	2 (0.3%)	1 (0.2%)

Note: there is no significant difference for all complications between the traditional protocol and enhanced protocol (Chi-square test).

There was a total observed complications rate of 6.0% in the TP group and 4.5% in the ER group, which is illustrated in Table 5. The spread of complications was comparable across both groups. There was no difference in VTE related complications between the groups. During the study period 7 patients died within 90 days after surgery. In the TP group, two patients died of pneumonia, one patient died of the complications after a severe stroke, and one patient died of a cardiac arrest. In the ER group, two patients had a cardiac arrest and one patient died of pneumonia.

4. Discussion

This study demonstrates that, since the introduction of our local ER protocol, blood transfusion for patients undergoing elective total hip or total knee replacement has been significantly reduced, without increasing the number of VTE complications. Furthermore, there was a reduction in mean LOS, especially for the patients undergoing a THR, without an increase in the number of readmissions.

The number of blood transfusions dropped significantly in the ER group, with an odds ratio of 0.45 (95% CI: 0.27 to 0.74). This is most likely the result of the combination of tranexamic acid and local adrenaline infiltration. There are multiple studies reporting the benefits of tranexamic acid for reducing blood transfusion rates for patients undergoing elective arthroplasty [12–14]. Although blood transfusions do not seem to be related to an increased mortality rate [15], they are related to a higher rate of wound infection and can lead to severe transfusion reactions [16, 17]. Furthermore, blood transfusion has a significant associated cost (£125 per unit, ref. NHS Blood and Transplant 2012).

The postoperative haemoglobin drop was equal in both the TP group and the ER group. The number of units transfused was also comparable between the groups. This supports the fact that transfusion practice did not change in the study period.

The LOS significantly reduced in the ER group. We found that LOS was associated with certain patient characteristics. In the ER group, patients undergoing a THR stayed for an equal period of time in hospital compared with the TKR group. Before implementation of the protocol the length of stay was, on average, a day longer compared to the TKR patient group. Patients whose postoperative recovery was complicated with severe blood loss requiring a blood transfusion stayed longer in hospital (mean of 10.5 days), compared to the patients who did not receive blood (5.2 days) ($P \leq 0.001$). Increasing age was directly correlated to prolonged hospital stay; this is in line with other comparable studies [1, 18, 19]. This is most likely directly related to the increased incidence of comorbidities with age and social circumstances. Whilst occupational therapists are members of our arthroplasty MDT, their role between pre-ER protocol and post-ER protocol did not change. They routinely assess patients in the postoperative period to facilitate discharge. This was the case for both patient cohorts. A potential area of improvement to bring down LOS would be to see if this process could be any more efficient. Nevertheless, this study shows clearly that the elderly patient has more benefit from the ER protocol compared to the younger patient.

Females had a longer LOS compared to males, which has been previously shown in other studies [1, 18]. There is no clear explanation for this finding. Both females and males benefitted equally from the ER approach.

Readmission rates in our study were low (3.3% in TP group and 2.7% in ER group) and there was no difference in the number of readmissions between the two groups ($P = 0.327$). Compared to similar study designs our readmission rate was remarkably lower (2.7% versus 5%, Husted et al., 2008 [1], and 4.8%, Malviya et al., 2011 [3]). However, our mean LOS was longer compared to other similar studies (4.8 days, ER group, in our study versus 3.8 days, Husted et al., 2008 [1], and 3.7 days, Malviya et al., 2011 [3]).

During the study period the number of VTE complications did not differ between the TP group and the ER group. There are studies which reported a reduced incidence of VTE events in their ER group; this effect is most likely due to the early mobilisation and adequate VTE prophylaxis [2, 4]. There was no significant difference in the incidence of other complications between the TP group and the ER group. There may be a small trend towards fewer complications in the ER group, but this study is underpowered to properly assess this.

Limitations of our study are in the retrospective design. Furthermore, the TP group and the ER group are from different time periods. Although no differences in distribution of the patients were identified and no other changes in treatment for elective arthroplasty were made other than the implementation of the ER protocol, this may be a confounding factor. The reduction in the number of postoperative transfusions in the ER group is most likely due to a combination of local injection of adrenalin, tranexamic acid, and standardised wound management. Tranexamic acid is potentially, given the previously published results, the largest contributing factor to this reduction [6–8].

The enhanced recovery protocol compromises multiple factors of which perioperative tranexamic acid, early mobilisation, adequate analgesia monitored by a specialised "pain team," and start of anticoagulation immediately postoperatively are the most important. This study showed a reduction in LOS which is likely to be multifactorial.

In conclusion, our ER protocol led to a significant reduction in postoperative transfusion rate after elective TKR and THR, without an increased incidence of VTE complications. Furthermore, a significant reduction in LOS without an increase in the number of readmissions was seen in the ER group. The reduction in both LOS and blood transfusions has obvious beneficial cost implications.

Competing Interests

The authors declare that they have no competing interests.

References

[1] H. Husted, G. Holm, and S. Jacobsen, "Predictors of length of stay and patient satisfaction after hip and knee replacement surgery: fast-track experience in 712 patients," *Acta Orthopaedica*, vol. 79, no. 2, pp. 168–173, 2008.

[2] S. K. Khan, A. Malviya, S. D. Muller et al., "reduced short-term complications and mortality following enhanced recovery primary hip and knee arthroplasty: results from 6,000 consecutive procedures," *Acta Orthopaedica*, vol. 85, no. 1, pp. 26–31, 2014.

[3] A. Malviya, K. Martin, I. Harper et al., "Enhanced recovery program for hip and knee replacement reduces death rate: a study of 4,500 consecutive primary hip and knee replacements," *Acta Orthopaedica*, vol. 82, no. 5, pp. 577–581, 2011.

[4] M. S. Ibrahim, H. Twaij, D. E. Giebaly, I. Nizam, and F. S. Haddad, "Enhanced recovery in total hip replacement: a clinical review," *The Bone & Joint Journal*, vol. 95, no. 12, pp. 1587–1594, 2013.

[5] D. B. Auyong, C. J. Allen, J. A. Pahang, J. J. Clabeaux, K. M. MacDonald, and N. A. Hanson, "Reduced length of hospitalization in primary total knee arthroplasty patients using an updated enhanced recovery after orthopedic surgery (ERAS) pathway," *Journal of Arthroplasty*, vol. 30, no. 10, pp. 1705–1709, 2015.

[6] C. M. Duncan, B. P. Gillette, A. K. Jacob, R. J. Sierra, J. Sanchez-Sotelo, and H. M. Smith, "Venous thromboembolism and mortality associated with tranexamic acid use during total hip and knee arthroplasty," *Journal of Arthroplasty*, vol. 30, no. 2, pp. 272–276, 2015.

[7] Q. Wu, H.-A. Zhang, S.-L. Liu, T. Meng, X. Zhou, and P. Wang, "Is tranexamic acid clinically effective and safe to prevent blood loss in total knee arthroplasty? A meta-analysis of 34 randomized controlled trials," *European Journal of Orthopaedic Surgery and Traumatology*, vol. 25, no. 3, pp. 525–541, 2015.

[8] J. Xie, J. Ma, P. Kang et al., "Does tranexamic acid alter the risk of thromboembolism following primary total knee arthroplasty with sequential earlier anticoagulation? A large, single center, prospective cohort study of consecutive cases," *Thrombosis Research*, vol. 136, no. 2, pp. 234–238, 2015.

[9] S. Jones, M. Alnaib, M. Kokkinakis, M. Wilkinson, A. St Clair Gibson, and D. Kader, "Pre-operative patient education reduces length of stay after knee joint arthroplasty," *Annals of the Royal College of Surgeons of England*, vol. 93, no. 1, pp. 71–75, 2011.

[10] L. S. Moulton, P. A. Evans, I. Starks, and T. Smith, "Pre-operative education prior to elective hip arthroplasty surgery improves postoperative outcome," *International Orthopaedics*, vol. 39, no. 8, pp. 1483–1486, 2015.

[11] J. T. Machin, S. Phillips, M. Parker, J. Carrannante, and M. W. Hearth, "Patient satisfaction with the use of an enhanced recovery programme for primary arthroplasty.," *Annals of the Royal College of Surgeons of England*, vol. 95, no. 8, pp. 577–581, 2013.

[12] E. Irisson, Y. Hémon, V. Pauly, S. Parratte, J.-N. Argenson, and F. Kerbaul, "Tranexamic acid reduces blood loss and financial cost in primary total hip and knee replacement surgery," *Orthopaedics & Traumatology: Surgery & Research*, vol. 98, no. 5, pp. 477–483, 2012.

[13] M. Sukeik, S. Alshryda, F. S. Haddad, and J. M. Mason, "Systematic review and meta-analysis of the use of tranexamic acid in total hip replacement," *Journal of Bone and Joint Surgery B*, vol. 93, no. 1, pp. 39–46, 2011.

[14] S. Alshryda, P. Sarda, M. Sukeik, A. Nargol, J. Blenkinsopp, and J. M. Mason, "Tranexamic acid in total knee replacement: a systematic review and meta-analysis," *The Journal of Bone & Joint Surgery—British Volume*, vol. 93, no. 12, pp. 1577–1585, 2011.

[15] J. L. Carson, F. Sieber, D. R. Cook et al., "Liberal versus restrictive blood transfusion strategy: 3-year survival and cause of death results from the FOCUS randomised controlled trial," *The Lancet*, vol. 385, no. 9974, pp. 1183–1189, 2015.

[16] N. B. Frisch, N. M. Wessell, M. A. Charters, S. Yu, J. J. Jeffries, and C. D. Silverton, "Predictors and complications of blood transfusion in total hip and knee arthroplasty," *Journal of Arthroplasty*, vol. 29, no. 9, pp. 189–192, 2014.

[17] S. Engelbrecht, E. M. Wood, and M. F. Cole-Sinclair, "Clinical transfusion practice update: haemovigilance, complications, patient blood management and national standards," *Medical Journal of Australia*, vol. 199, no. 6, pp. 397–401, 2013.

[18] H. Husted, H. C. Hansen, G. Holm et al., "What determines length of stay after total hip and knee arthroplasty? A nationwide study in Denmark," *Archives of Orthopaedic and Trauma Surgery*, vol. 130, no. 2, pp. 263–268, 2010.

[19] J. H. Hayes, R. Cleary, W. J. Gillespie, I. M. Pinder, and J. L. Sher, "Are clinical and patient assessed outcomes affected by reducing length of hospital stay for total hip arthroplasty?" *Journal of Arthroplasty*, vol. 15, no. 4, pp. 448–452, 2000.

29

A Novel Technique for Proximal Hamstring Tendon Repair: High Reoperation Rate in a Series of 56 Patients

William Blakeney,[1,2] Simon Zilko,[1] Wael Chiri,[1] and Peter Annear[2,3]

[1] *Department of Orthopaedics, Royal Perth Hospital, Perth, WA 6000, Australia*
[2] *Department of Orthopaedics, Mount Hospital, Perth, WA 6000, Australia*
[3] *Perth Orthopaedics and Sports Medicine Centre, Perth, WA 6005, Australia*

Correspondence should be addressed to William Blakeney; blakeney@gmail.com

Academic Editor: Federico Canavese

This investigation looked at functional outcomes, following a novel technique of surgical repair using table staples. Patients underwent surgery for proximal hamstring rupture with table staples used to hold the tendon reapproximated to the ischial tuberosity. Functional outcomes following surgery were assessed. We also used a combined outcome assessment measure: the Perth Hamstring Assessment Tool (PHAT). A total of 56 patients with a mean age of 51 (range 15–71) underwent surgery. The mean follow-up duration was 26 months (range 8–59 months). A large proportion of patients (21/56, 37.5%) required reoperation for removal of the staple. Patients that did not require removal of the table staple did well postoperatively, with low pain scores (0.8–2 out of 10) and good levels of return to sport or running (75.8%). Those that required removal of the staple had a significantly lower PHAT score prior to removal, 47.8, but this improved markedly once the staple was removed, with a mean of 77.2 ($P < 0.001$). Although our patients achieved similar outcomes in terms of pain and function, we thought the reoperation rate was unacceptably high. We would not recommend proximal hamstring tendon repair using this technique.

1. Introduction

Proximal hamstring rupture from the ischial tuberosity occurs acutely following an injury involving sudden hip flexion with an extended knee. It is often seen in athletes with a peak incidence in middle-aged individuals [1]. Surgical repair results in significantly better outcomes, including greater rate of return to sport, greater strength/endurance, and better subjective outcomes than nonsurgical treatment [2]. There have been a number of proposed surgical methods for the treatment of proximal hamstring injuries. A well-described technique is using bioabsorbable or metal suture anchors [3]. Some surgeons use suture-only fixation with or without bone tunnels. Others have used headless metal interference screw fixation with Achilles allograft reconstruction [4]. A systematic review which included 298 patients found a rerupture rate of 2.7% [2].

Table staples have been extensively used in the past for ligament repairs and reconstructions. They have been used to augment Anterior Cruciate Ligament (ACL), Medial Collateral Ligament, and posterolateral corner repairs [5–7]. Repair of proximal hamstring tendon ruptures with table staples has not, that we are aware of, been reported in the literature.

The trial surgeon (PA) performed a number of repairs of proximal hamstring tendons with table staples over a two-year period. It was hoped that this technique would increase the strength of surgical repair and decrease rerupture rates. We noticed a high number of patients following surgery with ongoing localised pain related to the table staple. Many of these required surgery to remove the staple. We did a retrospective review of a series of proximal hamstring injuries that had repairs with table staples.

2. Methodology

2.1. Eligibility Criteria. Symptomatic patients, between the ages of 15 and 75, with MRI confirmed injuries of the proximal hamstring origin who were fit and willing to undergo

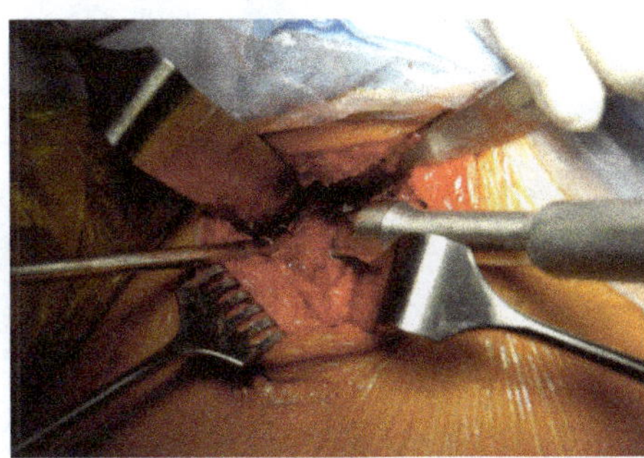

Figure 1

surgical repair were included. This included acute incomplete ruptures with retraction >2 cm or chronic incomplete ruptures which remained symptomatic. Chronic ruptures were defined as those presenting later than 3 months from injury (see Figure 6: treatment algorithm).

2.2. Setting and Location. The trial was undertaken at one metropolitan tertiary care hospital.

2.3. Surgical Procedure. The patient under general anaesthetic is positioned prone on the operating table. The affected limb is prepped and draped, allowing access to the surgical site and the ability to flex the knee. In the setting of an acute tear, a transverse incision of 6–8 cm in the line of the gluteal fold was used. With chronic tears or late presentations with retraction of the tendon, a longitudinal incision extending distally from the ischial tuberosity for 6–8 cm was used.

After dissection through superficial layers, the gluteus maximus muscle was elevated superiorly with a broad retractor, and the deep fascia was incised vertically. The sciatic nerve was identified and dissected free of any surrounding scar tissue. Often, especially in the chronic presentations, the sciatic nerve is densely adherent to the retracted tendon. Once the sciatic nerve was protected, the hamstring tendons were identified, debrided, and mobilised.

The ischial tuberosity is debrided to provide a fresh bed for the tendons. If the tendon ends were easily reapproximated to the ischial tuberosity, they were then held in place with stainless steel table staples. A medium-sized 4-prong staple was used for the semitendinosus and biceps femoris attachment and a small 2-prong staple for the semimembranosus attachment (see Figure 1). In patients with smaller anatomy such that the ischial tuberosity could not accommodate 2 staples, a single 4-prong staple was used to attach all tendons (see Figure 2). Where only one tendon was torn a single 2-prong staple was used. Patients with retracted tendons that were difficult to approximate to the ischial tuberosity had number 5 braided nonabsorbable sutures passed through the hamstring tendons and then through drilled bone tunnels in the ischial tuberosity. The tendons were then reapproximated and held with the table staples. The sutures were tied over the table staples.

Wound closure was performed in layers with a subcuticular skin suture. All patients followed a standard postoperative rehabilitation regime.

Table 1: PHAT scoring guide.

Category	Method	Score
(1) Pain (×3)	Patient marks on line	10-Ans
(2) Maximum times (×3)	0 mins	0
	1–10 mins	5
	11–30 mins	8
	31–60 mins	12
	>60 mins	15
(3) Activity grade	Full sport	15
	Can run, Cannot play full sport	10
	Cannot run pain free	5
	Pain with walking	0
(4) Local tenderness	None	10
	Mild	5
	More than mild	0
Maximum points		100

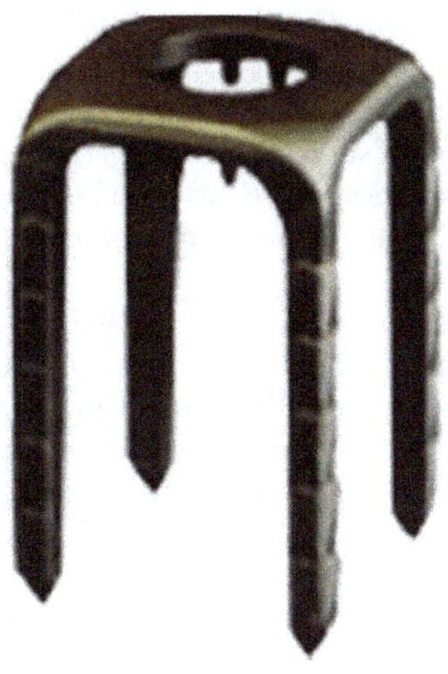

Figure 2

2.4. Outcomes. The main outcomes assessed were functional outcomes: rates of return to sport, return to other activities (sitting, driving a car, and running), and pain scores using a visual analog scale.

We created a combined outcome assessment measure: the Perth Hamstring Assessment Tool (see the appendix). The Perth Hamstring Assessment Tool (PHAT) is a score that looks at a range of functional outcomes. It includes pain scores at rest, sitting, and stretching out. It looks at return to activities from sitting, to driving a car, to running, and full preinjury level of sport. It provides a score out of 100, with a higher score corresponding to a higher function (see Table 1). We looked at total score as well as the individual components. Patients that required a second procedure were scored both before the surgery and then after surgery.

We also assessed our complications: in particular, the number of patients requiring a second surgical procedure for removal of table staple. In patients that had repeat surgery we

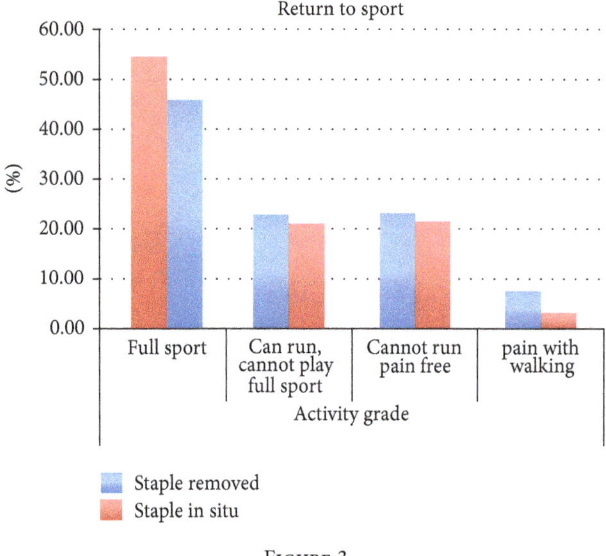

Figure 3

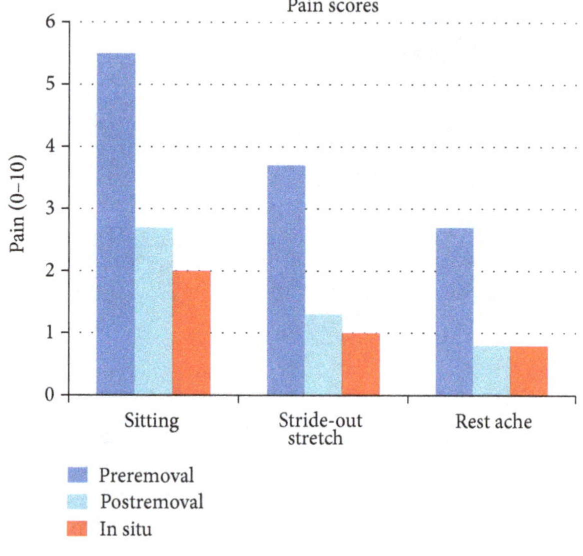

Figure 4

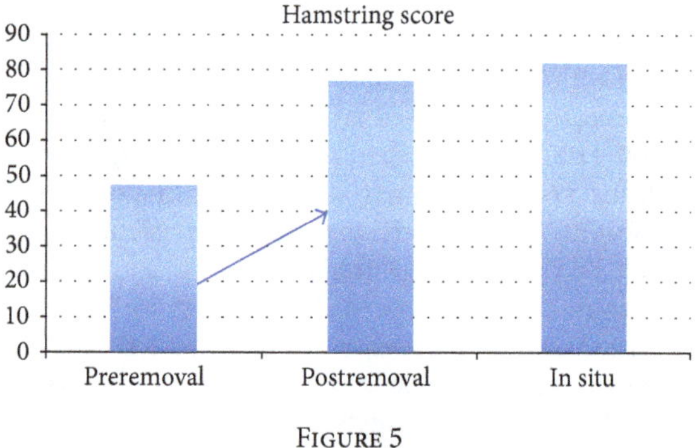

Figure 5

also looked at the state of repair of the proximal hamstring repair at the time of surgery and whether the staple was solid or had loosened. These outcomes were assessed by review of patient's clinical notes. Other complications were also noted.

2.5. Statistical Methods. The statistical analysis used independent Mann-Whitney U test to compare differences between mean values between patients requiring reoperation and those who did not. Wilcoxon T test was used to compare difference in means between patients' scores before and after reoperation. Fisher exact test was used to determine any significant difference in reoperation rate between the different staple sizes. A P value <0.05 was used to determine significance.

3. Results

A total of 56 patients underwent proximal hamstring tendon repair. The mean age was 51 (range 15–71) and there were 29 females and 27 males. The mean follow-up was 26 months (range 8–59 months). Thirty patients had an acute rupture and 26 patients had chronic ruptures. Only 46 of 56 patients (82.1%) completed the PHAT Questionnaire. All patients' clinical notes were available for review. Of the 10 patients that did not complete the questionnaire 5 had the staple in-situ and 5 had the staple removed.

Seventy-four point four per cent of patients (34/46) return to full sport or running. There was a higher number of patients that returned to sport in the group that did not require reoperation (see Figure 3). Only 2 of 46 patients (4.35%) had ongoing pain with walking.

A similar trend was seen with pain scores (at rest, with stride-out stretch, and sitting) significantly higher in those that required staple removal compared to those with the staple in situ ($P < 0.001$). These reduced to similar levels after staple removal, with no significant difference seen in mean pain scores in those with staple removed and those not requiring removal ($P = 0.517$) (see Figure 4).

The mean PHAT Score in all patients was 80.6. Patients with the staple left in situ had a mean score of 82.3. Those that required removal of the staple had a significantly lower score prior to removal, 47.8, but this improved markedly once the staple was removed, with a mean of 77.2 ($P < 0.001$) (see Figure 5). There was no significant difference in the PHAT Score between those that still had the staple in situ and those that had had it removed ($P = 0.38$).

Of the 56 patients, 21 (37.5%) underwent reoperation for removal of the staple. Of the 35 that have not had a reoperation, a further 4 are awaiting surgery to have the staple removed. Seven patients had a single 2-prong staples inserted (of which one required reoperation for removal), 29 had a single 4-prong staple inserted (of which 12 were removed), and 19 had both a 4-prong and a 2-prong staple, inserted (of which 8 were removed). There was no significant difference in the incidence of reoperation between any of the staple combinations ($P = 0.43$). At the time of surgery, the staple was noted to be loose in 5 cases, but in only one case had the repair failed when the staple loosened requiring rerepair. In

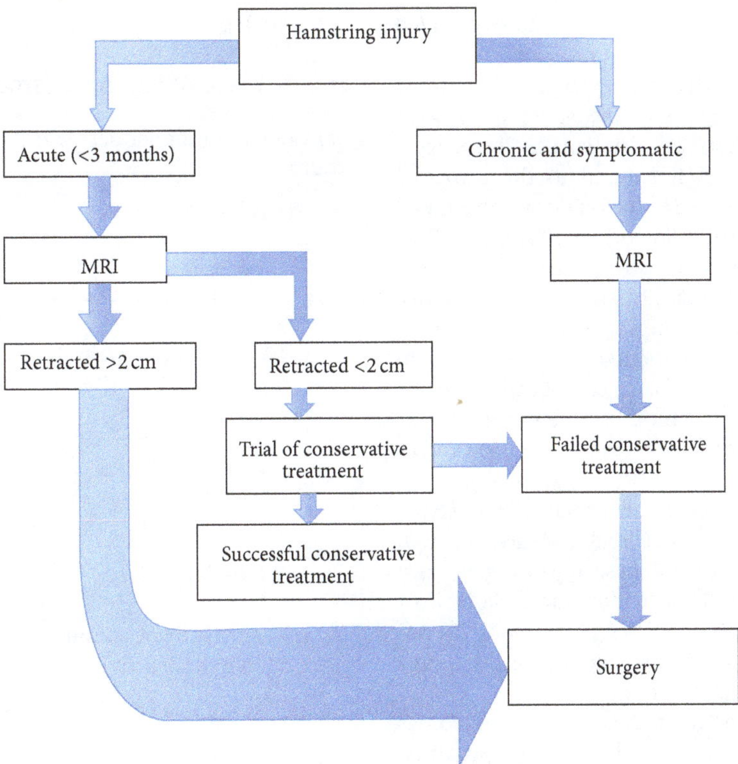

FIGURE 6: Treatment algorithm.

4 cases the surgeon noted that the staple was proud or had backed out. In the remaining cases, the staple was still in a good position.

Five other complications were seen overall. There were three deep infections, which required return to theatre for washout and debridement. One of these deep infections followed the second operation for removal of staple. There was one wound dehiscence.

4. Discussion

This study assessed patient functional outcomes following surgery for proximal hamstring tendon rupture. Patients that did not require removal of the table staple did well postoperatively, with low pain scores (0.8–2 out of 10) and good levels of return to sport or running (75.8%). Patients that required removal of table staple went on to achieve similar levels of return to sport and running (69.2%), as well as similarly low pain scores (0.8–2.7 out of 10).

A large proportion of patients (21/56, 37.5%) that underwent proximal hamstring repair with a table staple required reoperation for removal of the staple. This is an unacceptably high reoperation rate, with the inherent risks of a second operation. Most of the patients that required reoperation had localized pain over the ischial tuberosity and increased pain with all activities. Some of these problems were due to loosening of the staple or backing out. Some of these problems were due to loosening of the staple or backing out. In some patients the staple was still in the original position, suggesting the anatomy of the ischial tuberosity must not be amenable to table staples.

We find the Perth Hamstring Assessment Tool useful for assessing patients' pain and function after hamstring repair. High scores were achieved in both patients that had the staple left in situ (mean 82.3) and those that had the staple removed (mean 77.2). It is a useful tool for assessing those that require removal of the staple, with preremoval scores very low (mean 47.8).

A systematic review by Harris et al. in 2011 on the treatment of proximal hamstring ruptures, showed significantly better subjective outcomes ($P < 0.05$), return to sport ($P < 0.001$), and reduced risk of rerupture ($P < 0.05$) in patients treated surgically compared with patients treated nonsurgically [2]. Surgical techniques included bioabsorbable or metal suture anchors, suture only fixation; reconstruction plate internal fixation for bony avulsions, and Achilles tendon allograft augmentation. All surgical techniques were grouped together and not compared.

A 2008 study by Wood et al. looked at 72 consecutive reconstructions using three suture anchors. At the time of the six-month postoperative check, fifty-seven patients (80%) had returned to their preinjury level of sports [8].

Another 2008 study by Sallay et al. reported on 25 patients that underwent primary repair of proximal hamstring tendon to the ischium with two to four titanium suture anchors [9]. At a mean of 53 months follow-up, 23 of 25 patients (92%) reported minimal to no pain. Four patients reported increased stiffness following sports and 2 patients reported constant stiffness. There were no obvious reruptures or failed repairs.

Folsom and Larson reported on repair of 26 acute or chronic proximal hamstring tears. The acute tears were repaired using suture anchors [4]. The chronic tears were repaired using Achilles allograft sutured to the proximal hamstring tendons and then fixed to the ischium with a metal interference screw. At a mean follow-up of 20 months, 20% reported ongoing pain and 76% had returned to sporting activities. There was no statistically significant difference between the chronic and acute groups. However, numbers in the chronic group were low (5 patients) with low power to detect a difference. There were 3 major complications in the acute group: one rerupture at 4 months, one patient developed complex regional pain syndrome and one deep infection.

Orava and Kujala reported on 8 proximal hamstring ruptures repaired with heavy nonabsorbable sutures through drilled bone tunnels [10]. Two of these repairs were augmented with grafts from plantaris tendon and facia lata. At a mean of 5.7 years follow-up only 62% reported good overall outcome. Those operated on within 2 months of the injury did better than those operated on later.

Brucker and Imhoff reported on the functional outcomes of 8 patients that underwent surgical repair for proximal hamstring rupture [11]. They used a suture anchor repair with a mean of 3.5 anchors. At a mean of 20 months follow-up, half of the patients (4 of 8) reported localised pain and discomfort and 75% (6 of 8) had returned to sport. One patient required a second operation following pull-out of a metal suture anchor.

A recent trial by Birmingham et al. looked at 9 acute and 14 chronic repairs using suture anchors, with the average period of follow-up 43.3 months [12]. Twenty-one of twenty-three patients reported returning to activity at an average of 95% of their preinjury activity level at an average of 9.8 months. Eighteen patients reported excellent results, four, good results, and one, fair results.

The functional results of patients in the above studies are similar to the patients in this study, when looking at those who did not require staple removal and those who did once the staple was removed. One limitation of this study is that the Perth Hamstring Assessment Tool is not a validated outcome measure. There is no validated outcome measure, to our knowledge, that is used for this patient population. We have found it a useful tool for identifying patient progress following surgery. Taking the components of the score individually gives us many of the important clinical outcomes that we look for following proximal hamstring repair.

This study is one of the largest series of proximal hamstring tendon repairs in the literature. Although our patients achieved similar outcomes in terms of pain and function, we thought the reoperation rate was unacceptably high. The study surgeon has now changed operative fixation technique, using suture anchors as described by Carmichael et al. [3]. Our future direction is to compare the patients operated with this new technique with the patient population in this study. We are in the process of validating the Perth Hamstring Assessment Tool.

Appendix

Perth Hamstring Assessment Tool

(1) Choose a number between 0 and 10 which best describes your pain.

(i) When Sitting:

0 1 2 3 4 5 6 7 8 9 10

(No Pain) - - - - - - - - - (Unbearable Pain)

(ii) With Stride-out Stretch:

0 1 2 3 4 5 6 7 8 9 10

(No Pain) - - - - - - - - - (Unbearable Pain)

(iii) At Rest:

0 1 2 3 4 5 6 7 8 9 10

(No Pain) - - - - - - - - - (Unbearable Pain)

(2) What is the maximum amount of time for which you can perform these activities without resting?

(i) Sitting in a chair:

0 mins □
1–10 mins □
11–30 mins □
31–60 mins □
>60 mins □

(ii) Driving a car:

0 mins □
1–10 mins □
11–30 mins □
31–60 mins □
>60 mins □

(iii) Running:

0 mins □
1–10 mins □
11–30 mins □
31–60 mins □
>60 mins □

(3) What best describes your current level of activity?

Full Sport □
Can run, Can't play full sport □
Can't run pain free □
Pain with waking □

(4) Do you have any local tenderness over your hamstring?

None □
Mild □
More than Mild □

Conflict of Interests

The authors declare that there is no conflict of interests regarding the publication of this paper.

Acknowledgment

No financial support has been received in the production of this paper.

References

[1] S. Cohen and J. Bradley, "Acute proximal hamstring rupture," *Journal of the American Academy of Orthopaedic Surgeons*, vol. 15, no. 6, pp. 350–355, 2007, (Review).

[2] J. D. Harris, M. J. Griesser, T. M. Best, and T. J. Ellis, "Treatment of proximal hamstring ruptures a systematic review," *International Journal of Sports Medicine*, vol. 32, no. 7, pp. 490–495, 2011.

[3] J. Carmichael, I. Packham, S. P. Trikha, and D. G. Wood, "Avulsion of the proximal hamstring origin. Surgical technique," *The Journal of Bone and Joint Surgery. American Volume*, vol. 91, supplement 2, pp. 249–256, 2009.

[4] G. J. Folsom and C. M. Larson, "Surgical treatment of acute versus chronic complete proximal hamstring ruptures: results of a new allograft technique for chronic reconstructions," *American Journal of Sports Medicine*, vol. 36, no. 1, pp. 104–109, 2008.

[5] J. J. Lee, K. Otarodifard, B. J. Jun, M. H. McGarry, G. F. Hatch III, and T. Q. Lee, "Is supplementary fixation necessary in anterior cruciate ligament reconstructions?" *American Journal of Sports Medicine*, vol. 39, no. 2, pp. 360–365, 2011.

[6] N. Adachi, M. Ochi, M. Deie, Y. Izuta, and H. Kazusa, "New hamstring fixation technique for medial collateral ligament or posterolateral corner reconstruction using the mosaicplasty system," *Arthroscopy*, vol. 22, no. 5, pp. 571. e1–571. e3, 2006.

[7] P. F. Hill, V. J. Russell, L. J. Salmon, and L. A. Pinczewski, "The influence of supplementary tibial fixation on laxity measurements after anterior cruciate ligament reconstruction with hamstring tendons in female patients," *American Journal of Sports Medicine*, vol. 33, no. 1, pp. 94–101, 2005.

[8] D. G. Wood, I. Packham, S. P. Trikha, and J. Linklater, "Avulsion of the proximal hamstring origin," *Journal of Bone and Joint Surgery. American Volume*, vol. 90, no. 11, pp. 2365–2374, 2008.

[9] P. I. Sallay, G. Ballard, S. Hamersly, and M. Schrader, "Subjective and functional outcomes following surgical repair of complete ruptures of the proximal hamstring complex," *Orthopedics*, vol. 31, no. 11, p. 1092, 2008.

[10] S. Orava and U. M. Kujala, "Rupture of the ischial origin of the hamstring muscles," *American Journal of Sports Medicine*, vol. 23, no. 6, pp. 702–705, 1995.

[11] P. U. Brucker and A. B. Imhoff, "Functional assessment after acute and chronic complete ruptures of the proximal hamstring tendons," *Knee Surgery, Sports Traumatology, Arthroscopy*, vol. 13, no. 5, pp. 411–418, 2005.

[12] P. Birmingham, M. Muller, T. Wickiewicz, J. Cavanaugh, S. Rodeo, and R. Warren, "Functional outcome after repair of proximal hamstring avulsions," *Journal of Bone and Joint Surgery. American Volume*, vol. 93, no. 19, pp. 1819–1826, 2011.

30

The Impact of an Intact Infrapatellar Fat Pad on Outcomes after Total Knee Arthroplasty

Leigh White, Nicholas Hartnell, Melissa Hennessy, and Judy Mullan

School of Medicine, University of Wollongong, Wollongong, NSW 2522, Australia

Correspondence should be addressed to Leigh White; lw844@uowmail.edu.au

Academic Editor: Doron Norman

Background. The infrapatellar fat pad (IPFP) is currently resected in approximately 88% of Total Knee Arthroplasties (TKAs). We hypothesised that an intact IPFP would improve outcomes after TKA. *Methods.* Patients with an intact IPFP participated in this cross-sectional study by completing two surveys, at 6 and 12 months after TKA. Both surveys included questions regarding kneeling, with the Oxford Knee Score also included at 12 months. *Results.* Sixty patients participated in this study. At 6 and 12 months, a similar number of patients were able to kneel, 40 (66.7%) and 43 (71.7%), respectively. Fifteen (25.0%) patients were unable to kneel due to knee pain at 6 months; of these, nine (15%) were unable to kneel at 12 months. Moreover, at 12 months, 90.0% of the patients reported minimal or no knee pain. There was no correlation between the inability to kneel and knee pain ($p = 0.13$). There was a significant correlation between the inability to kneel and reduced overall standardised knee function scores ($p = 0.02$). *Conclusions.* This was the first study to demonstrate improved kneeling and descending of stairs after TKA with IPFP preservation. These results in the context of current literature show that IPFP preservation reduces the incidence of knee pain 12 months after TKA.

1. Introduction

The strongest predictor of osteoarthritis (OA) is increasing age; thus with increasing life expectancy there is an increasing incidence of OA [1]. One of the most common joints to be effected by OA is the knee, which inevitably leads to severe pain and immobility [1]. Total Knee Arthroplasty (TKA) is proven to be a cost-effective treatment for end-stage degenerative joint disorders including OA [2]. Each year the number of TKAs being performed continues to increase globally [3], predominately due to an increasing incidence of knee OA [1, 4–6].

Overall patient satisfaction with their TKA is very high, with as many as 81–89% of patients reporting that they are satisfied with their procedure [7–9]. Areas of highest satisfaction, among patients receiving TKAs, include improved knee stability, reduced pain after long periods of sitting, and the ability to complete basic activities of daily living, inclusive of bathing [7–10]. Despite the high level of patient satisfaction, there are also areas of patient dissatisfaction which need to be considered. The most common reasons for patient dissatisfaction include pain resulting from the procedure, an inability to kneel, and trouble descending stairs following the procedure [9]. Given that the number of patients undergoing TKA is increasing, it is important to explore strategies which could be used to improve patient satisfaction in these areas [8, 9]. One such strategy, currently being investigated, is to keep the infrapatellar fat pad (IPFP) intact during routine TKA. To date, there is a paucity of evidence regarding the post-TKA outcomes when the IPFP has not been removed during the procedure [11].

The IPFP has been traditionally removed in order to enhance surgical access during TKA [12]. Over the past few decades, some of the equipment required to perform a TKA has evolved and changed significantly, such as the tibial alignment guides. These guides have become much smaller and subsequently can be used without the need to resect and remove the IPFP for surgical access. However, even with the improvement and the reduction in size of these alignment guides, current literature indicates that the IPFP is still being partially or completely removed in up to 88% of TKAs [9].

Emerging evidence suggests that the IPFP may play an important role in reducing postoperative anterior knee pain

TABLE 1: The Oxford Knee Score [28, 29].

Question number	Question
1	Describe the pain you usually have from your knee? (Pain)
2	How much trouble do you have washing and drying yourself (all over) because of your knee (Function)
3	How much trouble do you have getting in/out of your car or using public transport because of your knee? (Function)
4	For how long have you been able to walk before pain from your knee becomes severe? (with or without a stick) (Pain)
5	After a meal (sat at a table), how painful has it been for you to stand up from a chair because of your knee? (Pain)
6	Have you been limping when walking, because of your knee? (Function)
7	Could you kneel down and get up again afterwards? (Function)
8	Have you been troubled by pain from your knee in bed at night? (Pain)
9	How much has pain from your knee interfered with your usual work (including housework)? (Pain)
10	Have you felt that your knee might suddenly "give way" or let you down? (Function)
11	Could you do household shopping on your own? (Function)
12	Could you walk down one flight of stairs? (Function)

following TKA [13–17]. Even though Maculé et al. [18] and Tanaka et al. [19] found that patients with an intact IPFP experienced the same or higher rates of knee pain in the short term (less than six months after TKA), other studies that considered the long-term effects (beyond six months) showed that patients with an intact IPFP experienced less pain than those with an IPFP resection after TKA [12, 19, 20].

In addition to the potential impact of IPFP resection on anterior knee pain after TKA, it may also have an impact on patients' ability to kneel. TKA alone can improve patients' ability to kneel, from approximately 2–4% prior to the procedure [21, 22] to between 41 and 73% following the procedure [9, 23–26]. Notably, however, some of these patients will experience some degree of difficulty with kneeling following the procedure [21, 23, 25]. This level of difficulty is important, because kneeling is a function that many people require in order to successfully perform everyday tasks, such as professional duties (e.g., carpet laying and plumbing) and recreational activities (e.g., gardening and playing lawn bowls) [21]. The ability to kneel holds an even greater level of importance in middle eastern and far eastern cultures where kneeling is integral to everyday activities, such as praying and sitting for meals [22]. Of all functional outcomes kneeling has been shown to have the least amount of improvement following a TKA [27]. It is therefore surprising that only a small number of studies have looked at kneeling after TKA [22–25] and that no studies have looked at the impact of an intact IPFP on kneeling. The aim of this study was to investigate the impact of an intact IPFP after TKA on knee pain and knee functions, such as the ability to kneel and descend stairs.

2. Material and Methods

2.1. Overview of Study Design. Following ethics approval from the University of Wollongong human research ethics committee, patients attending an outpatient clinic between July 2013 and May 2014, who did not have their IPFP removed during their routine TKA, were invited to participate in this cross-sectional study. Volunteering patient participants were asked to complete two surveys, which were mailed out to them at 6 and 12 months after TKA. Both surveys included demographic questions and kneeling survey questions, with the addition of the validated Oxford Knee Score [28, 29] in the 12-month survey. These procedures were all performed by the same surgeon at two different hospitals using a cemented, hydroxyapatite-coated posterior cruciate retaining prosthesis incorporated into their tibia. Each knee replacement included patellar resurfacing with a cemented polyethylene button. Surgical access for each operation was gained via a midline incision, with a medial parapatellar approach.

2.2. Kneeling Survey Questions. The four questions in both the 6-month and 12-month surveys which focused on kneeling included the following: (1) Are you able to kneel on your replaced knee? (2) Do you have pain with kneeling? (3) Do you have discomfort or increased pressure within the knee with kneeling? (4) Does pain stop/prevent you from kneeling. These questions were scored as yes or no answers and each question was analysed using descriptive statistical analysis.

2.3. Oxford Knee Score [28, 29]. In addition to the kneeling survey questions discussed above, at twelve months patients were also asked to complete validated and reliable Oxford Knee Score (OKS) [28, 29] as part of their 12-month postprocedure questionnaire. The OKS is a standardised questionnaire consisting of twelve questions, which is used to gauge overall knee pain and knee function after TKA, including the ability to descend stairs and kneel [28, 29] (Table 1).

Patients were asked to base their responses to the OKS on their experiences over the previous four weeks. The possible responses were given a numerical value from zero (worst) to four (best). Overall pain and function scores were calculated based on responses to the OKS [9]. The pain score was calculated by adding together the scores of the five questions related to pain (questions 1, 4, 5, 8, and 9; Table 1), an approach used by Baker et al. [9]. The overall function score was calculated by adding together the scores of the function based questions (questions 2, 3, 6, 7, 10, 11, and 12; Table 1) [9]. The overall pain and function scores were converted to standardised scores to allow for comparison. This was done

TABLE 2: Results of kneeling survey at 6 and 12 months after Total Knee Arthroplasty.

	6 months		12 months	
	Number of patients ($N = 60$)	%	Number of patients ($N = 60$)	%
Are you able to kneel?	40	66.7	43	71.7
Factors Deterring From Kneeling				
Does pain deter you from kneeling?	25	41.7	10	16.7
Does discomfort or pressure deter you from kneeling?	22	36.7	44	73.7
Factors Preventing Kneeling				
Are you unable to kneel due to knee pain?	15	25.0	9	15.0
Does discomfort or pressure stop you from kneeling?	5	8.3	8	13.3

by dividing the overall scores by the highest possible score for pain (20) or function (28), a technique used by other researchers in the literature [9]. For example, a pain score of 15 produced a standardised pain score of 0.75 (15/20 = 0.75) and a function score of 14 produced a standardised function score of 0.50 (14/28 = 0.50). The standardised scores were then grouped together to compare the overall pain and function of the patients that could kneel versus those who could not.

2.4. Statistical Analysis. The data was analysed using the statistics function of Microsoft Excel 2010. A multivariate logistic regression of the standardised knee pain and knee function scores were conducted to provide comparisons between the group of patients that could kneel and those that could not. A p value ≤ 0.05 was considered to be statistically significant.

3. Results

3.1. Patient Demographic Data. Seventy-nine eligible patients were mailed questionnaires at six and twelve months after TKA. Sixty patients returned both questionnaires (32 female, 28 male), indicating a response rate of 75.9%. The mean age of the patients at 6 and 12 months was 67 years.

3.2. Patient Kneeling Capabilities. At six months after TKA, 40 of the 60 respondents (66.7%) were able to kneel. Of the 20 patients unable to kneel, 5 (8.3%) reported that this was due to discomfort or knee pressure (Table 2). The remaining 15 (25%) reported that they were unable to kneel due to knee pain (Table 2). Pain was reported as a deterrent factor from kneeling in 41.7% (n = 25) of those surveyed (Table 2). Of the 60 respondents surveyed at 12 months after TKA, 43 (71.7%) reported that they were able to kneel. A total of 9 (15%) patients were unable to kneel due to pain, and 8 (13.3%) were unable to kneel due to discomfort and knee pressure (Table 2).

3.3. Overall Oxford Knee Score Results. At 12 months after TKA, the average OKS for the 60 patient participants was 42.7/48 (Figure 1). The overall OKS result is a validated indicator of how successful a TKA has been for the patient [28, 29]. The overall OKS can range from zero, which is an extremely poor result, to 48, which represents a knee with perfect function and no pain [28, 29]. In this study, the lowest overall OKS recorded was 13, which means that they scored on average one to two out of four for each question. In contrast, however, 90 percent of patients (n = 54) recorded a score of 36 or higher, which indicates that they had minimal to no problems with the TKA [27] (Figure 1).

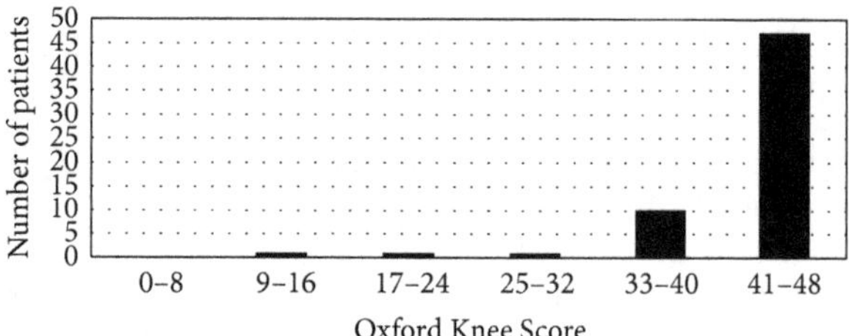

FIGURE 1: Overall Oxford Knee Score distribution in 60 patients at 12 months after Total Knee Arthroplasty.

TABLE 3: Frequency (%) of responses to the Oxford Knee Score questions for stair-descending, knee stability, and kneeling ability at 12 months after Total Knee Arthroplasty (n = 60).

	0 (worst)	1	2	3	4 (best)
Ability with stairs	0 (0.0)	1 (1.7)	5 (8.3)	15 (25.0)	39 (65.0)
Knee stability	0 (0.0)	0 (0.0)	1 (1.7)	9 (15.0)	50 (83.3)
Kneeling ability	5 (8.3)	5 (8.3)	16 (26.7)	20 (33.3)	14 (23.3)

3.3.1. Ability to Descend Stairs, Knee Stability, Kneeling, and Overall Knee Function from the OKS. At 12 months after TKA, the majority of patients reported on the OKS that they were able to descend stairs with minimal to no difficulty (90%), with a mean score of 3.5 out of a possible score of 4 for ability with stairs. Patients had minimal to no problems with their knee stability (3.8/4) and overall knee function (24.8/28). Kneeling was the only question where patients reported mild to moderate difficulty, with a mean score of 2.6 out of 4. The frequency of responses to each of these questions is featured in Table 3.

TABLE 4: Standardised pain and function scores in patients that could and could not kneel at 12 months after Total Knee Arthroplasty.

Score*	Overall		Able to kneel		Unable to kneel	
	Number	Standardised score (95% CI)	Number	Standardised score (95% CI)	Number	Standardised score (95% CI)
Pain	60	0.90 (0.86 to 0.94)	43	0.91 (0.87 to 0.95)#	17	0.85 (0.74 to 0.96)
Function	60	0.89 (0.86 to 0.92)	43	0.91 (0.88 to 0.94)¥	17	0.83 (0.74 to 0.90)

*Pain is the summation of questions 1, 4, 5, 8, and 9 of the OKS; function is the summation of questions 2, 3, 6, 7, 10, 11, and 12 of the OKS. #There was a nonsignificant difference between the pain scores of the patients that could kneel and those that could not ($p = 0.13$). ¥There was a significant difference in function scores between the group of patients that can kneel and those who cannot ($p = 0.02$).

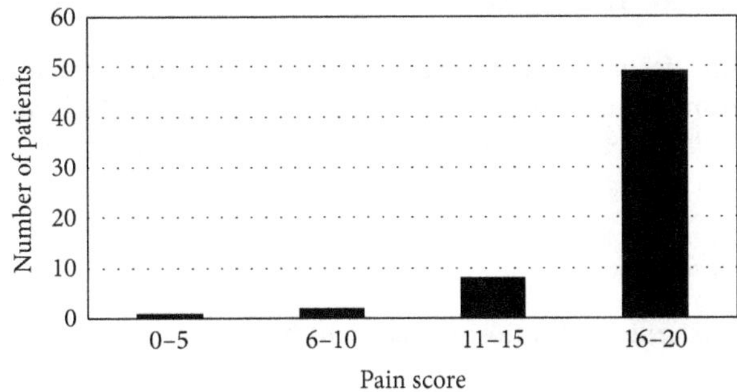

FIGURE 2: Postoperative pain scores derived from questions 1, 4, 5, 8, and 9 of the Oxford Knee Score at 12 months after Total Knee Arthroplasty ($n = 60$).

3.3.2. Knee Pain at 12 Months after TKA from the OKS. The mean pain score derived from the OKS was 17.9/20. Figure 2 shows the pain scores of each patient as calculated from the OKS. The majority of patients (90%) had overall pain scores between 15 and 20, indicating that they experience minimal to no pain at 12 months after TKA. Only six (10%) patients reported their overall knee pain to be in the mild to moderate range (10–14) (Figure 2).

3.4. Analysis of Ability to Kneel in Relation to Standardised Pain and Function Scores. The overall group of patients ($n = 60$) had a mean standardised pain score of 0.90 and mean standardised function score of 0.89 (Table 4). There was a significant difference in the standardised function scores between the patients that could kneel (0.91) and those that could not (0.82), as determined by multivariate regression modeling ($p = 0.02$). There was also a difference in the standardised pain score between those who could kneel (0.91) and those who could not (0.85). However, this difference was not significant ($p = 0.13$).

4. Discussion

Results of this study showed that a high proportion of patients with an intact IPFP after TKA could kneel at 6 and 12 months following the procedure (66.7% and 71.7%, resp.). At 12 months after TKA, 90.0% of patients reported minimal to no knee pain and that they had minimal to no difficulty descending stairs. Kneeling was the only question where patients reported mild to moderate difficulty (2.6/4). Of comparisons between patients who could and could not kneel at 12 months after TKA, it was found that the inability to kneel was significantly related to knee function ($p = 0.02$) rather than knee pain.

4.1. Knee Pain. At 12 months after TKA, 90% of patients reported their knee pain to be mild or nonexistent. The low incidence of knee pain shown in this current study agrees with the results of a number of other studies, which have shown a significant reduction in the incidence of knee pain beyond six months after TKA in patients with an intact IPFP [12, 19, 20]. The incidence of knee pain in the IPFP resection after TKA increased to almost twice that of the preservation group at 5.1 years after procedure [12].

The overall standardised pain score calculated in our study was 0.90 (0.86 to 0.94; 95% CI). Baker et al. (2007) conducted a study of 8,231 patients that had very similar demographics and used an almost identical surgical technique to our study [9]. They found that 84.1% of their patients had either a partial or complete IPFP resection which yielded standardised pain scores of 0.81 (0.81 to 0.82; 95% CI), which was a lower result than our findings. From this comparison of our study with the current literature, it could be proposed that an intact IPFP contributes to reduced medium to long-term knee pain after TKA. One of the most likely explanations may be that the IPFP mediates pain and inflammation while there is an arthritic, inflammatory process occurring in the knee joint [30, 31]. Therefore, once the inflammation in the joint is resolved through TKA, the stimulus for the IPFP to mediate pain and inflammation may no longer be present.

4.2. Ability to Descend Stairs. To our knowledge, this was the first study to examine the ability to descend stairs in patients with an intact IPFP after TKA. Hassaballa et al. completed the only previous study to investigate the impact of TKA on the patients' ability to descend stairs [22]. They found that 73.1% of patients were able to descend stairs with minimal or no difficulty at 12 months after TKA; however, their methodology did not disclose the rate of IPFP resections conducted as part of the study [22]. As removal of the IPFP was common practice in the United Kingdom during the time of Hassaballa et al.'s study, it is likely that resection occurred in the majority of these patients [9]. In our study, which looked exclusively at patients with an intact IPFP after TKA, it was found that 90.0% of the patients could descend stairs with minimal to no difficulty at 12 months following their procedure. This is an increase of approximately 17% from Hassaballa et al.'s study, which could suggest that an intact IPFP after TKA increases the patient's ability to descend stairs [22]. One of the reasons we believe that an intact IPFP may increase the patient's ability to descend stairs is due to the effect that resection has on the patellar tendon. Recent studies have shown that IPFP resection causes shortening of the patellar tendon, which causes a reduction in the range of motion (ROM) in the knee joint [11, 19, 32]. This is important because a reduction in knee ROM impairs patients' ability to descend stairs [33].

4.3. Ability to Kneel. Kneeling is a crucial knee function to many people around the world and is currently a functional outcome that shows the least amount of improvement following routine TKA procedures [21, 22, 27]. An important function of the IPFP is to cushion the interface between patellar tendon and the tibial plateau, especially during kneeling [34]. Of the small number of studies that have investigated the impact of TKA on the ability to kneel, only one has explicitly stated the rate of IPFP resection. Baker et al. investigated the ability to kneel in 8,231 patients who had TKA, with 84.1% of these subjects having the IPFP resected [9]. Results of Baker et al.'s study showed that 57% of patients found it extremely difficult to impossible to kneel at 12 months after TKA [9]. In contrast, our study, which exclusively looked at patients with an intact IPFP, found that only 16.6% of patients found it extremely difficult to impossible to kneel at 12 months following the procedure. This suggests that having an intact IPFP may increase the likelihood that a patient can kneel following TKA.

There are commonly a number of reasons why people are unable to kneel after TKA, including pain, skin hypoesthesia, and decreased ROM [22]. In order to gain a better understanding of why the patients in our study were unable to kneel, we divided the results of those that could and could not kneel for further analysis. In these groupings we then compared standardised pain and function scores. Through this analysis we found that those that could kneel had a significantly higher standardised function score ($p = 0.02$) than those who could not. However, we found no significant difference between groups in standardised pain scores ($p = 0.13$). Therefore, these results show that pain is unlikely to be a limiting factor in the ability to kneel in post-TKA patients with an intact IPFP. We believe that the IPFP reduces pain during kneeling as it acts as a cushion which protects the patellar tendon from pressing against the metal tibial plateau prosthesis.

Limitations. As this was a pilot study conducted in a limited time frame, several limitations need to be acknowledged. This study did not include a control group, did not look at preoperative scores, only included a small sample size, and only investigated patients treated by one surgeon in two hospitals. A randomised controlled trial (RCT) with preoperative scoring and patients treated by multiple surgeons would have provided much more robust and clinically applicable results. An RCT would have also allowed for a higher level comparison of the impact of an intact versus resected IPFP.

In conclusion, our results in combination with the evidence in the current literature showed that IPFP preservation may lead to more favourable outcomes after TKA in OA patients. We found a correlation between an intact IPFP and reduced rates of knee pain at 12 months after TKA. This is the first study to look at the impact of an intact IPFP on functional outcomes such as kneeling and descending stairs after TKA. The results of this study indicate that an intact IPFP may improve the ability to kneel and descend stairs after TKA. The results of this study are not substantial enough to justify new guidelines to state that the IPFP should be left in situ during TKA. For this reason a well-constructed RCT needs to be conducted.

Ethical Approval

Authorisation to perform this study was given by a local committee and was performed in accordance with the Ethical Standards of the 1964 Declaration of Helsinki as revised in 2000.

Consent

All patients gave informed consent prior to enrolling in the study.

Conflict of Interests

The authors declare that they have no conflict of interests (both personal and financial).

References

[1] N. Arden and M. C. Nevitt, "Osteoarthritis: epidemiology," *Best Practice & Research Clinical Rheumatology*, vol. 20, no. 1, pp. 3–25, 2006.

[2] NSW Agency for Clinical Innovation (NSW ACI), *Musculoskeletal Network: NSW Evidence Review Preoperative, Perioperative and Postoperative Care of Elective Primary Total Hip and Knee Replacement*, Agency for Clinical Innovation, Chatswood, Australia, 2012, http://www.aci.health.nsw.gov.au/__data/assets/pdf_file/0020/172091/EJR-Evidence-Review.PDF.

[3] S. M. Kurtz, K. L. Ong, E. Lau et al., "International survey of primary and revision total knee replacement," *International Orthopaedics*, vol. 35, no. 12, pp. 1783–1789, 2011.

[4] C. J. Lavernia, J. F. Guzman, and A. Gachupin-Garcia, "Cost Effectiveness and quality of life in knee arthroplasty," *Clinical Orthopaedics and Related Research*, vol. 345, pp. 134–139, 1997.

[5] Australian Orthopaedic Association (AOA), "Hip and Knee Arthroplasty: Annual Report 2013," National Joint Replacement Registry, 2013, https://aoanjrr.dmac.adelaide.edu.au/presentations-2013.

[6] L. M. March and H. Bagga, "Epidemiology of osteoarthritis in Australia," *Medical Journal of Australia*, vol. 180, no. 5, supplement, pp. S6–S10, 2004.

[7] O. Robertsson, M. Dunbar, T. Pehrsson, K. Knutson, and L. Lidgren, "Patient satisfaction after knee arthroplasty: a report on 27,372 knees operated on between 1981 and 1995 in Sweden," *Acta Orthopaedica Scandinavica*, vol. 71, no. 3, pp. 262–267, 2000.

[8] J. G. Anderson, R. L. Wixson, D. Tsai, S. D. Stulberg, and R. W. Chang, "Functional outcome and patient satisfaction in total knee patients over the age of 75," *Journal of Arthroplasty*, vol. 11, no. 7, pp. 831–840, 1996.

[9] P. N. Baker, J. H. van der Meulen, J. Lewsey, and P. J. Gregg, "The role of pain and function in determining patient satisfaction after total knee replacement. Data from the national joint registry for England and Wales," *The Journal of Bone & Joint Surgery—British Volume*, vol. 89, no. 7, pp. 893–900, 2007.

[10] D. A. Heck, R. L. Robinson, C. M. Patridge, R. M. Lubitz, and D. A. Feund, "Patient outcomes after knee replacement," *Clinical Orthopaedics and Related Research*, vol. 356, pp. 93–110, 1998.

[11] A. Van Beeck, S. Clockaerts, J. Somville et al., "Does infrapatellar fat pad resection in total knee arthroplasty impair clinical outcome? A systematic review," *The Knee*, vol. 20, no. 4, pp. 226–231, 2013.

[12] P. Pinsornsak, K. Naratrikun, and S. Chumchuen, "The effect of infrapatellar fat pad excision on complications after minimally invasive TKA: a randomized controlled trial," *Clinical Orthopaedics and Related Research*, vol. 472, no. 2, pp. 695–701, 2014.

[13] N. Popovic and R. Lemaire, "Anterior knee pain with a posterior-stabilized mobile-bearing knee prosthesis: the effect of femoral component design," *The Journal of Arthroplasty*, vol. 18, no. 4, pp. 396–400, 2003.

[14] T. S. Waters and G. Bentley, "Patellar resurfacing in total knee arthroplasty: a prospective, randomized study," *The Journal of Bone & Joint Surgery—American Volume*, vol. 85, no. 2, pp. 212–217, 2003.

[15] D. J. Wood, A. J. Smith, D. Collopy, B. White, B. Brankov, and M. K. Bulsara, "Patellar resurfacing in total knee arthroplasty: a prospective, randomized trial," *The Journal of Bone & Joint Surgery—American Volume*, vol. 84, no. 2, pp. 187–193, 2002.

[16] R. S. J. Burnett, J. L. Boone, K. P. McCarthy, S. Rosenzweig, and R. L. Barrack, "A prospective randomized clinical trial of patellar resurfacing and nonresurfacing in bilateral TKA," *Clinical Orthopaedics and Related Research*, vol. 464, pp. 65–72, 2007.

[17] A. J. Smith, D. J. Wood, and M.-G. Li, "Total knee replacement with and without patellar resurfacing: a prospective, randomised trial using the Profix total knee system," *The Journal of Bone & Joint Surgery—British Volume*, vol. 90, no. 1, pp. 43–49, 2008.

[18] F. Maculé, S. Sastre, S. Lasurt, P. Sala, J.-M. Segur, and C. Mallofré, "Hoffa's fat pad resection in total knee arthroplasty," *Acta Orthopaedica Belgica*, vol. 71, no. 6, pp. 714–717, 2005.

[19] N. Tanaka, H. Sakahashi, E. Sato, K. Hirose, and T. Isima, "Influence of the infrapatellar fat pad resection in a synovectomy during total knee arthroplasty in patients with rheumatoid arthritis," *Journal of Arthroplasty*, vol. 18, no. 7, pp. 897–902, 2003.

[20] R. M. Meneghini, J. L. Pierson, D. Bagsby, M. E. Berend, M. A. Ritter, and J. B. Meding, "The effect of retropatellar fat pad excision on patellar tendon contracture and functional outcomes after total knee arthroplasty," *The Journal of Arthroplasty*, vol. 22, no. 6, pp. 47–50, 2007.

[21] J. Dawson, R. Fitzpatrick, D. Murray, and A. Carr, "Questionnaire on the perceptions of patients about total knee replacement," *The Journal of Bone & Joint Surgery—British Volume*, vol. 80, no. 1, pp. 63–69, 1998.

[22] M. A. Hassaballa, A. J. Porteous, and I. D. Learmonth, "Functional outcomes after different types of knee arthroplasty: kneeling ability versus descending stairs," *Medical Science Monitor*, vol. 13, no. 2, pp. CR77–CR81, 2007.

[23] M. A. Hassaballa, A. J. Porteous, J. H. Newman, and C. A. Rogers, "Can knees kneel? Kneeling ability after total, unicompartmental and patellofemoral knee arthroplasty," *The Knee*, vol. 10, no. 2, pp. 155–160, 2003.

[24] M. Mardani Kivi, M. Karimi Mobarakeh, K. Hashemi Motlagh, and K. Saheb Ekhtiari, "Evaluation of kneeling ability after total knee replacement in patients with osteoarthritis of the knee," *Minerva Ortopedica e Traumatologica*, vol. 63, no. 3, pp. 177–184, 2012.

[25] S. H. Palmer, C. T. Servant, J. Maguire, E. N. Parish, and M. J. Cross, "Ability to kneel after total knee replacement," *The Journal of Bone & Joint Surgery—British Volume*, vol. 84, no. 2, pp. 220–222, 2002.

[26] P. F. Sharkey and A. J. Miller, "Noise, numbness, and kneeling difficulties after total knee arthroplasty. Is the outcome affected?" *Journal of Arthroplasty*, vol. 26, no. 8, pp. 1427–1431, 2011.

[27] D. P. Williams, C. M. Blakey, S. G. Hadfield, D. W. Murray, A. J. Price, and R. E. Field, "Long-term trends in the Oxford knee score following total knee replacement," *The Journal of Bone & Joint Surgery—British Volume*, vol. 95, no. 1, pp. 45–51, 2013.

[28] D. W. Murray, R. Fitzpatrick, K. Rogers et al., "The use of the Oxford hip and knee scores," *The Journal of Bone & Joint Surgery—British Volume*, vol. 89, no. 8, pp. 1010–1014, 2007.

[29] K. I. A. Reddy, L. R. Johnston, W. Wang, and R. J. Abboud, "Does the oxford knee score complement, concur, or contradict the american knee society score?" *Journal of Arthroplasty*, vol. 26, no. 5, pp. 714–720, 2011.

[30] É. Toussirot, G. Streit, and D. Wendling, "The contribution of adipose tissue and adipokines to inflammation in joint diseases," *Current Medicinal Chemistry*, vol. 14, no. 10, pp. 1095–1100, 2007.

[31] H. Dumond, N. Presle, B. Terlain et al., "Evidence for a key role of leptin in osteoarthritis," *Arthritis and Rheumatism*, vol. 48, no. 11, pp. 3118–3129, 2003.

[32] M. Bohnsack, A. Wilharm, C. Hurschler, O. Rühmann, C. Stukenborg-Colsman, and C. J. Wirth, "Biomechanical and kinematic influences of a total infrapatellar fat pad resection on the knee," *The American Journal of Sports Medicine*, vol. 32, no. 8, pp. 1873–1880, 2004.

[33] N. Shah, "Clinical suggestion: increasing knee range of motion using a unique sustained motion," *North American Journal of Sports Physical Therapy*, vol. 3, pp. 110–113, 2008.

[34] G. Hamarneh, V. Chu, M. Bordalo-Rodrigues, and M. Schweitzer, "Deformation analysis of Hoffa's fat pad from CT images of knee flexion and extension," in *Medical Imaging 2005: Physiology, Function, and Structure from Medical Images*, vol. 5746 of *Proceedings of SPIE*, pp. 703–710, April 2005.

31

The Influence of Psychiatric Comorbidity on Inpatient Outcomes following Distal Humerus Fractures

Leonard T. Buller,[1] Matthew J. Best,[2] Milad Alam,[1] Karim Sabeh,[1] Charles Lawrie,[1] and Stephen M. Quinnan[1]

[1] *University of Miami Miller School of Medicine, Department of Orthopaedic Surgery and Rehabilitation, 1400 NW 12th Avenue, Miami, FL 33136, USA*
[2] *Johns Hopkins Department of Orthopaedic Surgery, 1800 Orleans Street, Baltimore, MD 21287, USA*

Correspondence should be addressed to Leonard T. Buller; leonard.buller@jhsmiami.org

Academic Editor: Werner Kolb

Background. The influence of psychiatric comorbidity on outcomes following inpatient management of upper extremity fractures is poorly understood. *Methods.* The National Hospital Discharge Survey was queried to identify patients admitted to US hospitals with distal humerus fractures between 1990 and 2007. Patients were subdivided into 5 groups: depression, anxiety, schizophrenia, dementia, and no psychiatric comorbidity. Multivariable logistic regression analysis identified independent risk factors for adverse events, requirement of blood transfusion, and discharge to another inpatient facility. *Results.* A cohort representative of 526,185 patients was identified as having a distal humerus fracture. Depression, anxiety, and dementia were independently associated with higher odds of in-hospital adverse events ($P < 0.001$). Depression was associated with higher odds of inpatient blood transfusion ($P < 0.001$). Depression, schizophrenia, and dementia were associated with higher odds of nonroutine discharge to another inpatient facility ($P < 0.001$). Patients with a diagnosis of schizophrenia had a mean of 12 ($P < 0.001$) more days of care than patients with no psychiatric comorbidity. *Discussion.* Patients with comorbid psychiatric illness who are admitted to hospitals with distal humerus fractures are at increased risk of inpatient adverse events and posthospitalization care.

1. Introduction

Psychiatric comorbidity is associated with longer hospital stays, higher risk of suboptimal outcomes, and increased resource utilization among patients undergoing inpatient surgery [1–7]. Major depressive disorder and anxiety are the most common psychiatric diagnoses [1–5]. Schizophrenia is less common, with an estimated prevalence of one percent [8], but is associated with significant cognitive impairment [9]. Dementia is present in approximately six percent of the population over 60 years of age [6]. The rate of elderly individuals with psychiatric disorders is projected to double by 2030 [10].

In orthopaedics, psychiatric comorbidity has been associated with worse long-term outcomes (i.e., pain and disability) following total knee arthroplasty [11], major spine surgery [12], and orthopaedic trauma [13]. Psychiatric comorbidity with concurrent antipsychotic and antidepressant use are known risk factors for extremity fractures [14–16], postulated to be a result of decreased bone mineral density. While prior research in lower extremity fractures has demonstrated longer hospital stays, more in-hospital adverse events, and lower rates of discharge to home among patients with psychiatric comorbidity [17], there is a paucity of data on the influence of psychiatric illness on acute, inpatient outcomes among patients admitted with upper extremity fractures. This study sought to evaluate the influence of psychiatric illness on length of stay, mortality, in-hospital adverse events, requirement for blood transfusion, and nonroutine discharge to another inpatient facility among patients admitted with distal humerus fractures. Knowledge of the effects of psychiatric illness on inpatient outcomes may be used for planning and resource allocation for orthopaedic patients with psychiatric illness.

2. Materials and Methods

2.1. Data Source. The National Hospital Discharge Survey (NHDS) database, developed by the National Center for Health Statistics [18], was used to evaluate the influence of psychiatric comorbidity on outcomes following distal humerus fractures. The NHDS is a publically available survey providing demographic and medical data for inpatients discharged from nonfederal, short-stay hospitals in the United States [19]. It is the principal database used by the US government for monitoring hospital use and is thought to be the most comprehensive of all inpatient surgical databases in use [19]. The survey, which began in 1965 and has been collected annually since then, uses International Classification of Diseases, 9th Revision, Clinical Modification (ICD-9-CM) codes [20] for classifying medical diagnoses and procedures. Using a stratified, multistage probability design, the NHDS collects demographic information (age, gender, and race), expected source of payment (insurance status), medical information of up to seven discharge diagnoses and up to four procedures, length of care, hospital size, US region, and inpatient outcomes including discharge destination [21]. The NHDS uses a complex three-stage probability design to ensure an unbiased national sampling of inpatient records including inflation by reciprocals of the probabilities of sample selection and adjustment for no response and population weighting ratio adjustments [19]. Because the NHDS is a publically available database with no patient identifying information, this study did not require approval by the institutional review board.

2.2. Study Population. Using ICD-9-CM codes, we identified all patients admitted in the United States with a distal humerus fracture between 1990 and 2007. Discharges with a diagnosis code (ICD-9-CM) of closed fracture of lower end of humerus (812.4x) or open fracture of lower end of humerus (812.5x) were identified using previously described techniques [22]. Patients managed surgically with open reduction and internal fixation (ORIF) or closed reduction and internal fixation (CRIF) were identified using ICD-9 procedure codes 79.3x and 79.1x, respectively. To analyze their influence on inpatient outcomes, psychiatric comorbidities were divided into four groups: depression (ICD-9-CM 296.2, 296.3, 296.5, 296.9, 300.4, 301.12, 309.0, and 311.x), anxiety (ICD-9-CM 300.0x, 309.24, and 309.28), schizophrenia (ICD-9-CM 295.x), and dementia (ICD-9-CM 290.x). After obtaining our study population, demographic variables were collected including age, sex, primary diagnosis, type of fracture, prevalence of comorbidities, length of stay, and discharge destination. The complication screening package [23] was used to determine the incidence of complications and the variable of adverse event was created based on the variables: shock (998.0), bleeding (998.1), acute postoperative infection (998.5), acute postoperative anemia (285.1), acute renal failure (584), acute myocardial infarction (410), pulmonary embolism (415.1), induced mental disorder (293), pneumonia (480–486), pulmonary insufficiency (518.5), deep venous thrombosis (453.4), intubation (96.xx), and transfusion of blood (99.x).

2.3. Statistics. We assumed a normal distribution of the data because of the large sample size. Differences between categorical variables were compared using the Pearson chi-square test and the independent-samples t-tests were used to compare differences between continuous variables. To analyze whether depression, anxiety, schizophrenia, or dementia were independent predictors of a negative in-hospital outcome (adverse events, requirement for blood transfusion, or discharge to inpatient facility), all variables present in at least 2% of the population [24] were included in a multivariable binary logistic regression model; for in-hospital adverse events, a 1% cutoff was used due to their lower rates of occurrence, as previously described [25]. The dichotomous variables were (1) presence of adverse events, (2) need for blood transfusion, and (3) discharge to inpatient facility. The multivariable regression model allowed us to control for potential confounders and isolate the effect of psychiatric illness on inpatient outcomes. Notably, the cooccurrence of psychiatric comorbidity was rare with depression and anxiety in 33 patients (0.00%), depression and schizophrenia in 46 patients (0.01%), and no cooccurrence of other psychiatric comorbidities. Covariates accounted for in the regression model included gender, age, region of the country, and preexisting comorbidities (anemia, obesity, diabetes mellitus, hypertension, congestive heart failure, coronary artery disease, atrial fibrillation, prior myocardial infarction, osteoporosis, connective tissue disease, thyroid disease, and chronic obstructive pulmonary disease). Odds ratios and confidence intervals were calculated to assess the association between psychiatric comorbidities and inpatient outcomes. To correct for multiple comparisons, a P value of <0.001 was used to define statistical significance, as previously described [25]. All data were analyzed using the statistical package for social sciences [SPSS] software version 20 (Chicago, IL, USA).

3. Results

A cohort representative of 526,185 discharges with a diagnosis of distal humerus fracture, between 1990 and 2007, was retrieved from the NHDS database. The prevalence of depression was 1.27%, anxiety was 0.42%, schizophrenia was 0.2%, and dementia was 0.36%. The mean age of the cohort was 30.3 years (95% CI, 27.6 to 33.0 years) while those with psychiatric illness were significantly older ($P < 0.001$) (Table 1). Females comprised 50.2% of the total cohort, 67.5% of patients with depression and greater than 80% of patients with either dementia or anxiety (Table 1). The most common diagnosis was closed supracondylar humerus fracture (ICD-9-CM 812.41), followed by closed fracture of unspecified part of humerus (812.4), and closed fracture of lateral condyle of humerus (812.42). Length of hospital stay was significantly longer for patients with schizophrenia (16.12 days) compared with nonpsychiatric patients (3.96; $P < 0.001$) (Table 1). In-hospital mortality was lower in patients with depression ($P < 0.001$), but not statistically significantly different between patients with anxiety, dementia, or schizophrenia and no psychiatric comorbidity (Table 1).

The prevalence of comorbidities and adverse events with bivariate analyses are listed in Tables 2 and 3, respectively.

Table 1: Patient characteristics for patients with distal humerus fractures with bivariate analysis comparing those with a concomitant diagnosis of depression, anxiety, dementia, and schizophrenia to those not affected by any psychiatric diagnosis (SEM, standard error of mean).

Parameter	Total, percentage (%)	Psychiatric comorbidity								
		None, %	Depression, %	*P*	Anxiety, %	*P*	Schizophrenia, %	*P*	Dementia, %	*P*
N =	526,185	514,432	6,700		2,191		1,067		1,874	
% of total cohort	100.0%	97.8%	1.3%		0.4%		0.2%		0.4%	
Gender										
Male	49.8%	50.2%	32.5%	<0.001	13.6%	<0.001	73.1%	<0.001	19.8%	<0.001
Female	50.2%	49.8%	67.5%		86.4%		26.9%		80.2%	
Age										
<8	35.2%	36.0%	0.0%	<0.001	1.7%	<0.001	0.0%	<0.001	0.0%	<0.001
8–25	22.2%	22.5%	7.9%		16.0%		21.8%		0.0%	
26–50	14.6%	14.4%	14.9%		36.5%		74.0%		0.0%	
>50	28.0%	27.1%	77.2%		45.8%		4.2%		100.0%	
Primary diagnosis										
812.4 (fracture of lower end of humerus closed)	19.0%	18.6%	29.7%	<0.001	14.9%	<0.001	19.3%	0.577	75.9%	<0.001
812.41 (closed supracondylar fracture of humerus)	48.2%	48.7%	24.9%	<0.001	34.6%	<0.001	56.2%	<0.001	14.2%	<0.001
812.42 (closed fracture of lateral condyle of humerus)	9.5%	9.7%	1.6%	<0.001	4.4%	<0.001	5.0%	<0.001	0.0%	<0.001
812.43 (closed fracture of medial condyle of humerus)	5.3%	5.1%	16.9%	<0.001	31.8%	<0.001	0.0%	<0.001	0.0%	<0.001
812.44 (closed fracture of unspecified condyle(s) of humerus)	4.7%	4.8%	4.0%	0.002	0.0%	<0.001	6.1%	0.041	7.5%	<0.001
812.49 (other closed fractures of lower end of humerus)	4.0%	3.9%	16.0%	<0.001	7.8%	<0.001	5.4%	0.007	2.4%	0.001
812.5 (fracture of lower end of humerus open)	3.1%	3.2%	2.8%	0.109	0.0%	<0.001	8.0%	<0.001	0.0%	<0.001
812.51 (open supracondylar fracture of humerus)	3.9%	4.0%	0.0%	<0.001	0.0%	<0.001	0.0%	<0.001	0.0%	<0.001
812.52 (open fracture of lateral condyle of humerus)	0.9%	0.9%	0.9%	0.902	0.0%	<0.001	0.0%	0.002	0.0%	<0.001
812.53 (open fracture of medial condyle of humerus)	1.2%	1.2%	4.1%	<0.001	0.0%	<0.001	0.0%	<0.001	0.0%	<0.001
812.54 (open fracture of unspecified condyle(s) of humerus)	0.6%	0.6%	0.0%	<0.001	4.0%	<0.001	0.0%	0.009	0.0%	<0.001
812.59 (other open fractures of lower end of humerus)	1.2%	1.2%	1.0%	0.198	4.6%	<0.001	0.0%	<0.001	0.0%	<0.001
Comorbidities										
No	84.9%	85.5%	47.5%	<0.001	65.5%	<0.001	96.4%	<0.001	50.9%	<0.001
Yes	15.1%	14.5%	52.5%		34.5%		3.6%		49.1%	
Adverse events										
No	93.8%	94.1%	76.7%	<0.001	92.8%	0.013	100.0%	<0.001	75.2%	<0.001
Yes	6.2%	6.0%	23.3%		7.2%		0.0%		24.8%	

TABLE 1: Continued.

Parameter	Total, percentage (%)	Psychiatric comorbidity								
		None, %	Depression, %	P	Anxiety, %	P	Schizophrenia, %	P	Dementia, %	P
Discharge disposition										
Routine/home (1)	85.0%	85.7%	50.8%		97.8%		37.2%		25.2%	
Left AMA (2)	0.3%	0.2%	1.8%		0.0%		0.0%		0.0%	
Short-term fac (3)	2.8%	2.6%	19.6%		0.0%		4.0%		0.0%	
Long-term fac (4)	7.3%	6.9%	19.4%	<0.001	0.0%	<0.001	40.6%	<0.001	69.3%	<0.001
Alive, not stated (5)	3.2%	3.1%	5.6%		2.2%		18.2%		3.0%	
Dead (6)	0.2%	0.2%	0.0%		0.0%		0.0%		0.0%	
Not reported (9)	1.3%	1.3%	3.0%		0.0%		0.0%		2.4%	
Mortality	0.2%	0.2%	0.0%	<0.001	0.0%	0.036	0.0%	0.144	0.0%	0.053
Age (years), mean (SE)	30.3 (1.37)	29.54 (1.33)	65.16 (2.94)	<0.001	52.42 (2.36)	<0.001	38.04 (1.72)	<0.001	84.7 (3.82)	<0.001
Days of care, mean (SE)	3.98 (0.18)	3.96 (0.18)	4.11 (0.19)	0.924	2.49 (0.11)	0.595	16.12 (0.73)	<0.001	3.8 (0.17)	0.957

Table 2: Prevalence of comorbidities and bivariate analysis in patients with distal humerus fractures comparing those with a concomitant diagnosis of depression, anxiety, dementia, or schizophrenia to those with none of these diagnoses.

Parameter (ICD-9)	Total (N = 526,185) Percentage (%)	Psychiatric comorbidity None, %	Depression, %	P	Anxiety, %	P	Schizophrenia, %	P	Dementia, %	P
Thyroid disease (240–246)										
No	97.86%	97.90%	94.49%	<0.001	98.17%	<0.001	100.00%	<0.001	96.10%	<0.001
Present	2.14%	2.10%	5.51%		1.83%		0.00%		3.90%	
Diabetes mellitus (250)										
No	95.25%	95.29%	91.58%	<0.001	95.85%	0.22	100.00%	<0.001	94.88%	0.4
Present	4.75%	4.71%	8.42%		4.15%		0.00%		5.12%	
Obesity (278.00, 278.01)										
No	99.66%	99.66%	99.36%	<0.001	100.00%	0.006	100.00%	0.056	100.00%	0.011
Present	0.34%	0.34%	0.64%		0.00%		0.00%		0.00%	
Hypertensive disease (401–405)										
No	90.72%	90.94%	74.61%	<0.001	95.85%	<0.001	96.44%	<0.001	78.44%	<0.001
Present	9.28%	9.06%	25.39%		4.15%		3.56%		21.56%	
Old myocardial infarction (412)										
No	99.48%	99.52%	96.04%	<0.001	100.00%	0.001	100.00%	0.023	100.00%	0.003
Present	0.52%	0.48%	3.96%		0.00%		0.00%		0.00%	
Coronary artery disease (414.01)										
No	99.03%	99.14%	91.51%	<0.001	100.00%	<0.001	100.00%	0.002	94.40%	<0.001
Present	0.97%	0.86%	8.49%		0.00%		0.00%		5.60%	
Atrial fibrillation (427.31)										
No	98.04%	98.14%	90.58%	<0.001	100.00%	<0.001	100.00%	<0.001	94.29%	<0.001
Present	1.96%	1.86%	9.42%		0.00%		0.00%		5.71%	
Congestive heart failure (428)										
No	98.17%	98.21%	97.69%	0.001	100.00%	<0.001	100.00%	<0.001	85.06%	<0.001
Present	1.83%	1.79%	2.31%		0.00%		0.00%		14.94%	
Chronic pulmonary disease (490–496)										
No	99.93%	99.93%	99.58%	<0.001	100.00%	0.215	100.00%	0.387	100.00%	0.252
Present	0.07%	0.07%	0.42%		0.00%		0.00%		0.00%	
Connective tissue disease (710)										
No	99.93%	99.93%	100.00%	0.03	100.00%	0.215	100.00%	0.387	100.00%	0.252
Present	0.07%	0.07%	0.00%		0.00%		0.00%		0.00%	
Osteoporosis (733.0)										
No	98.46%	98.70%	90.51%	<0.001	71.52%	<0.001	100.00%	<0.001	89.49%	<0.001
Present	1.54%	1.30%	9.49%		28.48%		0.00%		10.51%	

Table 3: Prevalence of adverse events in patients with distal humerus fractures with bivariate analysis comparing those with a concomitant diagnosis of depression, anxiety, dementia, or schizophrenia to those with none of these diagnoses.

Parameter (ICD-9)	Total ($N = 526{,}185$)	Psychiatric comorbidity								
	Percentage	None, %	Depression, %	P	Anxiety, %	P	Schizophrenia, %	P	Dementia, %	P
Postoperative bleeding (998.1)										
No	99.76%	99.76%	100.00%	<0.001	100.00%	0.021	100.00%	0.109	100.00%	0.034
Present	0.24%	0.24%	0.00%		0.00%		0.00%		0.00%	
Acute postoperative infection (998.5)										
No	99.56%	99.55%	100.00%	<0.001	100.00%	<0.001	100.00%	0.028	100.00%	0.004
Present	0.44%	0.45%	0.00%		0.00%		0.00%		0.00%	
Acute postoperative anemia (285.1)										
No	97.90%	97.93%	96.27%	<0.001	84.84%	<0.001	100.00%	<0.001	100.00%	<0.001
Present	2.10%	2.07%	3.73%		5.16%		0.00%		0.00%	
Acute renal failure (584)										
No	99.79%	99.79%	99.34%	<0.001	100.00%	0.032	100.00%	0.134	100.00%	0.047
Present	0.21%	0.21%	0.66%		0.00%		0.00%		0.00%	
Acute myocardial infarction (410)										
No	99.82%	99.81%	100.00%	<0.001	100.00%	0.041	100.00%	0.154	99.25%	<0.001
Present	0.18%	0.19%	0.00%		0.00%		0.00%		0.75%	
Pulmonary embolism (415.1)										
No	99.89%	99.89%	100.00%	0.007	100.00%	0.12	100.00%	0.278	100.00%	0.151
Present	0.11%	0.11%	0.00%		0.00%		0.00%		0.00%	
Induced mental disorder (293)										
No	99.70%	99.70%	100.00%	<0.001	100.00%	0.01	100.00%	0.073	100.00%	0.018
Present	0.30%	0.30%	0.00%		0.00%		0.00%		0.00%	
Pneumonia (480–486)										
No	99.11%	99.33%	89.01%	<0.001	97.95%	<0.001	100.00%	0.007	76.57%	<0.001
Present	0.89%	0.67%	10.99%		2.05%		0.00%		23.43%	
Pulmonary insufficiency (518.5)										
No	99.74%	99.73%	100.00%	<0.001	100.00%	0.015	100.00%	0.089	100.00%	0.024
Present	0.26%	0.27%	0.00%		0.00%		0.00%		0.00%	
Deep venous thrombosis (453.4)										
No	99.99%	99.99%	100.00%	0.415	100.00%	0.641	100.00%	0.745	100.00%	0.666
Present	0.01%	0.01%	0.00%		0.00%		0.00%		0.00%	
Intubation (96.x)										
No	98.80%	98.80%	98.84%	0.789	97.95%	<0.001	100.00%	<0.001	100.00%	<0.001
Present	1.20%	1.20%	1.16%		2.05%		0.00%		0.00%	
Transfusion of blood (99.0)										
No	98.60%	98.66%	93.27%	<0.001	98.81%	0.533	100.00%	<0.001	99.36%	0.008
Present	1.40%	1.34%	6.73%		1.19%		0.00%		0.64%	

Table 4: Logistic regression for predictors of adverse events among patients hospitalized for distal humerus fracture (N = 526,185). CI, confidence interval; OR, odds ratio.

Variable	OR (95% CI)	P
Dementia	5.024 (4.522–5.583)	<0.001
Congestive heart failure	4.881 (4.660–5.113)	<0.001
Depression	4.742 (4.476–5.024)	<0.001
Atrial fibrillation	3.493 (3.323–3.673)	<0.001
Osteoporosis	3.111 (2.931–3.301)	<0.001
Coronary artery disease	3.055 (2.876–3.245)	<0.001
Diabetes mellitus	2.679 (2.580–2.781)	<0.001
History of myocardial infarction	2.264 (2.058–2.491)	<0.001
Hypertension	1.667 (1.614–1.773)	<0.001
Open reduction and internal fixation	1.499 (1.466–1.533)	<0.001
DOC	1.041 (1.040–1.043)	<0.001
Age	1.016 (1.016–1.017)	<0.001
Obesity	1.166 (1.009–1.348)	0.0373
Region	1.013 (1.002–1.024)	0.017
Connective tissue disease	1.357 (0.982–1.875)	0.0648
Anxiety	1.171 (0.995–1.377)	0.0571
Sex (M)	0.781 (0.762–0.800)	<0.001
Thyroid disease	0.578 (0.524–0.637)	<0.001
Closed reduction and internal fixation	0.115 (0.110–0.121)	<0.001
Schizophrenia	0.007 (0.004–0.113)	0.001

Omnibus χ^2 = 4746, P < 0.001.
Nagelkerke R^2 = 0.0663.

Table 5: Logistic regression for predictors of requirement for blood transfusion among patients with distal humerus fractures (N = 526,185). CI, confidence interval; OR, odds ratio.

Variable	OR (95% CI)	P
Postop anemia	14.145 (13.325–15.015)	<0.001
Osteoporosis	7.032 (6.479–7.632)	<0.001
Depression	5.334 (4.834–5.886)	<0.001
Diabetes mellitus	5.179 (4.887–5.488)	<0.001
Atrial fibrillation	3.966 (3.637–4.325)	<0.001
Congestive heart failure	3.913 (3.607–4.244)	<0.001
Hypertension	3.427 (3.263–3.598)	<0.001
Postoperative bleeding	2.928 (2.204–3.888)	<0.001
Open reduction internal fixation	2.750 (2.618–2.888)	<0.001
Sex (M)	2.216 (2.080–2.361)	<0.001
Coronary artery disease	2.091 (1.924–2.271)	<0.001
History of myocardial infarction	1.670 (1.319–2.116)	<0.001
Thyroid disease	1.466 (1.283–1.675)	<0.001
Age	1.041 (1.040–1.042)	<0.001
Region	0.960 (0.937–0.982)	0.001
Anxiety	0.843 (0.572–1.242)	0.3875
Obesity	0.639 (0.390–1.045)	0.0743
Closed reduction internal fixation	0.146 (0.133–0.161)	<0.0001
Pulmonary embolism	0.062 (0.004–0.997)	0.0497
Schizophrenia	0.033 (0.002–0.525)	0.0157

Omnibus χ^2 = 4746, P < 0.001.
Nagelkerke R^2 = 0.2062.

Hypertensive disease was the most common comorbidity at 9.28% followed by diabetes mellitus at 4.75%. Psychiatric comorbidity was associated with a higher rate of inpatient adverse events (depression, 23.27%, anxiety, 7.21%, and dementia, 24.81%) compared with no psychiatric comorbidity (6.23%) (Tables 1 and 3). For patients with depression and dementia, the most common adverse event was pneumonia at 10.99% and 23.43%, respectively. Multivariable logistic regression analysis showed dementia (OR 5.024, range: 4.522 to 5.583, P < 0.001), depression (OR 4.742, range: 4.476 to 5.024, P < 0.001), and those treated with ORIF (OR 1.499, range: 1.466 to 1.533, P < 0.001) to be independently associated with higher odds of inpatient adverse events, whereas there was a lower odds ratio of adverse event among those treated with CRIF (OR 0.115, range: 0.110 to 0.121, P < 0.001) (model fit: for omnibus test of model coefficients: χ^2 = 4746, P < 0.001, Nagelkerke R^2 = 0.0663; Table 4).

Among the total cohort, 2.1% of patients experienced acute postoperative anemia. In multivariable logistic regression analysis, patients with depression (OR 5.334, range: 4.834 to 5.886, P < 0.001) and those treated with ORIF (OR 2.75, range: 2.618 to 2.884, P < 0.001) had significantly higher odds of blood transfusion, while patients with schizophrenia (OR 0.033, range: 0.002 to 0.525, P < 0.001), dementia (OR 0.452, range: 0.256 to 0.797, P = 0.006), and those treated with CRIF (OR 0.146, range: 0.133 to 0.161, P < 0.001) had a lower odds ratio of requiring blood transfusion (model fit: omnibus test of model coefficients: χ^2 = 4746, P < 0.001, Nagelkerke R^2 = 0.2062; Table 5).

Patients with comorbid mental illness experienced a higher rate of discharge to inpatient short- or long-term facility (depression, 38.9%, schizophrenia, 44.6%, and dementia, 69.3%) compared with patients who had no psychiatric comorbidity (9.5%). In multivariable regression analysis, dementia (OR 20.609, range: 18.674 to 22.745, P < 0.001), schizophrenia (OR 7.232, range: 6.708 to 8.163, P < 0.001), and depression (OR 5.909, range: 5.621 to 6.212, P < 0.001) were independently associated with nonroutine discharge to another inpatient facility, while patients treated surgically with ORIF (OR 0.785, range: 0.771 to 0.800, P < 0.001) or CRIF (OR 0.197, range: 0.190 to 0.203, P < 0.001) had a lower odds ratio of nonroutine discharge (model fit: omnibus test of model coefficients: χ^2 = 4717, P < 0.001, Nagelkerke R^2 = 0.482; Table 6).

4. Discussion

Psychiatric comorbidity is a common cause of disability, a known contributor to poor quality of life and increased healthcare resource utilization [25–27]. Previously, groups

TABLE 6: Logistic regression for predictors of requirement for discharge to another inpatient facility among patients with distal humerus fractures ($N = 526{,}185$). CI, confidence interval; OR, odds ratio.

Variable	OR (95% CI)	P
Dementia	20.609 (18.674–22.745)	<0.001
Congestive heart failure	8.376 (8.081–8.682)	<0.001
Atrial fibrillation	7.330 (7.075–7.594)	<0.001
Schizophrenia	7.232 (6.408–8.163)	<0.001
Depression	5.909 (5.621–6.212)	<0.001
Diabetes mellitus	5.598 (5.446–5.754)	<0.001
Hypertension	5.419 (5.305–5.535)	<0.001
Transfusion	5.157 (4.939–5.386)	<0.001
Coronary artery disease	4.917 (4.682–5.164)	<0.001
Osteoporosis	4.704 (4.489–4.930)	<0.001
Thyroid disease	4.280 (4.108–4.458)	<0.001
History of myocardial infarction	3.974 (3.686–4.286)	<0.001
Chronic pulmonary disease	1.985 (1.534–2.567)	<0.001
Obesity	1.617 (1.420–1.840)	<0.001
Sex (M)	1.356 (1.319–1.394)	<0.001
Region	1.153 (1.139–1.167)	<0.001
DOC	1.059 (1.058–1.060)	<0.001
Thyroid disease	1.053 (1.052–1.054)	<0.001
Open reduction and internal fixation	0.785 (0.771–0.800)	<0.001
Closed reduction and internal fixation	0.197 (0.190–0.203)	<0.001
Anxiety	0.002 (0.000–0.032)	<0.001

Omnibus $\chi^2 = 4717$, $P < 0.001$.
Nagelkerke $R^2 = 0.4820$.

have demonstrated poor long-term outcomes after orthopaedic surgery for patients with psychiatric illness [26]. However, reports are conflicting on whether psychiatric comorbidities affect inpatient outcomes in patients with musculoskeletal injuries, as some studies have demonstrated decreased rates of major in-hospital complications and mortality [22]. The influence of psychiatric comorbidities on lower extremity fractures has previously been investigated [17]. In this study, we used nationally representative data collected over a 17-year period to evaluate the effect of psychiatric comorbidity on inpatient adverse events, requirement for blood transfusion, and discharge status for patients admitted with distal humerus fractures.

The findings of this study demonstrate that, in patients admitted with distal humerus fractures, diagnoses of depression and dementia are associated with higher odds of in-hospital adverse events. This finding is consistent with previous studies conducted by Hu et al. [28], Bot et al. [25], and Beresnevait et al. [7] who found increased complication rates among patients with psychiatric illness who are undergoing surgery. Of note, our study demonstrated a decreased risk of adverse events for patients with schizophrenia, which is contradictory to previous findings [17]. One reason for this discrepancy could be the small sample size of only 1,007 patients. Another reason could be due to the limited coding available in the database. The NHDS only allows for 7 diagnosis codes per weighted case, which may limit the amount of comorbidities and adverse events listed.

This study found depression to be associated with increased odds of requirement for blood transfusion in patients with distal humerus fractures. A possible explanation for this finding is that medications used for the treatment of depression, such as selective serotonin reuptake inhibitors, inhibit platelet activity and could result in increased bleeding [29, 30]. It is also possible that symptoms of depression, such as fatigue, may mimic symptoms of anemia leading to a higher rate of transfusion. Paradoxically, patients with anxiety had increased rates of postoperative anemia but lower rates of blood transfusion. In our study, patients with anxiety had the shortest hospital stay at 2.49 days, which may have limited their treatment options and could explain their decreased rate of transfusion despite increased rates of anemia.

This study demonstrated an increased risk for nonroutine discharge to another inpatient facility for patients with depression, schizophrenia, and dementia after hospitalization with a distal humerus fracture. In addition, in-hospital days of care were significantly greater for patients with depression and schizophrenia. These findings correlate with prior studies showing psychiatric illnesses, in patients with orthopaedic conditions, are independent risk factors for increased health-care resource utilization [25–27].

Interestingly, mortality rates were lower among patients with depression. This finding is in line with studies by previous groups and has been postulated to be due to increased attention from health care professionals due to heightened fear and awareness of pain and symptoms by these patients [31]. While the mechanism of fracture is unknown due to limitations of the database, our results demonstrate that patients with no comorbid psychiatric diagnoses were significantly younger. It is possible this cohort sustained a distal humerus fracture from a high-energy mechanism, possibly as part of a polytrauma, which may explain the higher morbidity.

The use of the NHDS database for this study allowed for a national analysis of a large number of patients over a 17-year period. However, despite the benefits of using a large, national database [32], this type of data collection poses several limitations [33]. Diagnosis codes and procedure codes were collected to compose all parts of the statistical analysis. Misclassification of ICD-9-CM codes poses an intrinsic source of error. However, misclassifications are likely distributed evenly among groups, preventing them from affecting our statistical analysis [34]. Additionally, the database only allows for seven diagnosis codes and four procedure codes per entry. As a result, the prevalence of comorbid conditions and adverse events may be underreported, as the prevalences found in this study are lower than other national estimates of depression, anxiety, and dementia [35–37]. This is similar to multiple prior administrative database studies [17, 25]. Another potential cause of the lower prevalence may be that patients with distal humerus fractures who have psychiatric comorbidities may not be admitted to the hospital and are selected to receive conservative treatment from initial presentation. It is also possible that the lower numbers among patients with distal humerus fractures and psychiatric comorbidities may be due to inequities in access to care, or they may be neglected and not present to the hospital or they may choose not to receive treatment at all. Regardless of the cause, because all cases undergo the same data collection process, potential underreporting should be equally distributed. Another limitation is that the database only provides inpatient data, so complications that arise after discharge are not obtainable. What is more, the large sample size may have resulted in the identification of statistically significant differences that may not be clinically relevant. Additionally, calculation of odds ratios by binomial logistic regression has been shown to result in an overestimate of effect when the outcome occurs in greater than 10 percent of the cohort [38] and thus should be interpreted as a trend instead of an absolute effect size. Finally, the influence of treatment status among patients with psychiatric illness is unknown, as medications are not listed in the database. Therefore, it is impossible to discern whether treatment of psychiatric illness influences outcomes in patients admitted with distal humerus fractures.

5. Conclusion

In conclusion, this study utilized the NHDS to analyze US national data over a 17-year period and showed that psychiatric illness poses an increased risk of in-hospital adverse events, requirement for blood transfusion, and nonroutine discharge to an inpatient facility for patients admitted with distal humerus fractures. These findings may aid healthcare providers in appropriately allocating resources to orthopaedic patients with psychiatric illness.

Ethical Approval

This study was conducted using the National Hospital Discharge Survey, a publically available database conducted by the Centers for Disease Control and Prevention, in which all data are deidentified and available for public use. As a result, this study was exempt from approval by the institutional review board.

Competing Interests

The authors report no financial, consultant, institutional, or other relationships that may lead to bias or competing interests.

References

[1] J. de Miguel-Díez, P. Carrasco-Garrido, J. Rejas-Gutierrez et al., "The influence of heart disease on characteristics, quality of life, use of health resources, and costs of COPD in primary care settings," *BMC Cardiovascular Disorders*, vol. 10, article 8, 2010.

[2] C. Enger, L. Weatherby, R. F. Reynolds, D. B. Glasser, and A. M. Walker, "Serious cardiovascular events and mortality among patients with schizophrenia," *The Journal of Nervous and Mental Disease*, vol. 192, no. 1, pp. 19–27, 2004.

[3] L. J. Graven and J. Grant, "The impact of social support on depressive symptoms in individuals with heart failure," *The Journal of Cardiovascular Nursing*, vol. 28, no. 5, pp. 429–443, 2013.

[4] A. H. Jakobsen, L. Foldager, G. Parker, and P. Munk-Jørgensen, "Quantifying links between acute myocardial infarction and depression, anxiety and schizophrenia using case register databases," *Journal of Affective Disorders*, vol. 109, no. 1-2, pp. 177–181, 2008.

[5] C. B. Nemeroff and P. J. Goldschmidt-Clermont, "Heartache and heartbreak-the link between depression and cardiovascular disease," *Nature Reviews Cardiology*, vol. 9, no. 9, pp. 526–539, 2012.

[6] B. Ruo, J. S. Rumsfeld, M. A. Hlatky, H. Liu, W. S. Browner, and M. A. Whooley, "Depressive symptoms and health-related quality of life: the Heart and Soul study," *The Journal of the American Medical Association*, vol. 290, no. 2, pp. 215–221, 2003.

[7] M. Beresnevait, R. Benetis, G. J. Taylor, K. Jurnien, Š. Kinduris, and V. Barauskien, "Depression predicts perioperative outcomes following coronary artery bypass graft surgery," *Scandinavian Cardiovascular Journal*, vol. 44, no. 5, pp. 289–294, 2010.

[8] J. Perälä, J. Suvisaari, S. I. Saarni et al., "Lifetime prevalence of psychotic and bipolar I disorders in a general population," *Archives of General Psychiatry*, vol. 64, no. 1, pp. 19–28, 2007.

[9] H. Kitchen, D. Rofail, L. Heron, and P. Sacco, "Cognitive impairment associated with schizophrenia: a review of the humanistic burden," *Advances in Therapy*, vol. 29, no. 2, pp. 148–162, 2012.

[10] C. F. Reynolds III, P. Cuijpers, V. Patel et al., "Early intervention to reduce the global health and economic burden of major depression in older adults," *Annual Review of Public Health*, vol. 33, pp. 123–135, 2012.

[11] D. A. Fisher, B. Dierckman, M. R. Watts, and K. Davis, "Looks good but feels bad: factors that contribute to poor results after total knee arthroplasty," *The Journal of Arthroplasty*, vol. 22, no. 6, supplement 2, pp. 39–42, 2007.

[12] C. L. Seebach, M. Kirkhart, J. M. Lating et al., "Examining the role of positive and negative affect in recovery from spine surgery," *Pain*, vol. 153, no. 3, pp. 518–525, 2012.

[13] R. J. Crichlow, P. L. Andres, S. M. Morrison, S. M. Haley, and M. S. Vrahas, "Depression in orthopaedic trauma patients: prevalence and severity," *Journal of Bone and Joint Surgery A*, vol. 88, no. 9, pp. 1927–1933, 2006.

[14] G. Cizza, S. Primma, M. Coyle, L. Gourgiotis, and G. Csako, "Depression and osteoporosis: a research synthesis with meta-analysis," *Hormone and Metabolic Research*, vol. 42, no. 7, pp. 467–482, 2010.

[15] T. Kishimoto, M. De Hert, H. E. Carlson, P. Manu, and C. U. Correll, "Osteoporosis and fracture risk in people with schizophrenia," *Current Opinion in Psychiatry*, vol. 25, no. 5, pp. 415–429, 2012.

[16] Y. Zhao, L. Shen, and H.-F. Ji, "Alzheimer's disease and risk of hip fracture: a meta-analysis study," *The Scientific World Journal*, vol. 2012, Article ID 872173, 5 pages, 2012.

[17] M. E. Menendez, V. Neuhaus, A. G. J. Bot, M. S. Vrahas, and D. Ring, "Do psychiatric comorbidities influence inpatient death, adverse events, and discharge after lower extremity fractures?" *Clinical Orthopaedics and Related Research*, vol. 471, no. 10, pp. 3336–3348, 2013.

[18] Centers for Disease Control and Prevention, National Hospital Discharge Survey, August 2013–June 2014, http://www.cdc.gov/nchs/nhds.htm.

[19] C. Dennison and R. Pokras, "Design and operation of the national hospital discharge survey: 1988 redesign," *Vital and Health Statistics*, no. 39, pp. 1–42, 2000.

[20] CDC/National Center for Health Statistics, *International Classification of Diseases, Ninth Revision, Clinical Modification (ICD-9-CM)*, 2013, http://www.cdc.gov/nchs/icd/icd9cm.htm.

[21] S. G. Memtsoudis, A. González Della Valle, M. C. Besculides, L. Gaber, and T. P. Sculco, "In-hospital complications and mortality of unilateral, bilateral, and revision TKA: based on an estimate of 4,159,661 discharges," *Clinical Orthopaedics and Related Research*, vol. 466, no. 11, pp. 2617–2627, 2008.

[22] O. Stundner, M. Kirksey, Y. L. Chiu et al., "Demographics and perioperative outcome in patients with depression and anxiety undergoing total joint arthroplasty: a population-based study," *Psychosomatics*, vol. 54, no. 2, pp. 149–157, 2013.

[23] L. I. Iezzoni, J. Daley, T. Heeren et al., "Using administrative data to screen hospitals for high complication rates," *Inquiry*, vol. 31, no. 1, pp. 40–55, 1994.

[24] S. Lemeshow, D. Teres, J. Klar, J. S. Avrunin, S. H. Gehlbach, and J. Rapoport, "Mortality probability models (MPM II) based on an international cohort of intensive care unit patients," *JAMA*, vol. 270, no. 20, pp. 2478–2486, 1993.

[25] A. G. J. Bot, M. E. Menendez, V. Neuhaus, and D. Ring, "The influence of psychiatric comorbidity on perioperative outcomes after shoulder arthroplasty," *Journal of Shoulder and Elbow Surgery*, vol. 23, no. 4, pp. 519–527, 2014.

[26] M. M. Vissers, J. B. Bussmann, J. A. N. Verhaar, J. J. V. Busschbach, S. M. A. Bierma-Zeinstra, and M. Reijman, "Psychological factors affecting the outcome of total hip and knee arthroplasty: a systematic review," *Seminars in Arthritis and Rheumatism*, vol. 41, no. 4, pp. 576–588, 2012.

[27] M. S. Walid and J. S. Robinson Jr., "Economic impact of comorbidities in spine surgery," *Journal of Neurosurgery: Spine*, vol. 14, no. 3, pp. 318–321, 2011.

[28] C. J. Hu, C. C. Liao, C. C. Chang, C. H. Wu, and T. L. Chen, "Postoperative adverse outcomes in surgical patients with dementia: a retrospective cohort study," *World Journal of Surgery*, vol. 36, no. 9, pp. 2051–2058, 2012.

[29] A. Dietrich-Muszalska, J. Rabe-Jablonska, P. Nowak, and B. Kontek, "The first- and second-generation antipsychotic drugs affect ADP-induced platelet aggregation," *World Journal of Biological Psychiatry*, vol. 11, no. 2, pp. 268–275, 2010.

[30] A. Flöck, A. Zobel, G. Bauriedel et al., "Antiplatelet effects of antidepressant treatment: a randomized comparison between escitalopram and nortriptyline," *Thrombosis Research*, vol. 126, no. 2, pp. e83–e87, 2010.

[31] J. I. Escobar, M. Gara, H. Waitzkin, R. C. Silver, A. Holman, and W. Compton, "Dsm-IV hypochondriasis in primary care," *General Hospital Psychiatry*, vol. 20, no. 3, pp. 155–159, 1998.

[32] D. D. Bohl, B. A. Basques, N. S. Golinvaux, M. R. Baumgaertner, and J. N. Grauer, "Nationwide inpatient sample and national surgical quality improvement program give different results in hip fracture studies," *Clinical Orthopaedics and Related Research*, vol. 472, no. 6, pp. 1672–1680, 2014.

[33] S. G. Memtsoudis, "Limitations associated with the analysis of data from administrative databases," *Anesthesiology*, vol. 111, no. 2, article 449, 2009.

[34] V. L. Tseng, F. Yu, F. Lum, and A. L. Coleman, "Risk of fractures following cataract surgery in medicare beneficiaries," *The Journal of the American Medical Association*, vol. 308, no. 5, pp. 493–501, 2012.

[35] R. C. Kessler, W. T. Chiu, O. Demler, K. R. Merikangas, and E. E. Walters, "Prevalence, severity, and comorbidity of 12-month DSM-IV disorders in the National Comorbidity Survey Replication," *Archives of General Psychiatry*, vol. 62, no. 6, pp. 617–627, 2005.

[36] R. C. Kessler, S. Aguilar-Gaxiola, J. Alonso et al., "The global burden of mental disorders: an update from the WHO World Mental Health (WMH) surveys," *Epidemiologia e Psichiatria Sociale*, vol. 18, no. 1, pp. 23–33, 2009.

[37] C. P. Ferri, M. Prince, C. Brayne et al., "Global prevalence of dementia: a Delphi consensus study," *The Lancet*, vol. 366, no. 9503, pp. 2112–2117, 2005.

[38] M. E. Menendez, V. Neuhaus, A. G. J. Bot, D. Ring, and T. D. Cha, "Psychiatric disorders and major spine surgery: epidemiology and perioperative outcomes," *Spine*, vol. 39, no. 2, pp. E111–E122, 2014.

Permissions

All chapters in this book were first published in AIOS, by Hindawi Publishing Corporation; hereby published with permission under the Creative Commons Attribution License or equivalent. Every chapter published in this book has been scrutinized by our experts. Their significance has been extensively debated. The topics covered herein carry significant findings which will fuel the growth of the discipline. They may even be implemented as practical applications or may be referred to as a beginning point for another development.

The contributors of this book come from diverse backgrounds, making this book a truly international effort. This book will bring forth new frontiers with its revolutionizing research information and detailed analysis of the nascent developments around the world.

We would like to thank all the contributing authors for lending their expertise to make the book truly unique. They have played a crucial role in the development of this book. Without their invaluable contributions this book wouldn't have been possible. They have made vital efforts to compile up to date information on the varied aspects of this subject to make this book a valuable addition to the collection of many professionals and students.

This book was conceptualized with the vision of imparting up-to-date information and advanced data in this field. To ensure the same, a matchless editorial board was set up. Every individual on the board went through rigorous rounds of assessment to prove their worth. After which they invested a large part of their time researching and compiling the most relevant data for our readers.

The editorial board has been involved in producing this book since its inception. They have spent rigorous hours researching and exploring the diverse topics which have resulted in the successful publishing of this book. They have passed on their knowledge of decades through this book. To expedite this challenging task, the publisher supported the team at every step. A small team of assistant editors was also appointed to further simplify the editing procedure and attain best results for the readers.

Apart from the editorial board, the designing team has also invested a significant amount of their time in understanding the subject and creating the most relevant covers. They scrutinized every image to scout for the most suitable representation of the subject and create an appropriate cover for the book.

The publishing team has been an ardent support to the editorial, designing and production team. Their endless efforts to recruit the best for this project, has resulted in the accomplishment of this book. They are a veteran in the field of academics and their pool of knowledge is as vast as their experience in printing. Their expertise and guidance has proved useful at every step. Their uncompromising quality standards have made this book an exceptional effort. Their encouragement from time to time has been an inspiration for everyone.

The publisher and the editorial board hope that this book will prove to be a valuable piece of knowledge for researchers, students, practitioners and scholars across the globe.

LIST OF CONTRIBUTORS

Derek Ochiai
Nirschl Orthopedic Center, Arlington, VA 22205, USA

Skye Donovan
Nirschl Orthopedic Center, Arlington, VA 22205, USA
Marymount University, Arlington, VA 22207, USA

Eric Guidi
Marymount University, Arlington, VA 22207, USA

Farshad Adib
University ofMaryland, Baltimore, MD 21201, USA

Metin Uzun
Maslak Hospital, Orthopaedic Department, Acibadem University, Darüşşafaka Street, Büyükdere Street No. 40, Maslak, Sarıyer,İstanbul, Turkey

Murat Çakar
Okmeydani Education and Training Hospital, Okmeydani, İstanbul, Turkey

Ahmet Murat Bülbül and Adnan Kara
Orthopaedic Department, Medipol University, İstanbul, Turkey

J. A. Kettunen
Arcada University of Applied Sciences, Jan-Magnus Janssonin Aukio 1, 00550 Helsinki, Finland

Y. Nietosvaara
Children's Hospital, Helsinki University Central Hospital, P.O. Box 281, 00029 Helsinki, Finland

S. Palmu
Children's Hospital, Helsinki University Central Hospital, P.O. Box 281, 00029 Helsinki, Finland
Tampere Center for Child Health Research (TACC), University of Tampere and Tampere University Hospital, Lääkärinkatu 1, 33014 Tampere, Finland

K. Tallroth
Orton OrthopaedicHospital, Orton Foundation, P.O. Box 29, 00281 Helsinki, Finland

M. Lohman
Department of Radiology, HUS Medical Imaging Center, Helsinki University Central Hospital and University of Helsinki, P.O. Box 340, 00029 Helsinki, Finland

Nicholas B. Robertson and TiborWarganich
1Harbor UCLA Medical Center, Department of Orthopaedics, 1000W. Carson Street Box 422, Torrance, CA 90245, USA

John Ghazarossian and Monti Khatod
KaiserWest Los Angeles, Department of Orthopaedics, 6041 Cadillac Avenue, Los Angeles, CA 90034, USA

Panagiotis Koulouvaris
Orthopaedic Clinic, Attikon Hospital, University of Athens, Olympic Village Polyclinic, 36122 Athens, Greece

David Sherr
New York Hospital, Cornell University, NY 10021, USA

Thomas Sculco
Hospital for Special Surgery, Cornell University, NY 10021, USA

Thomas Hester
Guys and StThomas' NHS Trust, Department of Orthopaedics,Westminster Bridge Road, London SE1 7EH, UK

Shoib Mahmood and Farid Moftah
Department of Orthopaedics, Darent Valley Hospital, Dartford DA2 8DA, UK

Nikolaos Davarinos
Department of Trauma & Orthopaedics, The Adelaide & Meath Hospital, Tallaght, Dublin 24, Ireland

Barry James O'Neill and William Curtin
Department of Trauma & Orthopaedics, Galway Regional Hospitals, Galway, Ireland

Anthony C. Levenda and Natalie R. Sanders
Lakeshore Bone and Joint Institute, 601 Gateway Boulevard, Chesterton, IN 46304, USA

Pradeep Jain, Parthapratim Dutta, Prabal Goswami, Amol Patel and Shammi Purwar
Department of Plastic Surgery, Institute of Medical Sciences, Banaras Hindu University, Varanasi 221005, India

Vaibhav Jain
Department of Plastic Surgery, Institute of PostgraduateMedical Education & Research, Kolkata 700020, India

Simon Tiziani, Georg Osterhoff, Max J. Scheyerer, Gian-Leza Spinas, Guido A.Wanner, Hans-Peter Simmen and Clément M. L. Werner
Department of Surgery, Division of Trauma Surgery, University Hospital Zurich, Raemistrasse 100, 8091 Zurich, Switzerland

Stephen J. Ferguson and Gregor Spreiter
Institute for Biomechanics, ETH Zurich, HCI-E355.2Wolfgang-Pauli-Strasse 10, 8093 Zurich, Switzerland

Manish Kiran
University Department of Orthopaedics and Trauma Surgery, TORT Centre, Ninewells Hospital, Dundee DD1 9SY, UK

Arpit Jariwala and Carlos A. Wigderowitz
NHS Tayside, Dundee DD1 9SY, UK

Zuned Hakim, Claire Rutherford, Elizabeth Mckiernan and Tony Helm
Royal Preston Hospital, Sharoe Green Lane North, Fulwood, Preston PR2 9HT, UK

Ainhoa Toro-Ibarguen, Ismael Auñón-Martín, Emilio Delgado-Díaz, Jose Alberto Moreno-Beamud, Miguel Ángel Martínez-Leocadio, Andrés Díaz-Martín and Luciano Candel-García
Orthopaedic and Traumatology Surgery, Hospital 12 de Octubre, 28041 Madrid, Spain

Masataka Uchino, Kouji Naruse, Noriko Hirakawa, Masahiro Toyama, Genyou Miyajima and Ken Urabe
Department of Orthopaedic Surgery, Kitasato University Medical Center, 6-100 Arai, Kitamoto, Saitama 364-8501, Japan

Ken Sugo
HOYA Technosurgical Corporation, 1-1-110 Tsutsujigaoka, Akishima, Tokyo 196-0012, Japan

Kentaro Uchida
Department of Orthopaedic Surgery, Kitasato University School of Medicine, 1-15-1 Kitasato, Minami-ku, Sagamihara, Kanagawa 252-0375, Japan

Juliann Kwak-Lee and Elke R. Ahlmann
Los Angeles County + University of Southern California Medical Center, 1200 N. State Street, GNH 3900, Los Angeles, CA 90033, USA

Lingjun Wang
Department of Orthopedics, Los Angeles County + University of Southern California Medical Center, 1200 N. State Street, GNH 3900, Los Angeles, CA 90033, USA

John M. Itamura
Keck School of Medicine, Kerlan-Jobe atWhite Memorial Medical Center, 1700 Cesar E. Chavez Avenue, Suite 1400, Los Angeles, CA 90033, USA

John Wang, James DiPietro, Mathias Bostrom, Bryan Nestor, Douglas Padgett and Geoffrey Westrich
Hospital for Special Surgery, 535 East 70th Street, New York, NY 10021, USA

Christine L. Farnsworth and Michael T. Rohmiller
Division of Orthopedics, Rady Children's Hospital-San Diego, 3020 Children'sWay, MC 5054, San Diego, CA 92123, USA

Peter O. Newton
Division of Orthopedics, Rady Children's Hospital-San Diego, 3020 Children's Way, MC 5054, San Diego, CA 92123, USA
Department of Orthopaedic Surgery, University of California San Diego, San Diego, CA 92103, USA

Eric Breisch
Department of Pathology, Rady Children's Hospital San Diego, San Diego, CA 92123, USA

Jung Ryul Kim
Department of Orthopaedic Surgery, Chonbuk National University Hospital, Jeonbuk 561-712, Republic of Korea

Behrooz A. Akbarnia
Department of Orthopaedic Surgery, University of California San Diego, San Diego, CA 92103, USA
San Diego Center for Spinal Disorders, La Jolla, CA 92037, USA

Mohammed S. Arshad, Shashi Godey, Arun Kumar and Martyn Lovell
University Hospital of South Manchester, Southmoor Road, Manchester M23 9LT, UK

Evalina L. Burger, Andriy Noshchenko Vikas V. Patels and EmilyM. Lindley
The Spine Center, Department of Orthopaedics, University of Colorado Denver, Aurora, CO 80045, USA

Andrew P. Bradford
Division of Basic Reproductive Sciences, Department of Obstetrics & Gynecology, University of Colorado Denver, Aurora, CO 80045, USA

G. Shyamalan and R. W. Jordan
Birmingham Heartlands Hospital, Bordesley Green East, Birmingham,West Midlands B9 5SS, UK

A. Jarvis
Worthing Hospital, Lyndhurst Road,Worthing,West Sussex BN11 2DH, UK

William J. Long
Insall Scott Kelly Institute, New York, NY 10065, USA
New York University, New York, NY 10065, USA
Hospital for Joint Disease, NYU, New York, NY 10065, USA
St. Francis Hospital, Roslyn, NY 11548, USA

Joseph W. Greene
Norton Healthcare, Louisville, KY 40207, USA
Department of Orthopaedic Surgery, University of Louisville, Louisville, KY 40202, USA

Fred D. Cushner
Southside Hospital, Bay Shore, NY 11706, USA

Lenox Hill Hospital, Northwell Health System, New York, NY 10065, USA

M. Jason Palmer Stephanie L. Tanner and Rebecca G. Snider
Greenville Health System Department of Orthopaedics, 701 Grove Road, Greenville, SC 29605, USA

Thomas B. Pace
Greenville Health System Department of Orthopaedics, 701 Grove Road, Greenville, SC 29605, USA
University of South Carolina SOM, Greenville Health System, P.O. Box 27114, Greenville, SC 29616, USA

James C. Karegeannes
Blue Ridge Bone and Joint, 129 McDowell Street, Asheville,NC 28801,USA

RamK. Shah and Sujit R. Shrestha
1Nepal Medical College, Jorpati, Kathmandu, Nepal

Raju Rijal and Rosan P. Shah Kalawar
B.P. Koirala Institute of Health Sciences, Dharan, Nepal

Niraj Kumar Shah
Department of General Surgery, PGIMER, Chandigarh, India

Raffaele Russo and Fabio Cautiero
Orthopaedic and Traumatology Department, Ospedale dei Pellegrini, 80134 Napoli, Italy

Giuseppe Della Rotonda
Royal BerkshireHospital, London Road, Reading RG1 5AN, UK

Hayat Ahmad Khan, Younis Kamal, Mohammad Ashraf Khan, Munir Farooq Naseemul Gani Adil Bashir Shah and Mohammad Shahid Bhat
Department of Orthopaedics, B & J Hospital, GMC Srinagar, Kashmir 190005, India

Nazia Hassan
GMC Srinagar, Kashmir, India

Avishai Reuven, Grigorios N.Manoudis, Olga L. Huk, David Zukor and John Antoniou
Department of Orthopaedics, McGill University, Jewish General Hospital, 3755 Cote-St.-Catherine Road, Room E-003, Montreal, QC, Canada H3T 1E2

Ahmed Aoude
Medical School, University of Montreal, P.O. Box 6128, Station Centre-Ville, Montreal, QC, Canada H3C 3J7

Mark Eidelman, Alexander Katzman and Michael Zaidman
Pediatric Orthopedic Surgery Unit, Rambam Health Care Campus, P.O. Box 9602, 31096 Haifa, Israel

Yaniv Keren
Department of Orthopedic Surgery, Rambam Health Care Campus, P.O. Box 9602, 31096 Haifa, Israel

Kirsten Juliette de Burlet, JamesWidnall, Cefin Barton and Stephen Duckett
Department of Orthopaedic Surgery, Leighton Hospital, Crewe CW1 4QJ, UK

Veera Gudimetla
Department of Anaesthetics, Leighton Hospital, Crewe CW1 4QJ, UK
Correspondence should be addressed to Kirsten Juliette de Burlet; kjdeburlet

William Blakeney
Department of Orthopaedics, Royal Perth Hospital, Perth,WA 6000, Australia
Department of Orthopaedics, Mount Hospital, Perth,WA 6000, Australia

Simon Zilko and Wael Chiri
Department of Orthopaedics, Royal Perth Hospital, Perth,WA 6000, Australia

Peter Annear
Department of Orthopaedics, Mount Hospital, Perth,WA 6000, Australia
Perth Orthopaedics and Sports Medicine Centre, Perth,WA 6005, Australia

Leigh White, Nicholas Hartnell, Melissa Hennessy and Judy Mullan
School of Medicine, University of Wollongong,Wollongong, NSW2522, Australia

Leonard T. Buller, Milad Alam, Karim Sabeh, Charles Lawrie and Stephen M. Quinnan
University of Miami Miller School of Medicine, Department of Orthopaedic Surgery and Rehabilitation, 1400 NW 12th Avenue, Miami, FL 33136, USA

Matthew J. Best
Johns Hopkins Department of Orthopaedic Surgery, 1800 Orleans Street, Baltimore, MD 21287, USA

Index

www.ingramcontent.com/pod-product-compliance
Lightning Source LLC
Chambersburg PA
CBHW080704200326
41458CB00013B/4965

* 9 7 8 1 6 3 2 4 2 5 2 2 5 *